Caregiving

Studies in Health, Illness, and Caregiving
Joan E. Lynaugh, Series Editor

A complete list of books in the series
is available from the publisher

Caregiving

Readings in Knowledge, Practice, Ethics, and Politics

edited by
Suzanne Gordon,
Patricia Benner, and
Nel Noddings

PENN

University of Pennsylvania Press

Philadelphia

Copyright © 1996 University of Pennsylvania Press
All rights reserved
Printed in the United States of America on acid-free paper

10 9 8 7 6 5 4 3 2

Published by
University of Pennsylvania Press
Philadelphia, Pennsylvania 19104-4011

Library of Congress Cataloging-in-Publication Data

Caregiving : readings in knowledge, practice, ethics, and politics / edited by Suzanne
Gordon, Patricia Benner, and Nel Noddings.
         p.   cm.—(Studies in health, illness, and caregiving)
    Includes bibliographical references and index.
    ISBN 0-8122-1582-6 (pbk. : alk. paper)
    1. Caregivers. 2. Home care services. 3. Institutional care. 4. Caring.
I. Gordon, Suzanne, 1945- .   II. Benner, Patricia E.   III. Noddings, Nel.
IV. Series.
HV40.C3595   1996
362'.0425—dc20   96-19693
                                                             CIP

Contents

Introduction   vii

Part I. Caring as a Way of Life   1

1. In the Gloaming
Alice Elliott Dark   5

2. The Cared-For
Nel Noddings   21

3. Caring Practice
Patricia Benner and Suzanne Gordon   40

4. Caring: A Negotiated Process That Varies
Barbara Tarlow   56

5. Facing Up to Moral Perils:
The Virtues of Care in Bioethics
Alisa L. Carse   83

Part II. Family Caregiving   111

6. *The Heather Blazing*
Colm Tóibín   115

7. Mothering as a Practice
Victoria Wynn Leonard   124

8. Nursing Loved Ones with AIDS:
Knowledge Development for Ethical Practice
Richard MacIntyre   141

Part III. Professional Caregiving 153

9. Hearing the Whole Story
Jeannie Chaisson 157

10. The Caring Professional
Nel Noddings 160

11. Ella
Suzanne Gordon 173

12. Two Stories of Caring in Teaching
James G. Henderson 189

13. The Phenomenology of Knowing the Patient
Christine A. Tanner, Patricia Benner, Catherine Chesla, and Deborah Gordon 203

Part IV. The Politics of Caregiving 221

14. Money Managers Are Unraveling the Tapestry of Nursing
Ellen D. Baer and Suzanne Gordon 226

15. The Rationality of Caring
Kari Waerness 231

16. Feminism and Caring
Suzanne Gordon 256

17. The Mormon Caregiving Network
Judith Dushku 278

18. Let Me Take a Listen to Your Heart
Rita Charon 292

List of Contributors 307

Index 310

Introduction

For the past several decades a growing number of scholars, researchers, activists, and practitioners in the caregiving professions and in moral philosophy, feminism, sociology, history, and religion have developed a rich body of thinking in the field of caring. This reader presents some of their best work. Unlike some major collections in the field, such as Finch and Groves, *Labour of Love: Women, Work and Caring* (1983), which focuses on the exploitative structures imposed on traditional women's work, and Larabee's *An Ethic of Care: Feminist and Interdisciplinary Perspectives* (1993), which concentrates on moral philosophy, this volume emphasizes the role of the practice and politics of caregiving and the ethics embedded therein.

Professional caregivers like nurses, teachers, and social workers have written a number of the essays in this reader. Scholars and researchers have written others. These complementary selections present some of the latest practical and theoretical thinking about caregiving practice, and amplify our understanding by placing us directly inside the daily realities of caregiving through first person stories and fiction. They bring to life the knowledge, skill, and notions of the good embedded in caring practices, relationships, and activities, poignantly illustrating the larger theoretical and human issues that are inevitably engaged when individuals care for each other.

The book has four sections. The introductory section, "Caring as a Way of Life" presents the book's conceptual framework. "Family Caregiving" considers the largest group of those who care for others. "Professional Caregiving" examines the practice of nurses, teachers, social workers, and others in the caregiving professions. Finally, "The Politics of Caregiving" focuses on the kinds of political strategies and public policies that support and advance caregiving both in the home and community.

Selections have been chosen because they best exemplify the book's goals. Our first goal is to illuminate the complexity of caregiving and to locate caregiving in a specific historical and personal context. Because the content of caregiving—while valued privately and romanticized publicly—remains invisible in our society, an appreciation of these practices, skills, and knowledge is essential. To borrow a phrase from the great social historian E. P. Thompson different cultures must not only be situated "in the thin air of meanings, attitudes and values," but located within a "particular equilibrium of social relationships" (1993, p. 7).

Thus, we locate the cultures of caregiving in the context of an advanced technological society. Such societies have, not surprisingly, created complex caregiving needs through the very accomplishments that were supposed to solve or eradicate such needs. By the year 2040 the elderly—many of them disabled and dependent—will comprise 13 million people (Longino 1988). Today people over 75 and dependent adults between the ages of 18 and 65 are the fastest growing segments of our society (Gordon 1991).

Men and women in contemporary America live longer than ever before in human history, but more than 80 percent of those 65 and over have one or more chronic illness and an estimated 30 percent of those over 85 suffer from some form of dementia (Gordon 1991). Most of the elderly will require some form of temporary or full-time family or institutional caregiving. Some will need complex and costly care for decades. The same is true for those dependent adults whose lives have been prolonged by modern technology.

Not only the ill, elderly, and disabled are in need of care. Healthy, vigorous children also need care. For example, while schools are concentrating on narrow academic goals, children—especially teenagers—are protesting that "nobody cares!" To make matters worse, an increasing proportion of our country's children live in poverty.

These care-related problems are complicated by the fact that women—who have been charged with caring for the young and old, sick and vulnerable—now work outside the home in greater numbers than ever before. By the year 2000, 64 percent of all women in the United States will be in the workforce. An estimated three-quarters of all children will have mothers who work outside the home. About 14.6 million preschool and 37.4 million school age children will, therefore, need some kind of infant, preschool, and after-school care (Gordon 1991).

In spite of increased female labor force participation, women still shoulder the main caregiving burden in our society. Most of the seven million family caregivers in America are women. Of these, 1.8 million women care for dependent children and dependent parents at the same time, and 33 percent of the women who care for chronically ill or infirm elderly parents are in the workforce. Today, in fact, technology has exacerbated rather than alleviated women's caregiving responsibilities.

In 1900 the average woman spent 18 to 20 years caring for children and 9 years caring for elderly parents or relatives. Today, the average woman still spends 18 to 20 years caring for children and *18 years* caring for elderly relatives ("Mothers Bearing," 1989). This dramatic statistic highlights the urgent necessity of creating community support for these caregivers, and of increasing men's participation in caregiving in the home and community.

Although caregiving remains primarily a woman's burden, more men are becoming caregivers in contemporary America. An increasing number are responding to family demands and their own growing desire to be more involved in domestic life, child-rearing, and the care of the elderly. More are single fathers. In fact, the fastest growing family category in American society, in relative terms, is that of families headed by single fathers. Men—as spouses and sons—are estimated to be about a quarter of those who are family caregivers of the elderly (U.S. Department of Labor, 1993).

Because of their socialization, however, men have very specific, gender-related caregiving problems. Because of gender ideology, traditional stereotypes, and the formal identification of men only with public life and economic activity, their caring practices are overlooked and understudied. These activities suffer a legitimization crisis and are constantly said to contradict current definitions of power and status. Thus men's nurturing practices of coaching, fostering independence, mentoring, and sponsorship in the public and economic world as well as other more direct caregiving are as hidden as the caring practices more closely associated with traditional women's work. These problems deserve greater articulation and research attention if men are to be educated into the skill of involvement from the earliest ages. They get that attention in the pages of this reader.

The book's second purpose is to discuss the ethics and politics of caregiving and to examine some of the controversies and discussions that have emerged in attempts to analyze caring and caregiving. In Western individualistic societies the ethical ideals and self-definitions embodied in caregiving conflict with longstanding beliefs in the primacy of an individual who is independent, self-determined, and self-created. We have been taught to imagine that the fully developed individual constructs him- or herself around an inner core conceived of as a kind of unique personal possession. Thus we have difficulty paying respect and homage to those who create and constitute our lives and make possible the very self we worship. Giving public attention to the constituting powers of caregiving challenges our notions of human power and responsibility. Because of this, it is necessary to understand the current realities that jeopardize both private and public caregiving.

In our contemporary world caregiving is under attack on several fronts. An increasingly market-oriented culture has imposed increasingly heavy burdens and irrational systems of delivery on both family and professional caregivers. For example, we pour increasing funds into high-tech health care that is often necessary because of a lack of low-tech preventive care. A homeless person will be admitted to a tertiary care hospital to receive multiple surgeries to correct the ravages of poor nutrition, exposure, and social isolation. We spend thousands of dollars on remedial tutorials for a young child but nothing on correcting the social or family conditions that have made it difficult for the child to learn to read.

Our enlightenment dream of shedding cumbersome obligations and our definition of freedom as negative freedom—freedom from rather than freedom to—make us fear and avoid caregiving both individually and socially. Ironically, this very flight from caregiving makes the provision of caregiving all the more difficult and burdensome. When caregiving needs have been long neglected, the crisis-like conditions which ensue impose great personal and financial costs on individual caregivers and the system in which they may work, and, ultimately, on the society as a whole.

Similarly, this flight from caregiving makes it almost impossible for us to address the question how we can pool resources to fund rational systems of care delivery in the home, community, or public sector. Because we live in an advanced technological society, caregiving often imposes great financial demands on individuals and their families. Whether those who require care are male or female, old or young, many of their caregiving needs have become so expensive to provide that neither individuals nor families can possibly shoulder them without a well developed system for pooling individual and social resources.

Yet whenever Americans are asked to implement, expand, and fund programs and policies that would help citizens fulfill their care related responsibilites, what should be considered a profound act of community and self-support is transformed into an ideological tug-of-war. Citizens of our advanced, industrial, liberal democracy have been so well schooled to view themselves as taxpayers who are being asked to provide gifts to the selfish and indigent that most cannot even imagine themselves—as C. B. MacPherson might have put it—as equal in their need to give and receive care (MacPherson 1962). Thus when it comes to making decisions about allocating individual time and societal resources, most Americans have no common theory of political obligation to direct their economic choices and no code of moral obligation to guide their personal ones.

The editors and essays in this book confront the market challenge to caregiving. Similarly, we confront questions about caregiving posed by those on the left. For the purposes of this volume, this challenge comes primarily from within feminism. Many feminists are understandably concerned that any discussion of caregiving or an ethic of care will once again entrap women in the home and caregiving professions. Essays, therefore, address questions like: Does a clear and cohesive explication of caring necessarily invite the domination and oppression of women by men and patriarchy? Is caregiving necessarily a conservative activity? Can caregiving ever be "freely chosen"? What are the problems with conceptualizing care in economic terms? These essays contend that an understanding of caregiving and a care ethic are central to women's search for equality, men's full participation in caregiving, and human society's continued survival.

The book's third purpose is to articulate an analysis of caregiving that makes distinctions among professional, public, and family caregiving. In the public imagination, we tend to think of caregiving as one vast and undifferentiated activity, mostly performed by women. In fact, each different culture produces a great variety of different kinds of caregivers. In our culture we have the nurse, educator, or child care or social worker as compassionate stranger, the helpful neighbor, the good Samaritan or volunteer, the paid rescue worker, and many more. As one who lives outside the intimate circle of a family or individual who must care for a loved one who is vulnerable, ill, dying, or in trouble, the compassionate stranger, for example, plays an enormously important role. But this role is very different from that played by an intimate family caregiver for whom the joys and losses involved in caregiving are far more personal.

What is the difference between the activities and demands of different kinds of caregiving? How are obligations and commitments conceptualized in the different spheres of caregiving? What is the difference between professional and family caregiving? How should private caregiving affect public caregiving, and public and professional caregiving influence private caregiving? Again, our essays consider these themes.

The book's fourth mission, articulated most explicitly in its final section, is to present a politics of caregiving. The networks of relationships in which human beings are inevitably entangled are often considered to be inherently conservative. But we believe that they can also be transformative. To understand the imperatives of caregiving and grasp what makes caregiving a special activity that differs dramatically from instrumental activities undertaken in the marketplace helps one to analyze politics, to undertake action, and not only to preserve but to create and transform. A multi-dimensional analysis of caregiving can provide practical and political proposals about the delivery of care in complex technological societies and offer a way to understand broader social and political issues.

By bringing together the multiple voices of care and caregiving, this collection of essays does more than provide a comprehensive introduction to the field. It expands the knowledge of scholars, activists, and researchers who may not be familiar with one another's work. The collection as a whole, moreover, demonstrates that areas of inquiry often deemed of little interest to a broader public do, in fact, contain practical wisdom and theoretical insights of great relevance to that public. Thus, for example, an examination of the ethical importance of nurses' relationships to patients highlights far more than caring practices in one profession. It makes it clear that so-called parochial concerns can expand the vision of a moral philosopher or developmental psychologist. Or a discussion of nontraditional family caregiving may enhance the ability to deal with the increasing cultural diversity in our society.

The book's organization, therefore, creates a dialogue between the readings and ultimately across disciplines. Our hope is that it will help to construct and strengthen life-sustaining public and private institutions in which caregiving activities are neither relegated to the margins nor deemed so heroic and unusual as to be beyond normal human beings. Our goal is to help promote a view that considers caring practice and theory as central components of institutional life and philosophy.

Before presenting the essays that are the heart of this work, we would like to clarify what we mean by caring and caregiving, how we understand the caregiving relationship and the significance of this field. First we want to distinguish caring from kindness, passion, involvement, or attention. Caring is often confused with an intent or emotional attribute that exists in particular human beings absent the skills necessary to put it into practice. But we argue that caring practices involve skill, education, and community and social resources.

Because caregiving has been women's traditional work, those working on caregiving often focus on women's experiences. We believe, however, that the capacity to care resides in all human beings. It is determined not by gender but rather by experience and relationships, societal expectations, and social and economic arrangements. These govern caring behavior and the conditions under which caregiving is performed both inside and outside the home.

Because caring involves skill, not hormones, we contend that not all who take care of the young, old, vulnerable, and infirm have actually mastered the moral, emotional, and intellectual practices necessary for expert caring. Moreover, distinctions must be made between the energy, skills, and level of commitment required in different kinds of caregiving. Similarly, rigorous analysis is often necessary to uncover caregiving practices that are concealed because of our individual and historical attitudes toward caregiving and because much of the reflection and education necessary to caregiving is hidden from those who receive care.

Briefly then, we define caring not as a psychological state or innate attribute but as a set of relational practices that foster mutual recognition and realization, growth, development, protection, empowerment, and human community, culture, and possibility. As defined above, these practices are required in relationships that are devoted—for however short or long a period of time—to helping educate, nurture, develop, and empower, assisting others to cope with their weaknesses while affirming their strengths. Caring relationships are also those that foster well-being in the midst of change, crisis, vulnerability, or suffering.

Caring practices always involve receptivity, engrossment ("to make large or visible, to show up"), attunement, engagement, intelligence, skill, shrewdness, and knowledge. All these elements have, unfortunately, been made invisible in our society. Leery of any rigorous discussion and exploration of caregiving, we fear that it may invite subservience, oppression, and dependence. Obsessed with theoretical knowledge and abstract reasoning, we do not recognize the practical knowledge, skilled know-how, and relational expertise of caregivers *as* knowledge, skill, and expertise. But caregiving in fact demands an intricate combination not only of abstract learning and reasoning but of relational intelligence, social learning, and skilled knowledge as well.

Caregiving is often described as too amorphous and vague to focus on—and certainly too fuzzy actually to write about—because it cannot be accomplished without relational intelligence. Caring demands that one *dwell*—as Martin Heiddeger would have described it—with another. Such dwelling does not produce the kinds of tangible products or services—a car, a takeover deal, an income tax return, a by-pass operation —that take a certain predictable amount of time to create or perform and can thus be neatly quantified and priced. The product of care is embedded in the person who is cared for and cannot be segregated from that human life. Caring is not dependent on what I do *to* you, but on what I do and how *you receive or respond to it.* The quality of any caregiving relationship, furthermore, depends not solely on the skills and receptivity of the caregiver but on the receptivity and response of the one cared for. Timing, context, and the ability to perceive a range of human possibilities is central both to caregiving and receiving. This individual relationship is, in turn, dependent on a social context that supports it.

Learning how to navigate caring relationships and acquire relational intelligence, the essays in this volume eloquently explain, is not at all simple. The human connections demanded of caregiving work are far more complex than patting someone on the head, passive listening, or ceaseless production of soothing utterances. The caregiving relationship requires the interplay of intricate emotional and intellectual work, distance and closeness, letting go as well as holding on. The learning that directs caregiving thus comes not only from the study of the liberal arts and science but from social and experiential learning as well. Caregivers learn from each other, from those they care for, from embodied intelligence, and from their own reflections and experience.

Caregiving is *extensive* as well as *intensive* work. Caregiving can sometimes be accomplished in a short period of time—a 15-minute diagnostic visit to the doctor, an hour-long English class, a 50-minute hour—but it is often captured in a relationship that lasts over a longer period of time. Moreover, the caregiving relationship is often interrupted with a variety of different activities and demands, and may encompass intimate domestic tasks—washing a bottom, feeding an elderly man or woman, emptying a bedpan. These tasks represent occasions for connection and assessment in caregiving. Yet, they have been consistently devalued. Writing in the seventeenth-century the playwright William D'Avenant expressed attitudes on this subject quite succinctly. "Kings who move within a lowly sphere of private loves are too domestic for any throne" (Oxford English Dictionary, 1971).

The assumption that domestic work is inherently too lowly for anyone of importance to perform infects our entire society. Indeed, many commonly believe that caregiving inherently involves more tedious drudgework than other personal or professional activities. This in spite of the fact that all work—no matter how elevated we deem it to be—contains a share of routine and tedium.

Caring also requires being with another human being, not necessarily doing for him or her. In a culture which values doing, not being, *being* is considered *doing nothing.* This profound misunderstanding of the *doing-ness* of being may be a result of our cultural apprehension that it is, in fact, sometimes far harder to *be* with, to demonstrate compassion for (i.e., suffer with) people at a moment of crisis than to *do* for them.

Finally, caregiving in a radically individualistic society fundamentally challenges the illusory nature of some of our most cherished beliefs about individual autonomy and independence. As nurses Donna Diers and Claire Fagin have written,

Nursing is a metaphor for intimacy. Nurses are involved in the most private aspects of people's lives and they cannot hide behind technology or a veil of omniscience as other practitioners or technicians in hospitals may do. Nurses do for others publicly what healthy persons do for themselves behind closed doors. Nurses, as trusted peers, are there to hear secrets, especially the ones borne of vulnerability. Nurses are treasured when these interchanges are successful, but most often people do not wish to remember their vulnerability and loss of control, and nurses are indelibly identified with those terribly personal times. (Diers and Fagin 1983, p. 116)

One could easily substitute the word caregiver for nurse. Caregivers are stained with shame because our society rejects any concept of interdependence and fears that even the short-term need for assistance will produce chronic dependence. In a radically individualistic society such dependence is thought to be illegitimate, and those who need care the most are often considered morally defective. As the political philosopher Adam Smith wrote in 1787, in *The Wealth of Nations,*

Man has almost constant occasion for the help of his brethren, and it is in vain for him to expect it from his benevolence only. It is not from the benevolence of the butcher, the brewer, or the baker that we expect our dinner, but from their regard to their own interest. We address ourselves not to their humanity but to their self love and never talk to them of our own necessities but of their advantages. *Nobody but a beggar chuses to depend chiefly upon the benevolence of their fellow citizens.* (Smith 1787/1976, p. 18)

Or as Michael Douglas said to Charlie Sheen in the movie *Wall Street,* "If you need a friend get a dog."

And of course, it is not only the poor, the very young, the weak, the old, and ill who come to be considered morally defective. Anyone who associates with those who need care—"losers"—risks becoming a "loser" by association.

This book demystifies and then recasts our societal understandings of caregiving, caring practices, and the construction of caregiving work in the home, community, and institutions. It argues that we must uncover the hidden work, knowledge, and notions of good embedded in expert caring. By presenting and analyzing the experiences, insights and practices of caregivers, this collection names and analyzes the hitherto hidden and undervalued know-how and ethical expertise that creates people, families, communities, and societies. Only through disclosing and naming the practices that constitute human life can we create an expanded public discourse that integrates our private lives and our public policies and preoccupations. Only through making caregivers' invisible work visible can we understand and begin to address some of the most pressing issues our society faces and create a genuine politics that supports rather than subverts this fundamental human enterprise.

References

Diers, Donna and Claire Fagin. 1983. "Nursing as Metaphor." *New England Journal of Medicine* 309, 2 (July 14): 116–17.

Finch, Janet and Dulcie Groves, eds. 1983. *A Labour of Love: Women, Work and Caring.* London and Boston: Routledge and Kegan Paul.

Gordon, Suzanne. 1991. *Prisoners of Men's Dreams: Striking Out for a New Feminine Future.* New York: Little, Brown.

Larrabee, Mary Jeanne, ed. 1993. *An Ethic of Care: Feminist and Interdisciplinary Perspectives.* New York: Routledge.

Longino, Charles F. 1988. "Who Are the Oldest Americans?" *Gerontologist* 28: 515–23.

MacPherson, C. B. 1962. *The Political Theory of Possessive Individualism: Hobbes to Locke.* Oxford: Oxford University Press.

"Mothers Bearing a Second Burden." 1989. *New York Times,* May 14, p. 26.

Smith, Adam. 1787/1976. *An Inquiry into the Nature and Causes of the Wealth of Nations.* Chicago: University of Chicago Press.

Thompson, E. P. 1993. *Customs in Common: Studies in Traditional and Popular Culture.* New York: New Press.

U.S. Department of Labor, Bureau of Women's Affairs. 1993. Interview with Susan Schenck.

Part I
Caring as a Way of Life

The title of this introductory section expresses our belief that caregiving sustains life, and, that to do so, caregiving must be a way of life. This does not mean that caregiving is all of life. But it does mean that all human beings must take it seriously and that equitable caregiving arrangements are based on that attitude of seriousness about the project of giving and receiving care.

No contribution better evokes the power of this purposeful and reflective caregiving than Alice Elliott Dark's short story "In the Gloaming." It pulls the reader directly into the world of caregiving by dramatizing the meaning of reciprocal human relationships. It also highlights some of the central themes of this book—that there is a difference between caring as sentiment and caring as practice, that caring is crucial to the human community, and that it entails skills that can be taught and learned. For this reason, we have chosen it as the first story in our book.

Dark's short story sets the stage for an inquiry into caregiving that views this fundamental human activity as far more than technique, mere theory, or extraordinary saintliness. By illustrating that caregiving is a set of skills and practices that can be taught, expanded, and refined, it supports the view that caregiving is the very fabric of everyday life. Dealing as it does with the kinds of male and female differences that stymie attempts to equalize the burden of caregiving in the family, it also introduces some of the many gender dilemmas that are immediately engaged when one discusses caregiving practice.

The second selection advances the argument that reciprocity and learning are involved in caregiving. Taken from Nel Noddings's book, *Caring: A Feminine Approach to Ethics and Moral Education* (1984) the essay "The Cared-For" provides an analytical introduction to the idea that reciprocity is central to successful caregiving relationships. Caring is not just a virtue, an act that one person performs for or on another, but a relationship to which the cared for contributes in a variety of ways.

In "Caring Practice" Patricia Benner and Suzanne Gordon draw on Dark's short story and other caregiving experiences to elaborate further the difference between sentiment and practice. Benner and Gordon question the idea that a caring person is one who expresses generalized, abstract concern for other individuals. Caring practice lives in actual relationships and the kinds of historical and contemporaneous interactions and exchanges that nourish them. A dialogue between people in the present as well as between past and present, caregiving is a skill that is embodied and embedded in social practices. It cannot be codified or reified but must be viewed in a constantly evolving context. Emotional connection is the ground of caring practice, but that connection must be lived, rather than asserted.

Inspired by much of the theoretical and descriptive work in the field of caregiving, sociologist Barbara Tarlow's "Caring: A Negotiated Practice That Varies" adds this connection by investigating concrete caregiving relationships. Interviews with people in three different settings—families, a vocational school, and a volunteer organization—inform her analysis. Through interviews with teachers and students, family members and volunteers, and those for whom they provide care, she identifies the non-negotiable characteristics of caregiving relationships. This lived geography of the world of caregiving expands our knowledge of what caregiving means to people who view this human activity as a positive force in their lives.

The last essay in this section, philosopher Alisa Carse's, "Facing Up to Moral Perils: The Virtues of Care in Bioethics," distinguishes between engaged and disengaged ethical reasoning and between the care and justice perspectives. This essay describes the difference between the justice and care approaches to moral thinking and separates out generality and particularity. It is particularly relevant to debates about the care ethic that have arisen within feminism because of the work of Carol Gilligan. Carse's contribution examines the difference between the "justice" and "care" orientations. Her subtle and sophisticated analysis argues for a conception of mutual interdependence and insists that the care ethic must supplement, rather than replace, the dispassionate and detached justice orientation to moral problems. To suggest how this approach can enrich moral debates, she investigates the challenges the care ethic poses to bioethical discussions that have tended to be framed by the justice orientation.

Chapter 1
In the Gloaming

Alice Elliott Dark

Her son wanted to talk again, suddenly. During the days, he still brooded, scowling at the swimming pool from the vantage point of his wheel chair, where he sat covered with blankets in spite of the summer heat. In the evenings, though, he became more like his old self; his *old* old self, really. He became sweeter, the way he'd been as a child, before he began to gird himself with layers of irony and clever remarks. He spoke with an openness that astonished her. No one she knew talked that way—no man at least. After he was asleep, Janet would run through the conversations in her mind, and realize what it was she wished she had said. She knew she was generally considered sincere, but that had more to do with her being a good listener than with how she expressed herself. She found it hard work to keep up with him, but it was the work she had pined for all her life.

A month earlier, after a particularly long and grueling visit with a friend who'd come up on the train from New York, he had declared a new policy: no visitors, no telephone calls. She didn't blame him. People who hadn't seen him for a while were often shocked to tears by his appearance, and rather than having them cheer him up, he felt obliged to comfort them. She'd overheard bits of some of those conversations. The final one was no worse than others, but Laird was fed up. He had said more than once that he wasn't cut out to be the brace one, the one who would inspire everybody to walk away from a visit with him feeling uplifted, shaking their heads in wonder. He had liked being the most handsome and missed it very much; he was not a good victim. When he had had enough he went into a self-imposed retreat, complete with a wall of silence and other ascetic practices that kept him busy for several weeks.

Then he softened. Not only did he want to talk again; he wanted to talk to *her*.

It began the night they ate outside on the terrace for the first time all summer. Afterward, Martin—Laird's father—got up to make a telephone call, but Janet stayed in her wicker chair, resting before clearing the table. It was one of those moments when she felt nostalgic for cigarettes. On nights like this, when the air was completely still, she used to blow her famous smoke rings for the children, dutifully obeying their commands to blow one through another or three in a row, or to make big, ropey circles that expanded as they floated up to the heavens. She did exactly what they wanted, for as long as they wanted, sometimes going through a quarter of a pack before they allowed her to stop. Incredibly, neither Anne nor Laird became smokers. Just the opposite; they nagged at her to quit, and were pleased when she finally did. She wished they had been just a little bit sorry; it was a part of their childhood coming to an end, after all.

Out of habit, she took note of the first lightning bug, the first star. The lawn darkened, and the flowers that had sulked in the heat all day suddenly released their perfumes. She laid her head back on the rim of the chair and closed her eyes. Soon she was following Laird's breathing, and found herself picking up the vital rhythms, breathing along. It was so peaceful, being near him like this. How many mothers spend so much time with their thirty-three year old sons? she thought. She had as much of him now as she had had when he was an infant; more, because she had the memory of the intervening years as well, to round out her thoughts about him. When they sat quietly together she felt as close to him as she ever had. It was still him in there, inside the failing shell. *She still enjoyed him.*

"The gloaming," he said, suddenly.

She nodded dreamily, automatically, then sat up. She turned to him. "What?" Although she had heard.

"I remember when I was little you took me over to the picture window and told me that in Scotland this time of day was called the 'gloaming.'"

Her skin tingled. She cleared her throat, quietly, taking care not to make too much of the event that he was talking again. "You thought I said it was 'gloomy'."

He gave a smile, then looked at her searchingly. "I always thought it hurt you somehow that the day was over, but you said it was a beautiful time because for a few moments the purple light made the whole world look like the Scottish highlands on a summer night."

"Yes. As if all the earth was covered with heather."

"I'm sorry I never saw Scotland," he said.

"You're a Scottish lad nonetheless," she said. "At least on my side."

She remembered offering to take him to Scotland once, but Laird hadn't been interested. By then, he was in college and already sure of his own destinations, which had diverged so thoroughly from hers. "I'm amazed you remember that conversation. You couldn't have been more than seven."

"I've been remembering a lot, lately."

"Have you?"

"Mostly about when I was very small. I suppose it comes from having you take care of me again. Sometimes, when I wake up and see your face, I feel I can remember you looking in on me when I was in my crib. I remember your dresses."

"Oh no!" She laughed lightly.

"You always had the loveliest expression," he said.

She was astonished, caught off-guard. Then, she had a memory, too — of her leaning over Laird's crib and suddenly having a picture of looking up at her own mother. "I know what you mean," she said.

"You do, don't you?"

He regarded her in a close, intimate way that made her self-conscious. She caught herself swinging her leg nervously, like a pendulum, and stopped.

"Mom," he said. "There are still a few things I need to do. I have to write a will, for one thing."

Her heart went flat. In his presence she had always maintained that he would get well. She wasn't sure she could discuss the other possibility.

"Thank you," he said.

"For what?"

"For not saying that there's plenty of time for that, or some similar sentiment."

"The only reason I didn't say it was to avoid the cliché, not because I don't believe it."

"You believe there is plenty of time?"

She hesitated; he noticed, and leaned forward slightly. "I believe there is time," she said.

"Even if I were healthy, it would be a good idea."

"I suppose."

"I don't want to leave it until it's too late. You wouldn't want me to suddenly leave everything to the nurses, would you?"

She laughed, pleased to hear him joking again. "All right, all right, I'll call the lawyer."

"That would be great." There was a pause. "Is this still your favorite time of day, Mom?"

"Yes, I suppose it is," she said, "although I don't think in terms of favorites anymore."

"Never mind favorites, then. What else do you like?"

"What do you mean?" she asked.

"I mean exactly that."

"I don't know. I care about all the ordinary things. You know what I like."

"Name one thing."

"I feel silly."

"Please?"

"All right. I like my patch of lilies-of-the-valley under the trees over there. Now can we change the subject?"

"Name one more thing."

"Why?"

"I want to get to know you."

"Oh, Laird, there's nothing to know."

"I don't believe that for a minute."

"But it's true. I'm average. The only extraordinary thing about me is my children."

"All right," he said. "Then let's talk about how you feel about me."

"Do you flirt with your nurses like this when I'm not around?"

"I don't dare. They've got me where they want me." He looked at her. "You're changing the subject."

She smoothed her skirt. "I know how you feel about church, but if you need to talk, I'm sure the minister would be glad to come over. Or if you would rather a doctor . . ."

He laughed.

"What?"

"That you still call psychiatrists 'doctors.' "

She shrugged.

"I don't need a professional, Ma." He laced his hands and pulled at them as he struggled for words.

"What can I do?" she asked.

He met her gaze. "You're where I come from. I need to know about you."

That night she lay awake, trying to think of how she could help, of what, aside from time, she had to offer. She couldn't imagine.

*   *   *

She was anxious the next day when he was sullen again, but the next night, and on each succeeding night, the dusk worked its spell. She set dinner on the table outside, and afterward, when Martin had vanished into the maw of his study, she and Laird began to speak. The air around them seemed to crackle with the energy they were creating in their effort to know and be known. Were other people so close, she wondered. She never had been, not to anybody. Certainly she and Martin had never really connected, not soul to soul, and with her friends, no matter how loyal and reliable, she always had a sense of what she could do that would alienate them. Of course, her friends had the option of cutting her off, and Martin could always ask for a divorce, whereas Laird was a captive audience. Parents and children were all captive audiences to each other; in view of this, it was amazing how little comprehension there was of one another's story. Everyone stopped paying attention so early on, thinking they had figured it all out. She recognized that she was as guilty of this as anyone. She was still surprised whenever she went over to her daughter Anne's house and saw how neat she was; in her mind, Anne was still a sloppy teenager who threw sweaters into the corner of her closet and candy wrappers under her bed. It still surprised her that Laird wasn't interested in girls. He had been, hadn't he? She remembered lying awake listening for him to come home, hoping that he was smart enough to apply what he knew about the facts of life, to take precautions.

Now she had the chance to let go of these old notions. It wasn't that she liked everything about Laird—there was much that remained foreign to her—but she wanted to know about all of it. As she came to her senses every morning in the moment or two after she awoke, she found herself aching with love and gratitude, as if he were a small perfect creature again and she could look forward to a day of watching him grow. Quickly, she became greedy for their evenings. She replaced her daily, half-facetious, half-hopeful reading of the horoscope in the daily newspaper with a new habit of tracking the time the sun would set, and drew satisfaction from seeing it come earlier as the summer waned; it meant she didn't have to wait as long. She took to sleeping late, shortening the day even further. It was ridiculous, she knew. She was behaving like a girl with a crush, behaving absurdly. It was a feeling she thought she'd never have again, and now here it was. She immersed herself in it, living her life for the twilight moment when his eyes would begin to glow, the signal that he was stirring into consciousness. Then her real day would begin.

"Dad ran off quickly," he said one night. She had been wondering when he would mention it.

"He had a phone call to make," she said automatically.

Laird looked directly into her eyes, his expression one of gentle reproach. He was letting her know he had caught her in the central lie of her life, which was that she understood Martin's obsession with his work. She averted her gaze. The truth was that she had never understood. Why couldn't he sit with her for a half an hour after dinner, or, if not with her, why not with his dying son?

She turned sharply to look at Laird. The word "dying" had sounded so loudly in her mind that she wondered if she had spoken it, but he showed no reaction. She wished she hadn't even thought it. She tried to stick to good thoughts in his presence. When she couldn't, and he had a bad night afterward, she blamed herself, as her memory efficiently dredged up all the books and magazine articles she had read emphasizing the effect of psychological factors on the course of the disease. She didn't entirely believe it, but she felt compelled to give the benefit of the doubt to every theory that might help. It couldn't do any harm to think positively. And if it gave him a few more months . . .

"I don't think Dad can stand to be around me."

"That's not true." It was true.

"Poor Dad. He's always been a hypochondriac—we have that in common. He must hate this."

"He just wants you to get well."

"If that's what he wants, I'm afraid I'm going to disappoint him again. At least this will be the last time I let him down."

He said this merrily, with the old, familiar light darting from his eyes. She allowed herself to be amused. He had always been fond of teasing, and held no subject sacred. As the de-facto authority figure in the house—Martin hadn't been home enough to be the real disciplinarian—she had often been forced to reprimand Laird, but, in truth, she shared his sense of humor. She responded to it now by leaning over to cuff him on the arm. It was an automatic response, prompted by a burst of high spirits that took no notice of the circumstances. It was a mistake. Even through the thickness of his terry cloth robe, her knuckles knocked on bone. There was nothing left of him.

"It's his loss," she said, the shock of Laird's thinness making her serious again. It was the furthest she would go in criticizing Martin. She had always felt it her duty to maintain a benign image of him for the children. He had become a character of her invention, with a whole range of postulated emotions whereby he missed them when he was away on a business trip and thought of them every few minutes when he had to work late. Some years earlier, when she was secretly seeing a doctor—a psychiatrist—she had finally admitted to herself that Martin was never going to be the lover she had dreamed of. He was an ambitious, competitive, self-absorbed man who probably should never have gotten married. It was such a relief to be able to face it that she had wanted to share the news with her children, only to discover that they were dependent on the myth. They could hate his work, but they could not bring themselves to believe he had any choice in the matter. She had dropped the subject.

"Thank you, Ma. It's his loss in your case, too."

A throbbing began behind her eyes, angering her. The last thing she wanted to do was cry. There would be plenty of time for that. "It's not all his fault," she said when she had regained some measure of control. "I'm not very good at talking about myself. I was brought up not to."

"So was I," he said.

"Yes, I suppose you were."

"Luckily, I didn't pay any attention." He grinned.

"I hope not," she said, and meant it. "Can I get you anything?"

"A new immune system?"

She rolled her eyes, trying to disguise the way his joke had touched on her prayers. "Very funny. I was thinking more along the lines of an iced tea or an extra blanket."

"I'm fine. I'm getting tired, actually."

Her entire body went on the alert, and she searched his face anxiously for signs of deterioration. Her nerves darted and pricked whenever he wanted anything; her adrenaline rushed. The fight-or-flight response, she supposed. She had often wanted to flee, but had forced herself to stay, to fight with what few weapons she had. She responded to his needs, making sure there was a fresh, clean set of sheets ready when he was tired, food for his hunger. It was what she could do.

"Shall I get the nurse?" She pushed her chair back from the table.

"O.K.," Laird said weakly. He stretched out his hand to her, and the incipient moonlight illuminated his skin so it shone like alabaster. His face had turned ashy. It was a sight that made her stomach drop. She ran for Maggie, and by the time they returned Laird's eyes were closed, his head lolling to one side. Automatically, Janet looked for a stirring in his chest. There it was; his shoulders expanded; he still breathed. Always, in the second before she saw movement, she became cold and clinical as she braced herself for the possibility of discovering that he was dead.

Maggie had her fingers on his wrist and was counting his pulse against the second hand on her watch, her lips moving. She laid his limp hand back on his lap. "Fast," she pronounced.

"I'm not surprised," Janet said, masking her fear with authority. "We had a long talk."

Maggie frowned. "Now I'll have to wake him up again for his meds."

"Yes, I suppose that's true. I forgot about that."

Janet wheeled him into his makeshift room downstairs and helped Maggie lift him into the rented hospital bed. Although he weighed almost nothing, it was really a job for two; his weight was dead weight. In front of Maggie, she was all brusque efficiency, except for the moment when her fingers strayed to touch Laird's pale cheek and she prayed she hadn't done any harm.

*   *   *

"Who's your favorite author?" he asked one night.

"Oh, there are so many," she said.

"Your real favorite."

She thought. "The truth is there are certain subjects I find attractive more than certain authors. I seem to read in cycles, to fulfill an emotional yearning."

"Such as?"

"Books about people who go off to live in Africa or Australia or the South Seas."

He laughed. "That's fairly self-explanatory. What else?"

"When I really hate life I enjoy books about real murders. 'True crime,' I think they're called now. They're very punishing."

"Is that what's so compelling about them? I could never figure it out. I just knew that at certain times I loved the gore, even though I felt absolutely disgusted with myself for being interested in it."

"You need to think about when those times were. That will tell you a lot." She paused. "I don't like reading about sex."

"Big surprise!"

"No, no," she said. "It's not for the reason you think, or not only for that reason. You see me as a prude, I know, but remember, it's part of a mother's job to come across that way. Although perhaps I went a bit far . . ."

He shrugged amiably. "Water under the bridge. But go on about sex."

"I think it should be private. I always feel as though these writers are showing off when they describe a sex scene. They're not really trying to describe sex, but to demonstrate that they're not afraid to write about it. As if they're thumbing noses at their mothers."

He made a moue.

Janet went on. "You don't think there's an element of that? I *do* question their motives, because I don't think sex can ever be accurately portrayed—the sensations and the emotions are—beyond language. If you only describe the mechanics, the effect is either clinical or pornographic, and if you try to describe intimacy instead, you wind up with abstractions. The only sex you could describe fairly well is bad sex—and who wants to read about that, for God's sake, when everyone is having bad sex of their own?"

"Mother!" He was laughing helplessly, his arms hanging limply over the sides of his chair.

"I mean it. To me it's like reading about someone using the bathroom."

"Good grief!"

"Now who's the prude?"

"I never said I wasn't," he said. "Maybe we should change the subject."

She looked out across the land. The lights were on in other people's houses, giving the evening the look of early fall. The leaves were different, too, becoming droopy. The grass was dry, even with all the watering and tending from the gardener. The summer was nearly over.

"Maybe we shouldn't," she said. "I've been wondering. Was that side of life satisfying for you?"

"Ma, tell me you're not asking me about my sex life."

She took her napkin and folded it carefully, lining up the edges and running her fingers along the hems. She felt very calm, very pulled together and all of a piece, as if she'd finally got the knack of being a dignified woman. She threaded her fingers and laid her hands in her lap. "I'm asking about your love life," she said. "Did you love, and were you loved in return?"

"Yes."

"I'm glad."

"That was easy," he said.

"Oh, I've gotten very easy, in my old age."

"Does Dad know about this?" His eyes were twinkling wickedly.

"Don't be fresh," she said.

"You started it."

"Then I'm stopping it. Now."

He made a funny face, and then another, until she could no longer keep from smiling. His routine carried her back to memories of his childhood efforts to charm her: watercolors of her favorite vistas (unrecognizable without the captions), bouquets of violets self-consciously flung into her lap, a chore performed without prompting. He had always gone too far, then backtracked to regain even footing. She had always allowed herself to be wooed.

Suddenly she realized: Laird had been the love of her life.

*   *   *

One night it rained hard. She decided to serve the meal in the kitchen, as Martin was out. They ate in silence; she was freed from the compulsion to keep up the steady stream of chatter that she used to affect when Laird hadn't talked at all; now she knew she could save her words for afterward. He ate nothing but comfort foods lately: mashed potatoes, vanilla ice cream, rice pudding. The days of his strict macrobiotic regime, and all the cooking classes she had taken in order to help him along with it, were long past. His body was essentially a thing of the past, too; when he ate, he was feeding what was left of his mind. He seemed to want to recapture the cosseted feeling he'd had when he was sick as a child and she would serve him flat ginger ale, and toast soaked in cream, and play endless card games with him, using his blanket-covered legs as a table. In those days, too, there'd been a general sense of giving way to illness: then, he let himself go completely because he knew he would soon be better and active and have a million things expected of him again. Now he let himself go because he had fought long enough.

Finally, he pushed his bowl toward the middle of the table, signaling that he was finished. (His table manners had gone to pieces. Who cared?) She felt a light, jittery excitement, the same jazzy feeling she got when she was in a plane that was just picking up speed on the runway. She arranged her fork and knife on the rim of her plate and pulled her chair in closer. "I had an odd dream last night," she said.

His eyes remained dull.

She waited uncertainly, thinking that perhaps she had started to talk too soon. "Would you like something else to eat?"

He shook his head. There was no will in his expression; his refusal was purely physical, a gesture coming from the satiation in his stomach. An animal walking away from its bowl, she thought.

To pass the time, she carried the dishes to the sink, gave them a good, hot rinse, and put them in the dishwasher. She carried the ice cream to the counter, pulled a spoon from the drawer and scraped together a mouthful of the thick, creamy residue that stuck to the inside of the lid. She ate it without thinking, so the sudden sweetness caught her by surprise. All the while she kept track of Laird, but every time she thought she noticed signs of his readiness to talk and hurried back to the table she found his face still blank.

She went to the window. The lawn had become a floodplain and was filled with broad pools; the branches of the evergreens sagged, and the sky was the same uniform greyish yellow it had been since morning. She saw him focus his gaze on the line where the treetops touched the heavens, and she understood. There was no lovely interlude on this rainy night, no heathered dusk. The grey landscape had taken the light out of him.

"I'm sorry," she said aloud, as if it were her fault.

He gave a tiny, helpless shrug.

She hovered for a few moments, hoping, but his face was slack, and she gave up. She felt utterly forsaken, too disappointed and agitated to sit with him and watch the rain. "It's all right," she said. "It's a good night to watch television."

She wheeled him to the den and left him with Maggie, then did not know what to do with herself. She had no contingency plan for this time. It was usually the one period of the day when she did not need the anesthesia of tennis games, bridge lessons, volunteer work, errands. She had not considered the present possibility. For some time, she hadn't given any thought to what Martin would call "the big picture." Her conversations with Laird had lulled her into inventing a parallel big picture of her own. She realized that a part of her had worked out a whole scenario: the summer evenings would blend into fall; then, gradually, the winter would arrive, heralding chats by the fire, Laird resting his feet on the pigskin ottoman in the den while she dutifully knitted her yearly Christmas sweaters for Anne's children.

She had allowed herself to imagine a future. That had been her mistake. This silent, endless evening was her punishment, a reminder of how things really were.

She did not know where to go in her own house, and ended up wandering through the rooms propelled by a vague, hunted feeling. Several times she turned around, expecting someone to be there, but, of course, no one ever was. She was quite alone. Eventually she realized she was imagining a person in order to give material properties to the source of her wounds. She was inventing a villain. There should be a villain, shouldn't there? There should be an enemy, a devil, an evil force that could be driven out. Her imagination had provided it with aspects of a corporeal presence so she could pretend, for a moment, that there was a real enemy hovering around her, someone she could have the police come and take away. But the enemy was part of Laird, and neither he nor she nor any of the doctors or experts or ministers could separate the two.

She went upstairs and took a shower. She barely paid attention to her own body any more, and only noticed abstractly that the water was too hot, her skin turning pink. Afterward, she sat on the chaise lounge in her bedroom and tried to read. She heard something; she leaned forward and cocked her head toward the sound. Was that Laird's voice? Suddenly she believed that he had begun to talk after all—she believed he was talking to Maggie. She dressed and went downstairs. He was alone in the den, alone with the television. He didn't hear or see her. She watched him take a drink from a cup, his hand shaking badly. It was a plastic cup with a straw poking through the lid, the kind used by small children while they are learning to drink. It was supposed to prevent accidents, but it couldn't stop his hands from trembling. He managed to spill the juice anyway.

*   *   *

Laird had always coveted the decadent pile of cashmere lap blankets she had collected over the years in the duty-free shops of the various British airports. Now he wore one around his shoulders, one over his knees. She remembered similar balmy nights when he would arrive home from soccer practice after dark, a towel slung around his neck.

"I suppose it has to be in the church," he said.

"I think it should," she said, "but it's up to you."

"I guess it's not the most timely moment to make a statement about my personal disbeliefs. But I'd like you to keep it from being too lugubrious. No lilies, for instance."

"God forbid."

"And have some decent music."

"Such as?"

"I had an idea, but now I can't remember."

He pressed his hands to his eyes. His fingers were so transparent that they looked as if he were holding them over a flashlight.

"Please buy a smashing dress, something mournful yet elegant."

"All right."

"And don't wait until the last minute."

She didn't reply.

*   *   *

Janet gave up on the idea of a rapprochement between Martin and Laird; she felt freer when she stopped hoping for it. Martin rarely came home for dinner anymore. Perhaps he was having an affair? It was a thought she'd never allowed herself to have before, but it didn't threaten her now. Good for him, she even decided, in her strongest, most magnanimous moments. Good for him if he's actually feeling bad and trying to do something to make himself feel better.

Anne was brave and chipper during her visits, yet when she walked back out to her car she would wrap her arms around her ribs and shudder. "I don't know how you do it, Mom. Are you really all right?" she always asked, with genuine concern.

"Anne's become such a hopeless matron," Laird always said, with fond exasperation, when he and his mother were alone again later. Once Janet began to tease him for finally coming to friendly terms with his sister, but she cut it short when she saw that he was blinking furiously.

They were exactly the children she had hoped to have; a companionable girl, a mischievous boy. It gave her great pleasure to see them together. She did not try to listen to their conversations but watched from a distance, usually from the kitchen as she prepared them a snack reminiscent of their childhood, like watermelon boats or lemonade. Then she would walk Anne to the car, their similar good shoes clacking across the gravel. They hugged, pressing each other's arms, and their brief embraces buoyed them up—forbearance and strength passing back and forth between them like a piece of shared clothing, designated for use by whoever needed it most. It was the kind of parting toward which she had aimed her whole life, a graceful, secure parting at the close of a peaceful afternoon. After Anne left, Janet always had a tranquil moment or two as she walked back to the house through the humid September air. Everything was so still. Occasionally there were the hums and clicks of a lawnmower or the shrieks of a band of children heading home from school. There were the insects and the birds. It was a straightforward, simple life she had chosen. She had tried never to ask for too much, and to be of use. Simplicity had been her hedge against bad luck. It had worked for so long. For a brief moment, as she stepped lightly up the single slate stair and through the door, her legs still harboring all their former vitality, she could pretend her luck was still holding.

Then she would glance out the window and there would be the heart-catching sight of Laird, who would never again drop by for a casual visit. Her chest would ache and flutter, a cave full of bats.

Perhaps she had asked for too much, after all.

*   *   *

"What did you want to be when you grew up?" Laird asked.

"I was expected to be a wife and mother. I accepted that. I wasn't a rebel."

"There must have been something else."

"No," she said. "Oh, I guess I had all the usual fantasies of the day, of being the next Amelia Earhart or Margaret Mead, but that was all they were—fantasies. I wasn't even close to being brave enough. Can you imagine me flying across the ocean on my own?" She laughed and looked over for his laughter, but he had fallen asleep.

*   *   *

A friend of Laird's had somehow gotten the mistaken information that Laird had died, so she and Martin received a condolence letter. There was a story about a time a few years back when the friend was with Laird on a bus in New York. They had been sitting behind two older women, waitresses who began to discuss their income taxes, trying to decide how much of their tip income to declare to sound realistic so they wouldn't attract an audit. Each offered up bits of folk wisdom on the subject, describing in detail her particular situation. During a lull in the conversation, Laird stood up.

"Excuse me, I couldn't help but overhearing," he said, leaning over them. "May I have your names and addresses, please? I work for the I.R.S."

The entire bus fell silent as everyone watched to see what would happen next. Laird took a small notebook and pen from the inside pocket of his jacket. He faced his captive audience. "I'm part of a new I.R.S. outreach program," he told the group. "For the next ten minutes I'll be taking confessions. Does anyone have anything he or she wants to tell me?"

Smiles. Soon the whole bus was talking, comparing notes—on when they'd first realized he was kidding, on how scared they'd been before they caught on. It was difficult to believe these were the same New Yorkers who were supposed to be so gruff and isolated.

"Laird was the most vital, funniest person I ever met," his friend wrote.

Now, in his wheelchair, he faced off against slow-moving flies, waving them away.

*   *   *

"The gloaming," Laird said.

Janet looked up from her knitting, startled. It was midafternoon, and the living room was filled with bright October sun. "Soon," she said.

He furrowed his brow. A little flash of confusion passed through his eyes, and she realized that for him it was already dark.

He tried to straighten his shawl, his hands shaking. She jumped up to help; then, when he pointed to the fireplace, she quickly laid the logs as she wondered what was wrong. Was he dehydrated? She thought she recalled that a dimming of the vision was a sign of dehydration. She tried to remember what else she had read or heard, but even as she grasped for information, facts, her instincts kept interrupting with a deeper, more dreadful thought that vibrated through her, rattling her and making her gasp as she often did when remembering her mistakes, things she wished she hadn't said or done, wished she had the chance to do over. She knew what was wrong, and yet she kept turning away from the truth, her mind spinning in every other possible direction as she worked on the fire, only vaguely noticing how wildly she made the sparks fly as she pumped the old bellows.

Her work was mechanical—she had made hundreds of fires—and soon there was nothing left to do. She put the screen up and pushed him close, then leaned over to pull his flannel pajamas down to meet his socks, protecting his bare shins. The sun streamed in around him, making him appear trapped between bars of light. She resumed her knitting, with mechanical hands.

"The gloaming," he said again. It did sound somewhat like "gloomy," because his speech was slurred.

"When all the world is purple," she said, hearing herself sound falsely bright. She wasn't sure whether he wanted her to talk. It was some time since he talked—not long, really, in other people's lives, perhaps two weeks—but she had gone on with their conversations, gradually expanding into the silence until she was telling him stories and he was listening. Sometimes, when his eyes closed, she trailed off and began to drift. There would be a pause that she didn't always realize she was making, but if it went on too long he would call out "Mom?" with an edge of panic in his voice, as if he were waking from a nightmare. Then she would resume, trying to create a seamless bridge between what she had been thinking and where she had left off.

"It was really your grandfather who gave me my love for the gloaming," she said. "Do you remember him talking about it?" She looked up politely, expectantly, as if Laird might offer her a conversational reply. He seemed to like hearing the sound of her voice so she went on, her needles clicking. Afterward, she could never remember for sure at what point she had stopped talking and had floated off into a jumble of her own thoughts, afraid to move, afraid to look up, afraid to know at which exact moment she became alone. All she knew was that at a certain point the fire was in danger of dying out entirely, and when she got up to stir the embers she glanced at him in spite of herself and saw that his fingers were making knitting motions over his chest, the way people did as they were dying. She knew that if she went to get the nurse Laird would be gone by the time she returned, so she went and stood behind him, leaning over to press her face against his, sliding her hands down his busy arms, helping him along with his fretful stitches until he finished this last piece of work.

*   *   *

Later, after the most pressing calls had been made and Laird's body had been taken away, Janet went up to his old room and lay down on one of the twin beds. She had changed the room into a guest room when he went off to college, replacing his things with guest-room decor, thoughtful touches such as luggage racks at the foot of each bed, a writing desk stocked with paper and pens, heavy wooden hangers and shoe trees. She made an effort to remember the room as it had been when he was a little boy; she had chosen a train motif, then had to redecorate when Laird decided trains were silly. He had wanted it to look like a jungle, so she had hired an art student to paint a jungle mural on the walls. When he decided *that* was silly, he hadn't bothered her to do anything about it, but had simply marked time until he could move on.

Anne came over, offered to stay, but was relieved to be sent home to her children.

Presently, Martin came in. Janet was watching the trees turn to mere silhouettes against the darkening sky, fighting the urge to pick up a true-crime book, a debased urge. He lay down on the other bed.

"I'm sorry," he said.

"It's so wrong," she said angrily. She hadn't felt angry until that moment; she had saved it up for him. "A child shouldn't die before his parents. A young man shouldn't spend his early thirties wasting away talking to his mother. He should be out in the world. He shouldn't be thinking about me, or what I care about, or my opinions. He shouldn't have had to return my love to me—it was his to squander. Now I have it all back and I don't know what I'm supposed to do with it," she said.

She could hear Martin weeping in the darkness. He sobbed, and her anger veered away.

They were quiet for some time.

"Is there going to be a funeral?" Martin asked finally.

"Yes. We should start making the arrangements."

"I suppose he told you what he wanted."

"In general. He couldn't decide about the music."

She heard Martin roll onto his side, so that he was facing her across the narrow chasm between the beds. He was still in his office clothes. "I remember being very moved by the bagpipes at your father's funeral."

It was an awkward offering, to be sure, awkward and late, and seemed to come from someone on the periphery of her life who only knew her slightly. It didn't matter; it was perfectly right. Her heart rushed toward it.

"I think Laird would have liked that idea very much," she said.

It was the last moment of the gloaming, the last moment of the day that her son died. In a breath, it would be night; the moon hovered behind the trees, already rising to claim the sky, and she told herself she might as well get on with it. She sat up and was running her toes across the bare floor, searching for her shoes, when Martin spoke again, in a tone she used to hear on those long-ago nights when he rarely got home until after the children were in bed and he relied on her to fill him in on what they'd done that day. It was the same curious, shy, deferential tone that had always made her feel as though all the frustrations and boredom and mistakes and rushes of feeling in her days as a mother did indeed add up to something of importance, and she decided that the next round of telephone calls could wait while she answered the question he asked her: "Please tell me—what else did my boy like?"

Chapter 2
The Cared-For

Nel Noddings

The One-Caring's Attitude and Its Effects

The "one-caring" comes across to the "cared-for" in an attitude. Whatever she does, she conveys to the cared for that she cares. If she is in conversation with a colleague, she listens, and her eyes reflect the seriousness, humor, or excitement of the message being spoken. If she tends the sick, her hands are gentle with the anticipation of pain and discomfort. If she comforts the night-terrored child, her embrace shields from both terror and ridicule. She feels the excitement, pain, terror, or embarrassment of the other and commits herself to act accordingly. She is present to the cared for. Her attitude is one of receptivity. But there is a receptivity required of the cared for also.

Suppose that a child of, say, eight years comes home from school angry. He storms into the kitchen and throws his books on the floor. His mother, startled, says, "What happened, honey?" (She resists the temptation to say something to the effect that "in this house we do not throw things.") The child says that his teacher is "impossible," "completely unfair," "mean," "stupid," and so on. His mother sympathizes and probes gently for what happened. Gradually, under the quiet influence of a receptive listener, the child calms down. As his mother sympathizes, he may even relax enough to say, "Well, it wasn't that bad," in answer to his mother's sympathetic outrage. Then the two may smile at each other and explore rational solutions; they can speculate about faults, mistakes, and intentions. They can plot a course of action for the future. The child,

An earlier version of this essay appeared as chapter 3, "The Cared-For," in Noddings, *Caring: A Feminine Approach to Ethics and Moral Education* (Berkeley: University of California Press, 1984), copyright © 1984 by Regents of the University of California. Reprinted by permission.

accepted and supported, can begin to examine his own role in the incident and, perhaps, even suggest how he might have behaved differently.

The receptivity of the one-caring need not lead to permissiveness nor to an abdication of responsibility for conduct and achievement. Rather, it maintains and enhances the relatedness that is fundamental to human reality and, in education, it sets the stage for the teacher's effort in maintaining and increasing the child's receptive capacity. As the teacher receives the child and works with him on cooperatively designed projects, as she resists the temptation—or the mandate—to manipulate the child, to squeeze him into some mold, she establishes a climate of receptivity. The one caring reflects reality as she sees it to the child. She accepts him as she hopes he will accept himself—seeing what is there, considering what might be changed, speculating on what might be. But the commitment, the decision to embrace a particular possibility, must be the child's. Her commitment is to him. While she expresses herself honestly when his vision of himself is unlovely and enthusiastically when it is beautiful, she never reflects a reality that pictures him detached, alone, abandoned. If her standards seem mysterious at times to outsiders, they are not so to the cared-for who has participated in their construction.

We shall return again and again to a discussion of receptivity. It is in the relaxation of detached and objective self, in this engrossment, that the one-caring assumes her full individuality in relatedness. The child who retains his receptivity can lose himself not only in others for whom he becomes one-caring, but also in ideas and objects. The teacher who encourages receptivity wants the child to look, to listen, to touch and, perhaps, to receive a vision of reality. When we speak of receiving reality, we do not deny that each human consciousness participates in the construction of reality, but we give proper emphasis to the relatedness that must be perceived and accepted before any coherent picture can be constructed. The other is received, his reality is apprehended as possibility for oneself. The object is received; its reality stands out against the background of its possibilities in the one receiving.

One learns to participate in cycles. At one stage, things are allowed to enter with little restriction; a reservoir of images and energy is stored up. Then a focusing takes place; the energies are made dense, brought sharply to focus on a point of interest. Then a diffusion may occur. The energy is converted to light and scattered over the entire field of interest illuminating elements and ground. The field is now characterized by coherence and grace. Both initial and final stages may be characterized as receptive. In the first we receive what is there; in the last, we receive what-is-there in relation to what-is-here. We see how we are related to this object to which we are related.

The cared-for responds to the presence of the one-caring. He feels the difference between being received and being held off or ignored. Whatever the one-caring actually does is enhanced or diminished, made meaningful or meaningless, in the attitude conveyed to the cared-for. This attitude is not something thought by either the one-caring or the cared-for although, of course, either one may think about it. It is a total conveyance of self to other, a continual transformation of individual to duality to new individual to new duality. Neither the engrossment of the one-caring nor the perception of attitude by the cared-for is rational; that is, neither is reasoned. While much of what goes on in caring is rational and carefully thought out, the basic relationship is not, and neither is the required awareness of relatedness. The essentially nonrational nature of caring is recognized by, for example, Urie Bronfenbrenner when he claims: "In order to develop, a chld needs the enduring, irrational involvement of one or more adults in care and joint activity with the child." In answer to what he means by "irrational," he explains: "Somebody has got to be crazy about that kid!" (1978, pp. 773–74).

The child about whom no one is "crazy" presents a special problem for teachers. Obviously, the teacher cannot be "crazy about" every child; the notion loses its force spread so thin. But the teacher can try to provide an environment in which affection and support are enhanced, in which children not passionately loved will at least receive attention and, perhaps, learn to respond to and encourage those who genuinely address them. Such a child may herself someday be "crazy about" some other child even though she herself was never the recipient of such affection.

Now, of course, philosophers are certain to point out that being "crazy" about a child is not necessarily irrational. But Bronfenbrenner's way of talking nevertheless makes an essential point about the caring relationship in which a child thrives. It is at bottom not rational; that is, it is fundamentally nonrational. However rational the decision making processes, however rational the investigation of means-ends relations, the commitment that elicits the rational activity precedes it and gives it personal meaning. We do not usually, as caring parents, select activities to share with our children on the basis of some "learning plan"; we do not, for example, take our children to the zoo so that they will be able to name and describe ten animals native to Africa. Rather, we decide more or less spontaneously to spend an afternoon at the zoo, because we remember our own childish pleasure in such occasions and anticipate delight in sharing the experience with our children. That our children learn things through visits to zoos, museums, national monuments, and the like is something we all take for granted but, for most of us, the potential learning is not what motivates the visits. We often find ourselves in teaching-learning situations with our children, but these arise naturally in the companionable relationship established through caring. We commit ourselves to our children.

Bronfenbrenner suggests, further, that children embraced in such nonrational relationships gain competence; that is, they become able to master situations of greater and greater complexity through their cooperative participation with adults. When parent and child work together on various projects over a period of time, the child gradually becomes competent in more and more tasks constituting the project. The parent who cares, who receives the child, allows him to take hold of what he can do. She does not keep him in a subservient position but welcomes his growing competence and independence.

We hear the word "competence" often these days. We hear it in the context of competency based education (CBE) and in reference to competence tests for high school graduation. But "competence" in these contexts refers more accurately to performance, to a demonstrated mastery of prespecified and discrete tasks. "Competence" as I am using it points to a global mastery of conditions in one's personal or professional environment and, indirectly, to the desire for such mastery. The psychologist Robert White suggests that the desire for competence is innate; that is, human beings naturally experience what may be termed "effectance motivation." He notes that activity thus engaged produces a feeling of efficacy:

. . . it is maintained that competence cannot be fully acquired simply through behavior instigated by drives. It receives substantial contributions from activities which, though playful and exploratory in character, at the same time show direction, selectivity, and persistence in interacting with the environment. Such activities in the ultimate service of competence must therefore be conceived to be motivated in their own right. (White 1959, p. 327)

Small children practice going up and down stairs, turning lights and faucets on and off, dropping things and retrieving them. All of these activities, which seem to adults repetitiously boring and even annoying, are engaged in for the sake of mastering the environment. The competent individual enjoys a sense of control over the objects and events with which he regularly comes in contact.

If this is right, we can see the importance of arranging the environment appropriately for growing children. To call forth a natural effectance motivation, the challenge must be within the optimal range. If the challenge is too great, the child may become frustrated and look for a way to avoid it entirely or to meet it—however unsatisfactorily—for the mere purpose of terminating it. Failing just to "get it over with" is not an unusual strategy in schools. If, on the other hand, the challenge is too slight, the child may become bored and, again, his approach may deteriorate—this time to perfunctory performance.

The one-caring receives the child and views that child's world through both sets of eyes. Martin Buber calls this relational process "inclusion" (Buber 1965, pp. 83–103). The one-caring assumes a dual perspective and can see things from both her own pole and that of the cared for. If this were not so, arranging an educational environment for the child would be very difficult. One would have to resort to descriptions of the child as abstraction and, indeed, many educators do exactly this. They say such things as "Children are interested in their own surroundings," and use this pronouncement as a reason for including a study of the neighborhood in beginning social studies and for excluding studies of foreign lands and ancient times. The result is often deadening. The one-caring, on the other hand, watches for incipient interest in the child— the particular, concrete child—and arranges the educational environment accordingly. Possibly no insight of John Dewey's was greater than that which reveals the vital importance of building educational strategy on the purposes of the child. The principle of the leading out of experience does not imply letting the child learn what he pleases; it suggests that, inescapably, the child will learn what he pleases. That means that the educator must arrange the effective world so that the child will be challenged to master significant tasks in significant situations. The initial judgment of significance is the teacher's task.

But there is another, vital aspect to "learning what one pleases." "Because it pleases me" is rarely our basic reason for acting. We might better think here of what we choose to do and consider the kinds of reasons we might give for our choices. A child—or anyone—can be forced to learn what he initially finds uninteresting or even repugnant. Indeed, we know that we may be forced to deny our principles and betray our loved ones if sufficiently terrible tactics are employed. How, then, can we support a position that insists that the child will learn what he chooses? The answer lies in recognizing that we sometimes choose against ourselves. We give way for reasons that do not make us proud of ourselves. We rationalize. We concoct reasons that are far removed from our normal pattern of motivation or, in the most dreadful situations, we act directly and unreflectively to preserve what we can of our physical or public selves. We deteriorate, and our ethical ideas are diminished. But we still choose, and recognition of the choice induces a new agony. I am in the sleazy motive, the panicked betrayal, the reluctant obedience.

The educator or parent, then, is not powerless. On the contrary, her power is awesome. Somehow the child must be led to choose for himself and not against himself, and this means that he will choose not only for his physical self but, more importantly, for his ethical self.

The child, as one cared-for, will often respond with interest to challenges proffered by the one-caring, if the one-caring is loved and trusted by the child. As an initial impulse to engage particular subject matter, love for the adult and the desire to imitate her are powerful inducements. Further, working together on tasks makes it possible for the child to accept greater challenges and to maintain a high level of effectance motivation. What is conveyed to the child is that there is something delightful about the companionship that continues through every stage of developing competence. At the earliest stages, a young child is not much help in, say, preparing meals. But he can do some things: he can hand me a spoon, poke the Jello to see if it has set, pat the hamburgers flat. He can share with me the sights, smells, sounds, tastes, and textures encountered in working with foods. As he watches me and helps me, he is learning the names of things, acquiring a sense of orderliness, learning to recognize phenomena such as boiling, thickening, and the like. After a while he can pour milk, crack eggs without squashing them, sift flour, and take turns stirring the batter. Eventually, he can prepare individual dishes and take responsibility for whole meals. Through all of these stages, there is mutual pleasure not only in the child's growing competence, but also in the shared activities and their products.

It would be easy to spend volumes talking about what children can learn through working with their parents in food preparation, but our main interest here is the attitude of the one-caring and how it affects the cared-for. The child is encouraged to try by the acceptance of the parent, and he is made to feel a partner in the enterprise. As we shall see later, the parent's attitude goes beyond acceptance to what Buber calls "confirmation." The one-caring sees the best self in the cared-for and works with him to actualize that self. The child is affected not only by his parent's attitude toward him, but also by her attitudes toward a multitude of objects and events. She may treat meals as celebrations or as duties. She may show an appreciation for the beauty of fresh fruits and vegetables or she may be indifferent to them. Cooking may be work or play or both. The kitchen may be clean or dirty, attractive or dreary. More important than anything else, however, is whether the child is welcome, whether he is seen as a contributing person.

Apprehension of Caring Necessary to the Caring Relationship; Unequal Meetings

This attitude of warm acceptance and trust is important to all caring relationships. We are primarily interested in parent-child and teacher-student relationships but it is clear that caring is completed in all relationships through the apprehension of caring by the cared-for. When this attitude is missed, the one who is the object of caretaking feels like an object. He is being treated, handled by formula. When it is present and recognized, the natural effectance motivation is enhanced.

A mother recounts the story of an upsetting experience with school counselors and administrators. She and her husband requested that their very bright daughter be skipped a grade. The child had suffered two serious illnesses and, during her long bed stay, had read, studied, and written well beyond her grade placement. On returning to school, she was bored with both the studies and the childishness of her classmates. The parents, quite naturally, feared that their child would lose interest in school entirely, and so they requested a special hearing. The school team received them in a physically cordial manner that quickly revealed a total lack of presence. They spoke patronizingly of how "all professional parents want to push their children," and how doting parents tend to "overestimate their children's abilities," of how the practice of skipping children "damages their social competence." The parents, of course, became more and more frustrated. The harder they tried to explain, the more quickly came smiling responses: "We understand." "Of course." "You think your child is exceptional." Finally, in utter frustration, the couple suggested that the matter be left to an evaluation of the school psychologist. Fortunately (things could have turned out differently), the school psychologist recommended that the child be advanced. Three reasons supported the recommendation: The child was large for her age, she was socially and emotionally advanced, and she exhibited a tested I.Q. over 160. These parents have never since been comfortable with school officials and school rulings, and they have assumed primary responsibility for the education of their children.

To be talked at by people for whom we do not exist, as Marcel points out, throws us back upon ourselves. To be treated as "types" instead of individuals, to have strategies exercised on us, objectifies us. We become "cases" instead of persons. Those of us who are able to escape such situations do so with alacrity, but escape is not always possible, and for some of us it is rarely possible. The fact is that many of us have been reduced to cases by the very machinery that has been instituted to care for us.

It is not easy for one entrusted with a helping function to care. A dif-

ference of status and the authorization to help prevent an equal meeting between helper and the one helped. In a dialogue with Carl Rogers,
Martin Buber emphasizes this point:

> . . . A man coming to you for help . . . . The essential difference between your
> role in this situation and his is obvious. He comes for help to you. You don't
> come for help to him. And not only this, but you are *able*, more or less, to
> help him. He can do different things to you, but not to help you. And not this
> alone. You *see* him, *really*. I don't mean that you cannot be mistaken, but you *see*
> him, . . . he cannot, by far, cannot *see you*. (Buber 1964, p. 487)

In this discussion, Buber was, of course, acknowledging the legitimacy and—more importantly—the sensitivity of Rogers's therapy. Not
every helper sees the patient or client. Indeed, we just reviewed a case
in which the counselors were totally absent to the struggling clients. But
even if the therapist is sensitive and receptive, Buber points out that
the fact of his or her authorization to help gets in the way of an equal
meeting. Social worker and client, physician and patient, counselor and
student in their formal roles necessarily meet each other unequally. Insofar as the client, patient, and student are part of their work load,
professionals may even find it desirable "to forget" them at the end of
the workday. To think of them, to be engrossed in them, would be to
take their "work" home. But to think this way is to misunderstand the
nature of engrossment in caring. It misses the potentiality and latency
that characterize caring.

It is not only the authorization to help or to instruct that makes unequal meetings in therapy or teaching inevitable. It is also the nature
of the cared-for's situation. The patient needs help; the student needs
instruction or information or interpretation. The teacher as one-caring
needs to see from both her own perspective and that of the student in
order to teach—in order to meet the needs of the student. Achieving
inclusion is part of teaching successfully, and one who cannot practice
inclusion fails as a teacher. The student, however, achieves his ends
without inclusion. He is freed by the teacher's engrossment in him and
his projects to pursue those projects without considering their significance for the personal development of the teacher. I think Buber is
right when he says that mutual inclusion moves a relationship away from
that of teacher-student toward friendship. Occasional equal meetings
may occur between teacher and student, of course, but the meetings
between teacher as teacher and student as student are necessarily and
generously unequal.

It is only through inclusion that the parent or teacher can practice
confirmation. I must see the cared-for as he is and as he might be—as
he envisions his best self—in order to confirm him. The attitude that is

perceived by the cared-for as caring is generated by efforts of the one-caring at inclusion and confirmation. It is an attitude that both accepts and confirms. It does not "accept" and shrug off. It accepts, embraces, and leads upward. It questions, it responds, it sympathizes, it challenges, it delights.

So far we have been discussing an attitude on the part of the one-caring which conveys the caring to the cared-for. We have spoken of acceptance and confirmation, of receiving, of inclusion, and of "unequal meetings," and we have considered some examples in the area of parent-child relationships and helper-client relationships. I have been proceeding in an informal phenomenological way, exploring situations and how the participants within them feel and see things. But it is important to keep sight of the logic of our concept of caring as it is being developed, and it is important, also, to recognize that there is empirical evidence for much of what has been claimed.

I have claimed that the cared-for "grows" and "glows" under the perceived attitude of the one-caring. Support for such claims can be found in many sources. It is especially impressive in the negative; that is, the evidence is clear that the rejection characteristic of noncaring has observable effects in the cared-for. Although the evidence from any one case cannot be conclusive, it is overwhelming in its collective form. Many researchers—among them, Sanger (1926), Montagu (1962), and Wengraf (1953)—present evidence that even the fetus is affected by the attitude of acceptance or rejection in its mother. A review of the undesirable effects that may be induced in children, both prenatal and postnatal, by maternal attitudes of rejection can be found in Edward Pohlman's discussion on birth planning (1969). Further, the attitude itself seems to be causal. Zilboorg says that it "has its rather mysterious ways of conveying itself to the child and provoking a considerable number of undesirable and at times directly pathological reactions" (1957, 73:308)

By "mysterious ways," Zilboorg and other researchers mean that it is an attitude that itself seems to do the mischief. Sears, for example, found few significant differences in child rearing practices between accepting and rejecting parents (1957), and a similar conclusion was reached by Schaefer and Bell (1957, pp. 391–5). But behavioral differences were found in the children. Hence a claim that attitude is crucial to an analysis of caring, that feeling is somehow conveyed directly, is partially supported empirically.

In addition to providing empirical support for what we see reflectively in a phenomenological view, I want to provide a logical analysis of the caring relation. I have claimed that the perception by the cared-for of an attitude of caring on the part of the one-caring is partially constitutive of caring. It and its successful impact on the cared-for are necessary to caring. Does this mean that I cannot be said to care for X if X does not recognize my caring? In the fullest sense, I think we have to accept this result. By looking closely at caring from the view of the one-caring, from the position of the cared for, and from the perspective of a third-person observer, we see pictures of caring that are potentially conflicting and yet, at bottom complementary. The third-person aspect will be important for us when we consider institutional problems of caring, but it does not enter or alter the essential description of caring. Caring involves two parties: the one-caring and the cared-for. It is complete when it is fulfilled in both. We are tempted to say that the caring attitude is characteristic of caring, that when one cares, she characteristically exhibits an attitude. But, then, it could be missed by the cared-for. Suppose I claim to care for X, but X does not believe that I care for him. If I meet the first-person requirements of caring for X, I am tempted to insist that I do care—that there is something wrong with X that he does not appreciate my caring. But if you are looking at this relationship, you would have to report, however reluctantly, that something is missing. X does not feel that I care. Therefore, sadly, I must admit that, while I feel that I care, X does not perceive that I care and, hence, the relationship cannot be characterized as one of caring. This result does not necessarily signify a negligence on my part. There are limits in caring. X may be paranoid or otherwise pathological. There may be no way for my caring to reach him. But, then, caring has been only partly actualized.

It may seem paradoxical to some that my caring should be in any way dependent on the other. A similar difficulty arises in the analysis of teaching. Some analysts find it unacceptable to pronounce teaching conceptually dependent on learning. Still, this position is clearly not a nonsensical one. Aristotle noted long ago that one process may find its actualization in another. So, that teaching is completed in learning and that caring is completed in reception by the cared-for should be neither incredible nor incomprehensible. We may still say, "I care," when we are prepared to care, and not every failure of caring is one to which blame attaches. But in recognizing that my use of "I care" in the incomplete relation is an ellipsis of sorts, I acknowledge that I am not alone—not solely to be credited or blamed—in the caring relation.

Logically, we have the following situation: (W, X) is a caring relation if and only if
   1) W cares for X (as described in the one-caring) and
   2) X recognizes that W cares for X.
When we say that "X recognizes that W cares for X," we mean that X receives the caring honestly. He receives it: he does not hide from it or deny it. Hence, its reception becomes part of what the one-caring feels when she receives the cared-for. We do not need to add a third condi-

tion and a fourth, as in, "W is aware that X recognizes," "X is aware that W is aware that . . . ," and so on.

Caring requires the typical engrossment and motivational displacement in W and, also, the recognition of caring by X. Now, of course, the relationship can be mutually (or doubly) caring if we can interchange W and X and retain true expressions. This seems the correct logical analysis of caring, and it has the merit that it accounts for the ambivalence that may arise in such a situation. By that, I mean that it allows me to say "I care for X," even if I must admit that (I, X) is not a fully caring relationship.

Reciprocity

We turn now to the problem of reciprocity. We are concerned with reciprocity in terms of the contribution of the human cared-for. We have already noted that the cared-for must "receive" the caring. But what is the nature of this reception?

What part does the cared-for play in caring? Clearly, in equal meetings, there may be mutual caring and, when this happens, we need not, in a practical sense, try to distinguish the roles of the one-caring and the cared-for. But we are interested in the logic of caring; further, in parent-child and teacher-student relations the meetings often are not equal. The child may like, even love, the parent or teacher, but he is incapable of the motivational displacement of caring and, usually, incapable of perceiving or understanding what the parent or teacher wants for herself. Now, obviously, this inequity is neither permanent nor invariant. Even a small child may have occasional equal meetings with an adult. But, by and large, it is the parent or teacher who is capable of inclusion; it is she who sees with two pairs of eyes.

We readily accept the inequality of meetings between adult and child, but we may wonder about the teacher-student relationship when both are adults. Are unequal meetings still likely? Is the inequality perhaps necessary to the relation? The teacher, because she is a teacher, must see things through the eyes of her student in order to teach him. She looks at and speaks about subject matter, of course, but she looks at it and speaks about it from two poles. She must interpret what she sees from one pole in the language that she hears at the other. Further, it is not only the subject matter that she must view dually. She must also grasp the effectance motivation of the student. What does he want to accomplish? Of what use may the proposed subject matter be to him in his striving for competence? What interests has he that may help her to persuade him to look at the subject matter? The teacher, I shall argue, is necessarily one-caring if she is to be a teacher and not simply a textbooklike source from which the student may or may not learn. Hence, when we look at "pedagogical caring" we shall begin not with pedagogy but with caring. Then we shall see what *form* caring takes in the teaching function.

Let us look at the student. Is it not true that he also sees things through his teacher's eyes as well as his own? We talk this way at times, but we can readily see that what we say so easily in metaphor is not possible. The student sees not what the teacher at her own pole sees but what the teacher presents by way of interpretation. This represents a kind of "seeing through the teacher's eyes," but it is a reflection that brightens the student's own vision.

The work of the teacher is facilitated by her dual vision. If, however, the student were to attempt inclusion with respect to the teacher, to discern her motives, to concentrate on what she was trying to accomplish, he would be distracted from his own learning task. Indeed, we often see this sort of thing happen in schools. Instead of concentrating on the objective elements of the problematic situation in, say, mathematics, the student focuses on what the teacher wants. The result is a catalog of nonmathematical heuristics that the student compiles in order to cope with the demands of schooling. John Holt, in *How Children Fail*, records many such incidents. Observing another teacher in a lesson using Cuisenaire rods, he observes:

It was Barbara who really made the dent on me, because she is usually such a thoughtful and capable student. You held up the black (7) and the blue (9), and reversing your previous procedure, said, "What is the blue of the black?" She said, "seven-ninths." You hesitated. Her face got red, she stared at you, not at the rods, for a second and then said, "Nine-sevenths." Nothing in her face, voice or manner gave me the feeling that she had the slightest idea why the first answer was wrong and the second right. (1964, p. 80)

The student may, then, to his ultimate disadvantage, make what seems to be an effort at inclusion. The inclusion is necessarily incomplete, however, because it is induced by the student's needs and not by engrossment in the teacher-as-subject. In the event that inclusion becomes actual, the relation is converted, as we have noted, from that of teacher-student to one of friendship. This may, of course, happen, but even if it does, when the teacher assumes her function as teacher, the relation becomes again, temporarily, unequal. Two friends may, indeed, assume the functions of teacher and student interchangeably.

We are trying to establish the role of the cared-for in caring. I have claimed that the recognition of caring by the cared-for is necessary to the caring relation. It is clear, however, that the cared-for need not be one-caring in order to constitute the relation. He does not have to receive the one-caring as she receives him. Yet he must respond to her somehow. There is, necessarily, a form of reciprocity in caring. How shall we describe this reciprocity?

A mother describes her two babies and the differences in responsiveness to her. As she holds one on her knee, the child looks right at her, responding to her smiles, frowns, and funny-faces. The other child, held in the same playful attitude, looks across the room. Both children are very bright and pleasant, but the mother confesses that she enjoys her responsive baby more. He is fun to be with. She is a bit baffled by the other.

Another mother describes typical differences in the behavior of two of her children. Let's say one of the children, about junior high age, comes home late for dinner. The mother, anxious, meets him at the door. This child spots the worry immediately and says, "Gee, I'm sorry to be so late but, Mother, I had the best time! Wait till you hear." And he spills over with a recitation of what he has been doing. The other child, in a similar situation, comes in, notes the time and says, "I'm sorry about being late. We didn't realize what time it was. There was a lot of traffic on the way home." He gives an explanation, sometimes a detailed one, but he neither responds to the worry and relief in his mother's eyes nor shares his experiences with her. The mother does not push the second child to share his life more fully with her, but she cannot help being drawn more to the first child. Now, of course, some mothers do demand that children share their lives with them. Some even profess to "live for" (and we might say through) their children. But that is not the case with the mother in our story. She sees and describes the difference with some surprise and with some chagrin because she realizes that she, in turn, feels differently toward the children.

The first child contributes to the caring relation in two ways. First, he acknowledges and responds to the particular form of his mother's present engrossment—worry and relief. Second, he shares his aspirations, appraisals, and accomplishments with her. This sharing enables her to care more easily. With a fuller knowledge of what he is striving for, of what pleases and delights him, she can readily contribute her support to his efforts. The motivational displacement of caring occurs naturally, supported by the buoyant responsiveness of the cared-for. The one-caring for a fully participating cared-for is sustained and invigorated, and her caring is unlikely to deteriorate to "cares and burdens."

To accept the gift of responsiveness from the cared-for is natural for the one-caring. It is consistent with caring. To demand such responsiveness is both futile and inconsistent with caring. The one-caring is motivated in the direction of the cared-for and she must, therefore, respect his freedom. She meets him as subject—not as an object to be manipulated nor a data source. Indeed, this recognition of the freedom-as-subject of the cared-for is a fundamental result of her genuine receiving of the cared-for. The responsive cared-for, in the fullness of the caring relation, feels the recognition of freedom and grows under its expansive support. The child genuinely cared for is free to respond as himself, to create, to follow his interests without unnecessary fear and anxiety. We are interested at this stage in developing a coherent account of the part played by the cared-for in caring, but it is worth noting, once again, that there is empirical support for what emerges in the logical component of our conceptual framework. In studies of the backgrounds of creative architects, Donald MacKinnon found that parental respect for the child's freedom seemed to support the creative impulse:

What appears most often to have characterized the parents of these future creative architects was an extraordinary respect for the child and confidence in his ability to do what was appropriate. Thus they did not hesitate to grant him rather unusual freedom in exploring his universe and in making decisions for himself—and this early as well as late. The expectation of the parent that the child would act independently but reasonably and responsibly appears to have contributed immensely to the latter's sense of personal autonomy which was to develop to such a marked degree. (1964, p. 104)

The cared-for is free to be more fully himself in the caring relation. Indeed, this being himself, this willing and unselfconscious revealing of self, is his major contribution to the relation. This is his tribute to the one-caring, but it is not delivered up as tribute. A mother is more drawn to the child who reveals himself spontaneously than to the one who presents formal explanations in response to what he takes to be her assessment of the problematic situation. A teacher is captivated by the student who thinks aloud and uses what his teacher has presented in his own way and for his own purposes. Obviously, when I say "a mother" and "a teacher" here I mean to point to a mother or a teacher as one-caring.

It is hard to overestimate the importance of what we are discussing now. The cared-for plays a vital role in the caring relation. Buber underscores the role of the one caring, that is, of the one-caring as the I in I-Thou relations, insisting: "The relation can obtain even if the human being to whom I say Thou does not hear it in his experience. For Thou is more than It knows. Thou does more, and more happens to it, than It knows. No deception reaches this far: here is the cradle of actual life" (1970 p. 60). But in other places, Buber emphasizes the reciprocity of relation: "One should not try to dilute the meaning of the relation: relation is reciprocity" (p. 58).

The problem that is raised here is precisely the one we must solve, for saying Thou—being engrossed—is a necessary condition for the one-caring to be in a relation of caring. The engrossment of caring is not necessarily typical of that of the lover, and I am not proposing a form of agapism or obligatory love. When one cares, there are active moments of caring in which the engrossment must be present. In those moments the cared-for is not an object. In Buber's words: "He is no longer He or She, limited by other Hes and Shes, a dot in the world grid of space and time, nor a condition that can be experienced and described, a loose bundle of named qualities. Neighborless and seamless, he is Thou and fills the firmament" (1970, 59).

The one-caring is engrossed; the cared for "fills the firmament." Does it make no difference how the cared-for responds to the one-caring? On the one hand, Buber insists that "relation is reciprocity"; on the other, that the relation may obtain even though the cared-for does not hear the Thou "in his experience." There must, then, be reciprocity, but what form does it take? Obviously reciprocity does not imply an identity of gifts given and received. Something, not necessarily identical to my engrossment as one-caring, is required of my Thou, the cared-for. The key lies in Buber's peculiar use of "experience." For him, "experience" points to the object-world of It. When we "experience" something, we have already made that which we experience into an object or thing. Thus the cared-for need not hear my Thou in his experience; that is, he need not acknowledge it propositionally. But he must respond to it. "Thou is more than It knows." The freedom, creativity, and spontaneous disclosure of the cared-for that manifest themselves under the nurture of the one-caring complete the relation. My Thou must be *in* the relation for the relation to obtain, but he need not acknowledge my Thou-saying in words so that others may discuss it. What the cared-for gives to the relation either in direct response to the one-caring or in personal delight or in happy growth before her eyes is genuine reciprocity. It contributes to the maintenance of the relation and serves to prevent the caring from turning back on the one-caring in the form of anguish and concern for self.

The Ethics of Being Cared-For

Is there a way in which we can move from the natural responsiveness of being cared-for in a genuine relation of caring to an ethical responsibility for behaving as cared-for in a situation where natural affection and receptivity break down? We have seen that caring arises naturally in the inner circles of human intercourse and that it must be summoned by a concern for the ethical self in situations where it does not arise naturally. Because I have come to care for my ethical self and not just my physical self, I behave as one-caring toward one for whom I feel no natural affection. Our question now is this: Is there a comparable ethical aspect for the cared-for to consider?

Suppose X and Y are in a relation that might be supposed on some formal criterion—X is Y's mother, let us say—to be a caring relation. Suppose, further, that X professes to care or, at least, does not deny that she cares. Y does not feel that X cares; the necessary attitude is not perceived by Y. Should Y respond as one cared-for?

So long as contact between X and Y must be maintained, our answer to this question must be, yes. Let us see how we may defend this answer. First, there is an argument from self-interest. In traditional wisdom, the "one-to-be-cared-for" in a standard caretaking situation—such as parent/child, physician/patient, teacher/student—acknowledges both the wisdom and motivational displacement of the "one-supposed-caring." Parents, doctors, and teachers do things for us and to us for our own good. In the Biblical commandment we are told to honor our fathers and mothers so that our days may be long upon the earth. Thus we are called upon to respond to the one-supposed-caring with respect and obedience. But obedience and respect may or may not be the sort of free, creative, and joyous response we expect of our genuinely cared-for. Indeed, they may be signs that we have abdicated our subjectivity and taken our indicated place in the It-World of the one-supposed-caring. If we have done this, we are not genuine cared-fors and cannot contribute to a caring relation.

To behave ethically in the potential caring relation, the cared-for must turn freely toward his own projects, pursue them vigorously, and share his accounts of them spontaneously. This is what the one-genuinely-caring wants but never demands. The one-supposed-caring, however, may not want freedom for the cared-for and may yet demand "spontaneous" accounts. The situation is very difficult for the cared-for. He must never feel guilt for the failed projects of the one-caring but only for his own failed projects. His contribution to the relation is not the same as that of the one-caring. But the one-supposed-caring may demand that he behave as cared-for when she really wants herself to be cared-for. This is the intolerable position the child is put into when the parent "lives for" her child. The child is not free to become more fully the self he aspires to be but must nevertheless behave as though he is.

It is easy to see that, in dependent relations, the greater responsibility belongs to the one-caring. As soon as the cared-for must consider the needs and motives of the one-caring, he becomes one-caring himself or he falls into a life of inauthenticity or he becomes an ethical hero—one who behaves as though cared-for without the sustenance of caring. I think that last is possible for a particular Y in relation to a particular X;

that is, I think it is possible for Y to behave as though cared-for by X even though the caring is not felt and perhaps not present. But I shall argue that it is not possible if *no* one comes through to Y as caring.

What we are exploring here is the possibility that one-to-be-cared-for may contribute genuinely as cared-for in a relation of caring even though the necessary reception of caring attitude is missing. Clearly, the relation in such cases is deficient and cannot properly be called caring, and the one-to-be-cared-for is not actually cared-for, but I am arguing that he may behave as cared-for. Why should he do this?

One possibility, as we have seen, is that he might behave as cared-for out of self-interest. Second, he may behave freely and spontaneously as cared for because he has a vision of self and ethical self and, if this is the case, he may strain to receive that which should come through in a caring relation. He feels the lack but maintains an intellectual doubt concerning it. He may consciously reach beyond the emptiness at the heart of the relation to fill it with induced caring. Every move of the one supposed-caring is interpreted in its best light, and each response is to that which should be meant.

It seems to me that there are two ways in which a potential cared-for might achieve such a state of magnanimous receptivity. First, he might have a long and rich history of being genuinely cared-for. As a result, he is already strong, receptive, expecting to be cared-for. He meets others with the expectation of genuine encounter. He is ingenuous—a loving innocent of sorts. This may happen even within a relation. X may, for example, have been in a genuine relation of caring to Y during infancy and early childhood and then, for whatever reason, she may lapse into caring and worrying for herself in such a way that the relation is filled with double messages, disavowed demands, and subtle pressures on Y to do what X wishes she might have done. The early love may, however, have contributed to Y's ability to see the relation as possibly-caring. It may also have made him strong enough to seek caring elsewhere and so contribute from a position of strength to the X-Y relation as cared for.

One behaving as cared-for may, of course, be doing so simply because he is enormously self-centered. He expects others to be engrossed in him, shares spontaneously to promote his own ego, and grows in his nonethical dimensions without even considering the relation. His show of cared-for behavior is not ethical but, interestingly, he may contribute just enough of what the genuine cared-for usually gives to maintain relations that either look like caring relations or are actually half-caring relations. It is possible, that is, for the one-caring in such a relation to be genuinely one-caring and for the one-to-be-cared-for to behave very like a genuine cared-for even though there is no recognition of the caring. In cases like this, the one-caring may eventually realize her irrelevance and withdraw. We see, then, that one may behave as cared-for in a relation where the necessary feeling is absent more or less accidentally and egocentrically.

But there is a second way in which one may ethically behave as cared-for when the necessary attitude is not detected, and I think this second way is more commonly taken than the first. The one-to-be-cared-for turns about and responds to the needs of the one-caring. In doing this, he consciously gives up his status as cared-for and, out of concern for the one supposed-caring, behaves as cared-for. Clearly, once again, the relation is not one of genuine caring (there is as yet no cared-for), but the external features of caring may be retained and, should the one-supposed-caring recognize the reversal of functions and respond to it, the relation may become fully caring with X and Y positionally exchanged. Our second way of behaving ethically as cared-for is, thus, not authentic. It puts such a burden on the one-to-be-cared-for turned one-caring that it may ultimately be very difficult for both parties. The fundamental deception, however generously initiated, warps the relation. In this care, one behaves ethically in a strict, narrow sense but diminishes the ethical ideal.

The first way is the way of hope and beauty. It gently turns toward the motives of the one-caring to satisfy them and, at the same time, to reflect them transformed to what they should have been. It generously assumes that the one-caring is caring, that the lack of feeling is (or may be) a lack in the cared-for or a result of accident or a product of too much effort—or anything that preserves the one-caring as one-caring. The cared-for lives as cared-for without the sustaining attitude and with persistent doubt strongly managed by his own commitment. This is a position of ethical heroism.

Our logic may be summarized. A caring relation requires the engrossment and motivational displacement of the one-caring, and it requires the recognition and spontaneous response of the cared-for. When caring is not felt in the cared-for, but its absence is felt, the cared-for may still, by an act of ethical heroism, respond and thus contribute to the caring relation. This possibility gives weight to our hope that one can learn to care and learn to be cared for.

References

Bronfrenbrenner, Urie. 1978. "Who Needs Parent Education?" *Teachers College Record* 79: 773–74.

Buber, Martin. 1964. "Dialogue Between Martin Buber and Carl Rogers." In *The Worlds of Existentialism*, ed. Maurice Friedman. Chicago: University of Chicago Press.

———. "Education." In Buber, *Between Man and Man*, trans. Ronald G. Smith. New York: Macmillan.

———. 1970. *I and Thou*, trans. Walter Kauffmann. New York: Scribner.

Holt, John. 1964. *How Children Fail.* New York: Dell Publishing.

MacKinnon, Donald W. 1964. "The Nature and Nurture of Creative Talent." In *Readings in Managerial Psychology*, ed. Harold J. Leavitt and Louis R. Ponti. Chicago: University of Chicago Press.

Montagu, M. F. Ashley. 1962. *Prenatal Influences.* Springfield, IL: Thomas.

Pohlman, Edward. 1969. *The Psychology of Birth Planning.* Cambridge, MA: Schenkmann.

Sanger, Margaret, ed. 1926. *Religious and Ethical Aspects of Birth Control.* Sixth International Neo-Malthusian and Birth Control Conference, vol. 4. New York: American Birth Control League.

Schaefer, E. S. and R. O. Bell. 1957. "Patterns of Attitudes Toward Child Rearing and the Famly." *Journal of Abnormal Social Psychology* 54: 391–95.

Sears, Robert R., Eleanor E. Maccoby, and Harry Levin with Edgar L. Lowell, Pauline S. Sears, and John W. M. Whiting. 1957. *Patterns of Child Rearing.* Evanston, IL: Row, Peterson.

Wengraf, Fritz. 1953. *Psychosomatic Approach to Gynecology and Obstetrics.* Springfield, IL: Thomas.

White, Robert W. 1959. "Motivation Reconsidered: The Concept of Competence." *Psychological Review* 66: 327.

Zilboorg, Gregory. 1957. "The Clinical Issues of Postpartum Psychopathological Reactions." *American Journal of Obstetrics and Gynecology* 73: 308.

Chapter 3
Caring Practice

Patricia Benner and Suzanne Gordon

The words "caring" and "to care" are some of the most heavily freighted in the English language. Like magnets, they attract the most noble images and concepts. Like veils, they conceal the most complex confusions and elisions.

Is there anyone who wants to be perceived of as "uncaring"? To say that someone is "uncaring" strikes at their very humanity. Indeed we have often coupled the terms "cold and uncaring", making the one synonymous with the other. It is not only humanly impossible not to care about something or someone, it is socially unacceptable to be without someone or something to care about. To say, however, that someone is a "caring person" seems to cloak them with a blanket of light. A sheath so thick we often fail to look underneath.

Because of the positive meaning of the word, it has become a cultural cliché and a vehicle of media manipulation. Hallmark Cards encourages us to buy its products because "you care enough to send the very best." A health insurance company whose market-oriented policies in fact negate the imperatives of caregiving urges us to enroll because it really "cares" about our health. A major American hospital—shrine to a medical model that often eliminates the human as it focuses on diseases—offers "a lifetime of caring."

Indeed, caring often becomes a kind of defense. A lawyer who is accused of being too greedy, insists he really "cares" about his clients; a doctor responding to attacks on his colleagues defends them because they really care about their patients. Because we view caring as an individual attribute that should somehow prevail against all odds, the very concept becomes a weapon used in all kinds of personal attacks. Children who are not allowed to take time off work to care for aging parents

An original essay.

are accused of not "caring" about them, as if sentiment were the only structure that supported human responsibility. A man who does not do hands-on caregiving for a dying son is immediately considered to be uncaring without any consideration of mitigating circumstances.

This burden of cultural weight and confusion must be directly addressed if we are to understand and analyze caring and caregiving. In this discussion of caring, we would like to highlight a central confusion in our society's vision of caring: the popular confusion between abstract sentiment and generalized intentions on the one hand and concrete caring practices embued with emotional connections to particular individuals, families and communities on the other. We want to make a distinction between a generalized feeling of benevolence for others or one particular other and a special set of skills, reflections and activities that allows one to be with and do for another—especially at inconvenient or uncomfortable moments, when another human being is needy, weak, vulnerable, recalcitrant and resistant to care, old, ill or dying. It is this that distinguishes abstract caring intentions from the practice of caregiving.

To illustrate the set of problems we wish to explore, consider the following example. For several months now, one of us has held a series of conversations about the contemporary medical system with a friend who is a general surgeon. When we discuss out-of-control medical treatment, callous behavior, impersonal treatment, and fragmentation of care, our friend sincerely laments what has happened to medicine, but nonetheless, insists that most of his colleagues—even the most highly specialized, disease oriented physicians—"really care about their patients."

Over the months, it has become clear that this statement—so often heard in so many different settings—illustrates a central dilemma in attempts to make visible to our society the complexity and importance of caring. Our friend is indeed right. Most of his colleagues do "care about their patients." That is to say that they wish them well, want them to be cured of whatever disease or disorder they might have, do not want to cause them pain, and will be sad if bad things happen to them and bad health outcomes result.

To our friend, however, this generalized sentiment of concern is too easily mistaken for the establishment of a set of practices and skills that make it possible for his colleagues to truly and consistently connect with, be with, attend to and do for their patients. It is this that distinguishes the sentiment of caring from the activity of caregiving.

This becomes apparent when we consider our friend's medical practice. From objective criteria, he is a genuine caregiver. He has deliberately established a set of practices that allow him to connect with and get to know patients. From the moment a patient enters his office, a caring frame is established. He never books four patients for 9:00, 9:15, and 9:30 slots. He does not have one patient in one exam room, another in the next, and a third in the next, so that while one undresses he can be taking the vital signs of another, and while one dresses he can—with his eyes on the clock and his mind on the patients in the other two rooms—try to listen to complaints. Thus, he creates a space for caring to exist even before the patient walks into the room.

When patients are with him, he gives them all the time they need. He lets patients talk, generally without interruption, and does not try to track their conversation into pathways with which he—rather than they—are comfortable. When he goes onto the hospital floor, he rarely visits one of his patients without consulting the nurse who has been with the patient for hours on end so he can find out the patient's concerns. When there is hands-on care to be given, he often rolls up his sleeves and cleans up a dirty stoma with the nurse, rather than standing aside to let her do it. He sets aside the time, puts in the energetic listening, and is able to *be with* patients when it is no longer enough to *do for* them. The construction of his practice in this case makes "care" a very apt word to define what he has consciously created. He has created a setting in which caring can take place and a style of being and communication that implicitly and explicitly tells patients that they are always, if not more important than he is, at least as important.

Contrast this with many other physicians who deny the space for more than cursory conversation and brief encounters that primarily center around advice giving: a doctor with an office full of patients, booked four per fifteen-minute slot, who must each endure one to three-hour waits before they even get into the exam room; a doctor who is running between two and three exam rooms, juggling two or three or more cases in his or her head; a doctor who, with body language, and impatient verbal interruptions signals that the patient has gotten "off track," because he or she is talking about what has meaning for the patient, rather than for the doctor. This doctor has created a space in which the primary metaphor is flight, not connection; where patients are distinctly informed of whose time and money and problems are more important, the doctor's not the patient's. This physician may want the best for his patients intellectually but has created an environment in which caregiving is impossible.

Caregiving is the operative word here. The central issue is not whether the doctor wishes the best for his patient; the central issue is whether the doctor can create a set of practices that must be triggered when an exchange centered around need, vulnerability, or infirmity is initiated.

The need to differentiate between caring as an abstract slogan or generalized sentiment and a practice is revealed quite distinctly not only in the hospital, but in the home, in the schoolroom, the welfare office, or the volunteer agency—anywhere that people are asking others to attend to their problems, dilemmas, or need for growth and empowerment. The difference between abstract sentiment and engaged relationships that evoke caring practices is revealed starkly in myriad encounters and examples gleaned not only from the caregiving professions but from literature, film, and life. In her short story, "In the Gloaming," included in this volume, Alice Elliott Dark recounts the story of a mother caring for a son with AIDS. The young gay man has come home to die. He sits day after day with his mother, as she drinks in all she can of a life she is soon to lose. She bathes and feeds him, gives him his medicines, shares his pain and anguish. As the story unfolds, the boy's father, her husband, appears only rarely. When he is present, he seems indifferent, uninterested, "uncaring."

In the story's most poignant moment, the mother recognizes that her son is about to die. When he begins to slip away, she realizes that she cannot leave his side but must be with him. Later that night the father returns home. The reader is prepared to dislike him, to accord him little sympathy because of his indifference. He approaches his wife and tries to comfort and question her. Then he begins to cry and says "Please tell me—what else did my boy like?"

There can be no better elaboration of the difference between the abstract sentiment of caring and the practice of engaged caregiving than that in that vivid moment of human anguish. Indeed, the father cared about his son. But without a set of caregiving skills and practices with which to embody his concern he could not join the boy's mother in being a caregiver to his son. He could not move from concern to presence, from emotional interest to attention or attunement, from distant observer to hands-on caregiver. The mother, on the other hand, was involved in a caregiving relationship until the end of her son's life. Because she was able to live her connection to her child even in his dying and beyond, he was not lost to her in the total and irretrievable manner in which the boy was lost, in life and death, to his father. It is oddly, the father, the one who could not connect, who seems the most tragic figure.

Practice and Caring Practices Defined

Countless other examples could be added to the two above. Contrasting the father and mother in the short story, or the hasty specialist with our friend the surgeon illustrates some of the fundamental characteristics of "practice."

A practice differs from discrete behaviors, strategies, or techniques in that it is a culturally constituted, socially embedded way of being in a situation and with others. It only makes sense to talk about being a good doctor, nurse, father, or mother because we have concrete practices and culturally transmitted visions that help us recognize and acknowledge excellence in these practices. Even though we may not be able completely to spell out the formal criteria for such roles, we can recognize another good practitioner, if we are ourselves practitioners, or appreciate and participate in caregiving with that practitioner because we are recipients of care.

Despite the fact that some teachers are able to relate better to some students than to others, most of us would be confident of our ability to recognize good teaching when we experience it. And, certainly, from first-hand experience we are confident we can definitively distinguish between a poor teacher or nurse and a good one.

The political philosopher Charles Taylor (1985) makes the distinction between the discrete behavior of raising the arm and the culturally constructed public human action of raising the hand in a voting practice. More than a collection of discrete behaviors, a practice is defined as a coherent, socially organized activity that has—internal to it—a notion of good and a variety of implicitly or explicitly articulated common meanings. (MacIntyre 1981). Located within a tradition and continually worked out in history and through ongoing development and refinement, a practice exists precisely because of this referential context of meanings, skills, and equipment. Human beings constantly refine practices in the differing contexts that permit and promote the actualization of those notions of good embedded within them. A practice has the capacity to be—indeed it must be—worked out in new situations. Thus practice itself is a source of innovation.

Carolyn Whitbeck identifies the core practices of women as follows:

> The practice that I consider to be the core practice is that of the (mutual) realization of people. I take this practice to have a variety of particular forms, most, if not all, of which are regarded as women's work and are therefore largely ignored by the dominant culture. Among these are the rearing of children, the education of children and adolescents, care of the dying, nursing of the sick and injured, and a variety of spiritual practices related to daily life.
> These practices are sometimes described as "nurturing." Although this language has the advantage of being familiar, it has often been used to evoke a sentimental picture of a woman doing a variety of mindless tasks in response to the demands of others, and for that reason I am reluctant to use it. The creativity and responsibility of all parties in the conduct of the practice in its full, liberated form is inconsistent with the sentimental picture of women's self-sacrifice. (1983, p. 65)

Caring requires sentiment and skills of connection and involvement, as well as caregiving knowledge and skills. Like the difference between the physician who reduced caring to a personal attitude and the physician who created a set of concrete practices and an environment that moved him from abstract intentions to activities that fostered caregiving, practice must be carried out in constantly evolving, living relationships that allow feelings and attitudes to guide meaningful human interactions. As is clear in Alice Elliott Dark's short story, to care—absent a complex social, practical, local and historical foundation in which one learns and refines caregiving skills—is not possible (Brown 1986).

That is why a practice cannot be completely objectified or formalized. It requires action and reasoning in transitions and transactions with the particular (Taylor 1993). The scientific evaluative strategies fashioned according to the various criteria of disengaged reasoning cannot replace being-in-relationship to particular persons/situations. Similarly, mastering specialized aspects of a practice will not necessarily qualify the practitioner to be recognized as an expert in his or her field. For example, if you need an operation, you might choose a physician who has done a great many of such operations and who is reputed to be a technical wizard in a particular surgical technique. Indeed, most of us would consider someone a fool who went to a surgeon who was trustworthy and caring but had no experience with the surgical procedure required.

This fact notwithstanding, if the entire medical profession and its practice were reduced to a collection of narrowly proficient technical wizards who had little or no skill in being with patients, then medicine would lack sufficient basis for carrying out the practice of doctoring. People would simply be unable to establish the kind of trusting relationships that allow them to put faith in diagnostic judgments, avoid manipulation or over- or under-treatment, and with some confidence choose the technical wizards for the specialized procedures. Interestingly, most medical practice recognizes this fact implicitly if not explicitly. It is the primary care physician who is the referral source. This is not only because he or she has more general knowledge and the clinical and ethical judgment to recognize when the services of the technically proficient specialist are warranted. It is also because he or she can develop trust, over time, with patients who need to—and because of that trust are willing to—be guided when making complex or life-threatening decisions. This doctor will also be more likely to listen to the patient's wishes. (Of course, those patients would probably be far happier if they were guided to the technical wizard who is also a compassionate listener and healer.)

The trust needed between providers and patients illustrates another characteristic of a practice—it is always socially situated and must relate to the particular person and situation as they evolve through time. In order to respond to the new and the particular, a practice or craft must be innovative, replete with skill, and carry within it a memory of past situations. In this way a practice differs from mechanical manufacturing processes, isolated techniques, and the criteria reasoning of science and technology (Taylor 1993). Because a practice is situated, particular, and responsive to another human being, it is always dialogical, existing in human interactions that demand responses. It cannot be defined separately from the being in and doing of the practice. This image is similar to Heidegger's vision of the excellent craftsman:

> A cabinetmaker's apprentice, someone who is learning to build cabinets and the like, will serve as an example. His learning is not mere practice, to gain facility in the use of tools. Nor does he merely gather knowledge about the customary forms of the things he is to build. If he is to become a true cabinetmaker, he makes himself answer and respond above all to the different kinds of wood and to the shapes slumbering within the wood—to wood as it enters into man's dwelling with all the hidden riches of its essence. In fact, this relatedness to wood is what maintains the whole craft. Without that relatedness, the craft will never be anything but empty busywork, any occupation with it will be determined exclusively by business concerns.
>
> Every handicraft, all human dealings, are constantly in that danger. (1954, 1993, p. 379).

When the craft is practiced in relationships with people, the identity of those involved in that relationship—like the grain of the wood—become determinants of the outcome of each encounter and of the caregiving relationship as a whole. Like the pliability of the wood, the skills and abilities of the person who is cared for—their openness and capacity to respond to care—are as important an influence on the success or failure of the caregiving relationship as the skills of the caregiver.

That expertise in caring practice is response-based, however, conflicts with our usual definitions of knowledge and expertise. We tend to think of expertise as traits and talents lodged in discrete individuals who then apply their wisdom—like a nail and hammer to wood—to practical situations. We emphasize the influence and power flowing from the expert and pay little attention to the responsive capacities of the one who is cared for. When, moreover, we focus on the expert caregiver, we try to disentangle and dis/integrate emotion, cognition and skill. What this unidimensional approach fails to grasp is the mutual synergistic, and often paradoxical, nature of expert practice.

Consider, for example, that in caring practices the timing and quality of the caring relationship often influences the outcome. There are only certain moments when it is possible to tell a friend you think she really should divorce her husband, or explain to a terminally ill patient that the treatment is not working and he should consider hospice care. At other times it is the trust, openness, and capacity of the one cared for that makes the relationship transformative. Thus nurses and doctors frequently speak about their "favorite patient," or educators of their "favorite student." Why is the patient or student so cherished? Perhaps because they more than others are able to receive and extend the care they are given or perhaps they can successfully call the doctor or nurse to account when the care is inadequate.

More importantly, sometimes "the outcome" is not the point, but rather the encounter and recognition, the ability to be with, see and hear who the other is. When the mother in "In The Gloaming" realizes her son is dying, she stops her activity to hold his hand. This decision to be with rather than do for does not delay his dying. Indeed, the inspiration and impact of that story sprang from the very fact that sometimes the most liberating, effective caring is based on letting the other be, letting go or allowing the other to show up. Thus in caring practice *being* with someone can be as important, or more important, than *doing* something to or for that person. Learning how to be with people, to respect where they are at and stop doing for them, is, in fact, an integral part of the education in caring practice.

This process of learning caring practices involves education into the various notions of good inherent in a practice. In a continuous dialogue with the historical understanding of the practice, these ideas of the good are continually being extended and elaborated. The distinction we are making here is between traditionalism—a dead or ritualistic repetition of past conventions—and a living tradition that is continually developed and worked out (Shils 1981). Dreyfus, drawing on Heidegger's (1926/1962) thinking about cultural practices, notes their interrelationship in a particular tradition or culture:

> In sum, the practices containing an interpretation of what it is to be a person, an object, and a society fit together. They are all aspects of what Heidegger calls an understanding of being. Such an understanding is contained in our know-how-to-cope in various domains rather than a set of beliefs that such and such is the case. Thus we embody an understanding of being that no one has in mind. We have an ontology without knowing it. (1991, p. 18)

Although in our highly individualistic society we constantly deny the importance of caring practice as we define it and emphasize instead mechanistic models of human behavior, societies that value individualism and individual freedom paradoxically require the most highly developed, interrelated caring practices. These are the only vehicles that can foster a high degree of responsible citizenship. It is because we view ourselves as separate and unique individuals that we cannot engage in meaningful encounters and generate genuine human responses without such caring practices. Charles Taylor (1991) traces this modern need for recognition to the ideal of authenticity as it was articulated in the writings of Herder and Rousseau. The ideal of authenticity calls the individual to discover his or her own original way of being:

> But in the nature of the case, there is no such thing as inward generation, understood as a monologue with oneself. In order to understand the close connection between identity and recognition, we have to take into account a crucial feature of the human condition that has been rendered almost invisible by the overwhelmingly monological bent of mainstream modern philosophy. The crucial feature of human life is its fundamentally *dialogical* character. We become full human agents, capable of understanding ourselves, and hence of defining our identity, through our acquisition of rich human languages of expression. . . . My own identity doesn't mean that I work it out in isolation, but that I negotiate it through dialogue, partly overt, partly internal, with others. That is why the development of an ideal of inwardly generated identity gives a new importance to recognition. My own identity crucially depends on my dialogical relations with others. . . . Inwardly derived, personal, original identity doesn't enjoy this recognition *a priori*. It has to win it through exchange, and the attempt can fail. (Taylor 1991, pp. 32, 34)

Caring practices provide the necessary preconditions for the creation of a separate, unique, autonomous individual. Ironically, however, we fail to acknowledge these recognition practices because our societal myth of the private self-constituted individual demands that we conceal or deny them. This is the only way we can prove that we are our "own person," one whose inner and outer life are unique and uninfluenced by others. Thus citizens in the United States argue that they don't need government because they have always "relied on their own initiative"; men deny the importance of "women's work" because they have become "independent" selves through forgetting their dependencies; or doctors insist that they alone cured the patient when in fact, patients, families, and nurses also participated in that curative process.

Being in relationship, feeling dependent on another, makes the individual who seeks unrealistic levels of control and autonomy feel vulnerable or like a failure. Nussbaum (1986) and Williams (1993) contrast this perspective with that of the early Greeks, who had a more nuanced vision about the limits of autonomy. Nussbaum notes:

For it is their [the early Greeks] instinct that some projects for self sufficient living are questionable because they ask us to go beyond the cognitive limits of the human being; and, on the other hand, that many attempts to venture, in metaphysical or scientific reasoning, beyond our human limits are inspired by questionable ethical motives, motives having to do with closedness, safety, and power. (1986, p. 8)

Extreme individualism and a disillusioned utilitarian view of the insular autonomous self undermine a sense of connectedness, community, and caring practices in all spheres, both public and private (Bellah et al. 1985; Hochschild 1983; Taylor 1991, Tronto 1993). If caring practices are to be sustained, the nature and content of those practices must be uncovered and the social-political conditions and institutional structures and environments that foster caring practices—and the strategies for nurturing them—will have to be worked out in a public discourse. Dominant views of morality that focus on autonomy as the condition for free moral choice instead inhibit this public conversation by concealing the need for care, and the skill, knowledge, and time required for care. Tronto notes:

Vulnerability has serious moral consequences. Vulnerability belies the myth that we are always autonomous, and potentially equal, citizens. To assume equality among humans leaves out and ignores important dimensions of human existence. Throughout our lives, all of us go through varying degrees of dependence and independence, of autonomy and vulnerability. A political order that presumes only independence and autonomy as the nature of human life thereby misses a great deal of human experience, and must somehow hide this point elsewhere. For example, such an order must rightly separate public and private life.

. . .

Care's absence from our core social and political values reflects many choices our society has made about what to honor. These choices, starting as far away as our conceptions of moral boundaries, operate to exclude the activities and concerns of care from a central place. Through that exclusion, those who are powerful are able to demand that others care for them, and they have been able to maintain their positions of power and privilege. (Tronto 1993, pp. 135, 179)

In our society, we think of ourselves as developing outside a web of human relationships that shape us. Our Enlightenment tradition of science is permeated with the view of the person as a private subject who stands over against the objective world (Dreyfus 1991). The knower and known are radically separated in our scientific procedures and practices. Reciprocity, mutuality, the impact and mutual influence of relationship between persons, and the larger context in which caring occurs is overlooked. Thus a new mother is told she can learn to care for her child by reading a book or seeing a video and that she no longer needs help from the community of mothers, from nurses in the hospital, or from friends or relatives. A teacher is told she should care for her students, even when society fails to provide her with the resources to do so. A social worker is castigated because she speaks harshly to a welfare mother, even though her workload has just been increased and her pay cut.

Ignoring the most important fact of human society—that we are constituted by other human beings (Marx 1992)—the duty to care is imposed on the individual with no social support. When caring is studied at all, it is turned into personal attributes such as attitudes, beliefs, abstract sentiments and intents and observable isolated behaviors. The technical promise is that caring can be produced by identifiable, discrete caring behaviors, that we can provide it without paying for it or supporting it, and that it can exist outside the human relationships that are its only fertile soil. Viewed as technique rather than a series of responsive relationships that create possibilities and constraints, caring is no more than another therapeutic technique that can be contractually arranged by separate individuals.

Caring thus becomes a free choice made by human beings who are depicted as rational choicemakers. These rational choicemakers can stand back and objectively choose whether or not to care for friends, loved ones, colleagues, or strangers. They are said to care because they "feel like it", and "get something out of it," just as they choose not to care for them if it "feels" inconvenient or doesn't feel good. This instrumental frame not only turns caring into a choice, it also transforms connectedness, responsiveness, and interdependence into signs of a moral lapse or sources of embarrassment or shame.

We tend to view care and caring practices as yet one more set of choices, until of course, we find ourselves in the position of caring or needing care (Taylor 1989). Then, we may realize that we "had no choice," that care always implies situated or bounded choice. If you are a mother or a father who loves his or her child, then your identity is shaped by that love and you cannot just freely choose to stop caring about that child, even though you may be separated physically. If you are vulnerable or incapacitated, you discover that your choices about being cared for and about how to respond to that caring are severely constrained.

The Centrality of Caring for Knowing

Caring practices contradict the central tenets of modern Western individualism. It is through our caring for and being cared for by others that we are able to live, to know, and to allow things to show up, to matter in the world. Caring practices cannot be separated from knowing or doing because, in the human world, caring practice is always bound up in knowing and doing (Benner and Wrubel 1989). Although the dominant Cartesian model insists that thought and reflection are most reliable when they take place in isolation—preferably in a warm dark room or ivory tower that is separated from the cares of the world—we reject this male view. That is because we recognize all too well that Descartes, and the many men who have followed in his footsteps, were able to escape from the cares of the world only because others shouldered their burdens.

This separation from the cares of the world has allowed men, and now many women, to believe that it is possible to segregate involvement from knowing, and detach theoretical knowledge—"knowing that"—from practical knowle ge,—"knowing how" (Polanyi 1958; Heidegger 1962; Guignon 1983; Benner 1984; Dreyfus and Dreyfus 1986; Benner and Wrubel 1989; Benner, Tanner, and Chesla 1995). But it is increasingly clear that reflection cannot exist without some level of involvement and that theoretical and practical knowledge are indeed interconnected.

Consider, for example, several recent studies of skill acquisition. They demonstrate that a certain level of involvement is essential if people are to move from a competent level of performance to a proficient or expert level (Dreyfus 1987; Dreyfus and Dreyfus 1986; Benner 1984; Benner, Tanner, and Chesla 1992; 1996). At the competent level of performance, clinicians realize that they must choose a plan of action based upon a perspective on the clinical situation—how old the patient is, his or her cultural background and life experience, his family connections, his education and so forth—and this realization causes them to feel a combination of risk and uncertainty. They now recognize that the outcomes will differ depending on the plan they choose. They feel responsible and deeply satisfied when the chosen plan works and the outcomes are good. Because they feel responsible for having chosen the plan of action they feel disappointed and sad when the plan fails (Dreyfus and Dreyfus 1996). This kind of involvement, caring about the outcomes, and having them matter, sets up an effective personal history, memory, and sense of salience that are central to human expertise (Dreyfus and Dreyfus 1986; Benner, Tanner, and Chesla 1996). No matter what the field, detached unemotional reasoning alone cannot provide the ground for the development of human expertise. Similarly, expertise does not develop well when the person is flooded or overwhelmed by emotion. Studies of skill acquisition in nursing, for example, demonstrate a coherent and ongoing dialogue about learning the right kind and level of involvement (Benner and Wrubel 1989; Benner, Tanner, Chesla 1996).

A Technological Self-Understanding

We have become increasingly confused and inarticulate about caring practices because, in our society, we are so enthralled by a technological self-understanding. Much like our modern view that the environment is made up of raw material to be converted to available power or into commodities, we have been taught to view ourselves as raw material that we spend a lifetime sculpting and refining. (Dreyfus 1991). Albert Borgmann characterizes the meanings taken up in a technological self-understanding as a device paradigm and argues against the futility of capturing caring practices in mere technical terms, or even polished scientific or formal theoretical accounts:

. . . the device paradigm . . . is designed to locate the crucial force that more and more detaches us from the persons, things, and practices that used to engage and grace us in their own right. . . . It first comes into relief when past and present are seen as times of toil, poverty, and suffering and when at the same moment a new natural science emerges from which great transformative power can be derived. On the basis of this power, a promise of liberation, enrichment, and of conquering the scourges of humanity is issued. The promise leads to the irony of technology when liberation by way of disburdenment yields to disengagement, enrichment by way of diversion is overtaken by distraction, and conquest makes way first to domination and then to loneliness. . . . Things in their depth yield to shallow commodities, and our once profound and manifold engagement with the world is reduced to narrow points of contact in labor and consumption. . . . It is the reduction of work to a mere means that has led to its degradation, and it is a certain understanding of means-ends distinction that sanctions that degradation. . . . The suggestion . . . is not that once having chosen ends we should be indifferent about means but that we do violence to things and events when we divide them into means and ends. The rule of instrumentality . . . allows us to take possession of things and to overpower them. But in the process we extinguish the life of things and lose touch with them (Borgmann 1984, pp. 59–75)

Separating means and ends causes one to de-value ordinary tasks and events and value select aspects like outcomes, while ignoring the caring means for achieving the outcomes. The strategic view of the person assesses performance in line with strategic aims (Taylor 1985; Benner and Wrubel 1989). It calls for heroic actions and sweeping breakthroughs — for example, leading us to experience health as a commodity and limiting our ability critically to question technological interventions. Outcomes are highlighted, while the skillful daily comportment required to achieve the outcomes is overlooked. Furthermore, means and outcomes are separated, which, as Borgmann (1984) points out, does violence to the coherence of caring practices.

The use of technology does not *necessarily* have to engender a technological self-understanding. If another practice-based self-understanding is available, it can offer an alternative self-understanding. For example, from our caring practices we can discern what is and what is not caring, as well as what is control or oppression. From a stance of care we can judiciously use or not use technology, subordinating technology appropriately to human concerns. We can value what technology can do to improve education or save lives and lessen suffering without taking up a technological self-understanding. From an ethic of care and responsibility, the distinguishing characteristics of persons cannot be identified as strategic powers and performance capacities alone, but on what matters to them and whether they can live out their concerns. Such a stance requires that we value human concerns such as dignity, integrity, and self worth. An ethic of care and responsibility calls for a discourse on means and ends as they relate to health, comfort, hope, dignity, shame, moral goodness, evil, dignity, suffering, and human forms of love (Taylor 1985). These human concerns determine the worth and approach to our strategic efforts toward education, child care, care of the ill and elderly, reproduction, health maintenance, and self-care. Outcome is no longer the only issue. Focusing on an ethic of care will make the merely negative agenda of care of diseases and warding off death yield to the more positive agenda of promoting health and well-being. From an ethic of care, maintaining ties, human connectedness, and human concerns are not just means but the very essence of being human.

An ethic of care and responsibility points out the limitation of the rational technical approach that considers efficiency of means while ignoring worthy ends and the reliable, ethical comportment required to reach these ends. The ethics of rights and justice (Rawls 1971, 1985) have similar limitations because they are primarily procedural. The ethics of rights and justice are based on a thin theory of good and are poorly designed to discuss worthy ends (Sandel 1982). In this sense, justice is always remedial. It is a necessary floor for a free society, but not an adequate vision for creating a good and full life. An adequate ethic of care and responsibility must contain a vision and possibility for an ongoing discourse about worthy ends.

We need a better understanding of the notions of good and skill embedded in the best of our caring practices so that we can redesign our public bureaucracies and economic structures to support them.

References

Bellah, Robert N. et al. 1985. *Habits of the Heart: Individualism and Commitment in American Life*. Berkeley: University of California Press.

Benner, Patricia. 1984. *From Novice to Expert: Excellence and Power in Clinical Nursing Practice*. Menlo Park, CA: Addison-Wesley.

Benner, Patricia E. and Judith Wrubel. 1989. *The Primacy of Caring: Stress and Coping in Health and Illness*. Menlo Park, CA: Addison-Wesley.

Benner, Patricia E., Christine A. Tanner, and Catherine Chesla. 1992. "From Beginner to Expert: Gaining a Differentiated Clinical World in Critical Care Nursing." *Advances in Nursing Science* 14, 3: 13–28.

———. 1996. *Expertise in Nursing Practice: Clinical Judgment, Ethics, and Caring*. New York: Springer.

Borgmann, Albert. 1984. *Technology and the Character of Contemporary Life: A Philosophical Inquiry*. Chicago: University of Chicago Press.

Brown, L. 1986. "The Experience of Care: Patient Perspectives." *Topics in Clinical Nursing* 8, 2: 56–62.

Dark, Alice Elliott. 1993. "In the Gloaming." *New Yorker*, May 3. Reprinted this volume, pp. 5–20.

Dreyfus, Hubert L. 1979. *What Computers Can't Do: The Limits of Artificial Intelligence.* Rev. ed. New York: Harper and Row.

———. 1991. *Being-in-the-World: A Commentary on Heidegger's Being and Time, Division I.* Cambridge, MA: MIT Press.

———. 1992. *What Computers Still Can't Do: A Critique of Artificial Intelligence.* Cambridge, MA: MIT Press.

Dreyfus, Hubert L. and Stuart E. Dreyfus. 1996. "The Relationship of Theory and Practice in the Acquisition of a Skill." In Benner et al. 1996.

Dreyfus, Hubert L. and Stuart E. Dreyfus, with Tom Athanasiou. 1986. *Mind over Machine: The Power of Human Intuition and Expertise in the Era of the Computer.* New York: Free Press.

Guignon, Charles B. 1983. *Heidegger and the Problem of Knowledge.* Indianapolis, IN: Hackett Publishing.

Heidegger, Martin. 1926/1962. *Being and Time,* trans. John Macquarrie and Edward Robinson. New York: Harper and Row.

———. 1954/1993. "What Calls for Thinking?" In *Basic Writings: From Being and Time to The Task of Thinking,* ed. David Krell, trans. F. Wieck and J. Gray. San Francisco: Harper.

Hochschild, Arlie Russell. 1983. *The Managed Heart: Commercialization of Human Feeling.* Berkeley: University of California Press.

MacIntyre, Alasdair C. 1981. *After Virtue: A Study in Moral Theory.* Notre Dame, IN: Notre Dame University Press.

Marx, Werner. 1992. *Towards a Phenomenological Ethics: Ethos and the Life-World,* trans. S. Heyvaert. SUNY Series in Contemporary Continental Philosophy. Albany: State University of New York Press.

Nussbaum, Martha C. 1986. *The Fragility of Goodness: Luck and Ethics in Greek Tragedy and Philosophy.* Cambridge: Cambridge University Press.

Polanyi, Michael. 1958. *Personal Knowledge: Towards a Post-Critical Philosophy.* Chicago: University of Chicago Press.

Rawls, John. 1971. *A Theory of Justice.* Cambridge, MA: Belknap Press of Harvard University Press.

———. 1985. "Justice or Fairness: Political not Metaphysical." *Philosophy and Public Affairs* 14, 3: 223–51.

Sandel, Michael J. 1982. *Liberalism and the Limits of Justice.* Cambridge: Cambridge University Press.

Shils, Edward A. 1981. *Tradition.* Chicago: University of Chicago Press.

Taylor, Charles. 1985. *Philosophical Papers.* 2 vols. Cambridge: Cambridge University Press.

———. 1989. *Sources of the Self: The Making of Modern Identity.* Cambridge, MA: Harvard University Press.

———. 1991. *The Ethics of Authenticity.* Cambridge, MA: Harvard University Press.

———. 1993. "Explanation and Practical Reason." In *The Quality of Life,* ed. Martha C. Nussbaum and Amartya Sen. Oxford: Clarendon Press.

———. 1994. *Multiculturalism: Examining the Politics of Recognition: An Essay,* ed. Amy Gutmann et al. Princeton, NJ: Princeton University Press.

Tronto, Joan C. 1993. *Moral Boundaries: A Political Argument for an Ethic of Care.* New York: Routledge.

Whitbeck, Carolyn. 1983. "A Different Reality: Feminist Ontology." In *Beyond Domination: New Perspectives on Women and Philosophy*, ed. Carol C. Gould. Totowa, NJ: Rowman and Allenheld.

Williams, Bernard Owen. 1993. *Shame and Necessity*. Berkeley: University of California Press.

Chapter 4
Caring: A Negotiated Process That Varies

Barbara Tarlow

Until the second wave of the women's movement, caring was a neglected area of social research. Like family life, caring is part of the world of women and has attracted few serious scholars and little academic interest. Family relationships are frequently the empirical starting place for researching and theorizing about caring. The household has been viewed as the locus of that activity and women as the primary or exclusive caring and nurturing agent. Social perceptions of caring have become closely identified with family life. Caring as experienced in family life has come to act as the metaphor and standard for all forms of caring.

The nature and location of care is changing and our ideas about caring are changing. Much of the research and writing on caring in the public sphere has been confined to the study of a single substantive area such as child or health care. The existing work on child and health care frequently focuses on generating or evaluating existing services, qualitative and quantitative studies of providers and consumers, and analysis of costs, benefits, and burdens. The resulting knowledge, although useful in the substantive area, contributes only modestly to a conceptualized understanding of care that could transcend boundaries of different settings. Little research looks at the relationships of caring.

The purpose of my research is to generate a full, grounded, and theoretically useful concept of caring. I have examined relationships in which a third person, along with the one caring and the one cared for, has identified the relationship as a successful caring one. To study caring in its vigorous form, I feel, is a productive approach to generating knowledge about the phenomenon. Researching caring in different contexts

An original essay.

helped me to understand both its unique and its universal characteristics. This essay, taken from a larger study of caring in family, schools, and voluntary agencies, explores the processes and caring concepts that my interview subjects identified as central to caring relationships.

Caring was researched in three subsamples—families, schools, and voluntary agencies—in order to generate a conceptual understanding of the phenomenon that included both particularistic and universal characteristics. I interviewed students and teachers at one urban and one rural vocational high school, and then drew the volunteer and family subsamples from the geographic locations served by each of the two schools. A total of 84 participant interviews were analyzed for this study. Five participant interviews were deleted from the analysis because they did not qualify as caring relationships. The total sample included 40 men and 44 women; 43 were married, 34 were single, and 7 other; 64 were between the ages of 15 and 60, with 6 being younger and 14 older. The family sample was initially recruited by me through friends and acquaintances. When the sample began to all resemble me, the researcher, I stopped and enlisted three clergy of different denominations to refer caring people, which did produce a more diverse sample. The school administration recommended caring teachers and the voluntary agencies' administrator or volunteer coordinator recommended volunteers. The caring person identified the care recipient for an interview. The interviews were taped in the respondent's home or at the agency, and varied in length from 45 minutes at the schools to 1–2 hours in people's homes. Interviewing took approximately nine months.

I assumed the recruitment process had generated a valid caring relationship if it was judged to be positive, satisfying, and valued by the referring person, the caregiver, care recipient, and myself. The interviews were transcribed and then analyzed using a grounded theory approach similar to that developed by Glaser and Strauss (1967).

In eighty-four interviews, caring was found to be a process best understood as a phenomenon with a past, present, and future. The eight caring concepts I developed constituted overlapping phases of the caring process: time; be there; talking; sensitivity; acting in the best interest of the other; caring as feeling; caring as doing; and reciprocity. To begin caring, there must be people present, time to do the tasks of caring, and a vehicle for facilitating the process—talking. Next, the caring person has to be sensitive to the needs of the other, act in the best interest of the other, be emotionally invested, and, most important, do helpful things for the other. The person cared for must then respond in such a way as to perpetuate the process, which involves reciprocity. What follows is a condensed summary of the eight caring concepts that emerged from my research interviews.

Time

[H]e spent quite a while helping me on a rock tune, and I was trying to figure it out and he made up the background music for it. He told me, helped me on how to count the beats for it. You know, he helped me with all this music stuff, and he spent a lot of time on it. I thought he really cared about them. It's like, he really was interested in what I was doing, and I think that was neat because he was, you know, he's this big shot, this big piano player and he is really helping me. I thought that was great. Now he does those things a lot, but . . . He does that a lot. Yah, that's one time I felt really cared about because he was willing to spend a lot of time you know, just helping me and letting me figure it out for myself. I thought that was good. (08-m-29-k-02)

As this thirteen-year-old boy described an encounter with his father, time appeared as both foreground and background in people's explanations of caring. Time as foreground was the primary subject of the participant's comments, as he referred to time in a direct and concrete way. As background, "time" was referred to casually and indirectly and nearly always as a prerequisite for something else to happen. Of the sample participants, 76 percent (64) identified time as being an integral part of caring relations. Time given was often depicted as evidence of another's caring. Caring required time and the presence of the caring person. Time might be needed on a continuous basis, intermittently or immediately to respond in a crisis. The amount of time people spent together was important and a reduction in their time together was noticed and often perceived as estrangement. Participants cited interesting negotiations of time as a scarce resource.

Time was a latent, necessary force underwriting all caring activities. Analogies between time and money were frequently made by both the caring person and the person cared about in all three subsamples. The thirteen-year-old boy speaking above understood time as a valuable thing. His father had apparently allocated a great deal of it as he helped his son with his music. Time was highlighted as a variable important to caring. How much time people got from one another was not trivial, but rather was a measure of the caring relationship.

One man provided a singularly exquisite account of the connections between time and caring. He spoke first of his wife and then referred back to a story he had about flying to Philadelphia, unexpectedly, to watch his son in a crew race.

You're communicating their importance by time. We all get twenty-four hours a day. Really the way that you show your priority in life is how you use that twenty-four hours. Nothing else really matters. You can say oh, my wife is the most important thing in my life, but if she and I only crawl into bed at night as the only time that we see each other then the message is there. So for my sons or my wife, it is when you make that commitment to spend time. That's the one thing that you can't get more of in a day. It's a tremendously powerful communication. My father is willing to fly down here to Philadelphia to see me row. There is nothing that you can do to ignore it. It's there. Of course my enthusiasm and my pride, kind of sharing in a good time, it's a good time! It's that kind of male bonding stuff. But that's why I say I kept looking around for where are all the parents? What can be more important than watching your son row? What else is there that is a higher priority? (11-m-07-k-17)

Families were especially sensitive to feeling time pressures. Not having enough time to spend with other family members along with absence was a common complaint.

Both teachers and students talked about the importance of time to caring relationships. One student, for example, confirmed the scarcity of time and its value when speaking of a teacher whom she identified as particularly caring.

Well, usually when I'm in the regular classes he doesn't have that much time because everybody else needs a lot of help too and stuff, so I just go to him on extra time. When he's not really busy I'll ask him to help me. I know the other kids need help too, and I pretty much knowing what I'm doing. . . . and when I was sick for a while. . . . Then we must have spent about a half an hour to 45 minutes just going over all that, just extra time that he put in with me. He likes putting in a lot of extra time to help me out, making sure I got my packet done on time, doing a good job. (05-m-15-a-118)

When time was talked about in the school sample, the concept was shaded differently. Unlike caring relationships in the family—relationships that were considered to be adaptable, flexible, and always available with no appointment necessary—in the schools teachers and students seemed to acknowledge and accept an implicit boundary to caring. Teachers expressed a felt obligation, and students expected that the teachers would be present and caring during the school day. Teachers did not have to be present at times other than the regular school day to be seen as caring, although some teachers were accessible beyond the scheduled school day. Although some were, teachers did not have to be present to meet this obligation at other times. The school day represented the institutionalized, formal place and time for that kind of caring to happen.

Parents were not assigned a time and place to be caring, but were on call twenty-four hours a day. Teachers, on the other hand, were released from their commitments at 2:00 P.M. This distinction however, did not make time a less important factor in schools. In the vocational school students had a full day of contact with their shop teachers that routinely continued for three or more years. For both the vocational students and their teachers, the increased frequency and duration of their time together was an integral part of student/teacher relationships. Everyone —administrators, staff, teachers and students—spoke about the close relationship between many students and their shop teachers. The importance of this fact in student/teacher relationships cannot be over emphasized. As one shop teacher explained:

Because academic teachers see them for 42–43 minutes. . . . Whereas a shop instructor sees them six hours a day, thirty hours a week. I see them more than their parents. (04-m-30-a-00)

And a resource teacher confirmed both shop teachers' claims:

Especially as a resource teacher, you get to keep the same student for the four years they are in high school . . . we keep the student from 9th grade through the 12th grade, which really allows you to get to know them. It's good. (05-f-01-a-008)

Students and teachers had similar ideas about caring and time. As one student put it:

It's related to your shop, but at shop during the class is all day long in the same room, I guess they learn to trust you. They learn to trust you. You spend so much time with them, six hours a day for a week, then you go to a school week, see them teachers for about forty-five minutes a day, then you go back to shop. Six hours with a teacher. You really get to know them. (05-m-16b-172)

Connections between caring and time were weakest in the voluntary setting. The data from the voluntary subsample provided confirmation about some of the connections between time and caring that had already been revealed in the other two subsamples. Participants openly and frequently acknowledged that time given and received was valuable. There was no evidence however that voluntary participants felt pressured for time. Volunteers negotiated in advance how often and for how long their time would be available to clients. Clients, in turn, called to request time or came and made use of a time-limited activity.

Caring relationships in the schools were marked by boundaries of time; caring happened during the school day and rarely extended beyond that. Time as a phenomenon in the voluntary setting was predictable and measured. Clients and volunteers came together to accomplish a task or engage in some prescribed activity.

No matter the setting, what was interesting about the identified relationship between time and caring was people's ability, within limits, to regularly and without fuss, tolerate and adjust for hiatuses in caring. Sometimes the cared for person had to wait. A student made clear how valuable and important it was for him to have gotten the extra help in order to succeed with a particular class project and explained that he could handle waiting to receive such help. A mother explained that she did not devote all her time to her children; clients and volunteers understood the parameters that defined their relationships. Yet with at least *enough* time dedicated to caring relationships, they could flourish.

Be There

"I was there for them." "She's always been there for me." "I want to be there for her." These remarks were repeated throughout my interviews. Of the participants, 48 percent (41) used this expression in their descriptions of caring. What participants meant by "be there" was that the caring person would be present and prepared to help the person cared for in whatever way he or she could. For participants in the school and voluntary subsamples particularly, be there meant the care giver was accessible, approachable, even welcoming for them to initiate a request for caring. The words elicited a sense of open-endedness. People could be called on for anything at any time. This limitless quality was a pronounced feature of family participants' caring descriptions. One woman speaking of her relation to her husband offered a typical and particularly clear notion of what "be there" meant:

He has to know that I am there for him, if he has a problem or if there is something with his job or something is bothering him, that I will not be preoccupied with something else. That I would put that aside to listen to him and try to help him. (11-f-12-k-22)

To be there—and of necessity, having the time to be there—often seemed to be a requirement for something else to happen. The essence of "be there" meant to be present. Being there seemed to be a special case of caring; it signaled commitment, especially in the family. A mother spoke about being there for her son:

If he needs my time, my efforts, my support I will give it to him; it's available. That's what I mean by "be there." And also, kind of like on his side, you know wanting what is best for him, not what's best for me, but really trying to be, do what's best for what he wants, what he needs. So I'm there for him, not for me or for anyone else's needs, or systems or needs. I feel my responsibility as a mother is to let them grow. (08-f-29-k-01)

And a father said:

Being tuned into what they are doing. What is of interest, where myself might fit in if need be, but I think that you have to be fully aware of what is going on within your family and participating when you can or if not participating, giving encouragement to who or whatever is going on. And it doesn't have to be in an obvious way. You can do this very quietly, just being there to lend and to me that's what it is. (11-m-06-k-15)

Retaining an identifiable core, the meaning of "be there" shifted with sample site. To students, "be there" had a singular meaning—to be physically present. When they were physically present, what caring teachers did to demonstrate caring varied. One student described a teacher's accepting and nonjudgmental manner; another described the teacher as present, as willing to take whatever time was required to do the teaching.

He was willing to spend all the time he needed to get you through this. He was always there and it didn't matter what it was that you needed him for, he was there and it was that way with . . . all you'd have to do is call his name and he's right there. (05-f-21-a-020)

Even though there is a discrepancy between a perception by the person cared for that a limitless quantity of time and energy is available and the reality that the one caring may not in fact have "all the time in the world" to devote to one relationship, successful caring relationships seem to be characterized by the feeling of an abundance of time for being there.

Perhaps this is because being there involves an ability to demonstrate that the one caring is poised and ready to help when called on or when noticing that the other needs help. This sense of being ready to help expresses a spirit of availability that in and of itself can provide comfort and security. To be there in caring relationships thus embraced a generous range of possibilities, as this teacher explains.

I care about them educationally, but I also care about what happens to them afterwards. You know before school, after school, I care that they get the most out of their education. That's what I am here for. . . . But that's what I'm here for. (05-f-24-b-043)

From a client in the voluntary subsample, another description, again similar to the family and school samples:

It's like when you go to the club, you know all the pool tables are taken up and you are just walking around and somebody comes up to you and says, "Hey, you want to go shoot some hoops?" or something like that, you know, that's like being there. When you are alone and you don't think anybody is around and all of a sudden somebody pops up and says, "hey, let's go shoot some hoops" or just walk around and talk. (12-f-20-v-19)

A distinguishing feature of the "be there" concept among the three subsamples was its diminution as it appeared in family, school, and voluntary agencies respectively. The family subsample participants gave rich, full descriptions and detailed examples of what they meant by "be there." The school participants talked about it less frequently, but it remained a strong, vigorous concept, also richly described. Few clients and no volunteer described "be there" as a relevant part of caring relationships, leaving this a conceptually weak part of the voluntary analysis. The concept seemed to lose its integrity in this context. It lost all connection to the sense of being available anytime for anything. In the voluntary setting "be there" meant that the volunteer would help with a specific task or activity at a specified time. Although altered, "be there" continued to refer to relations that were caring, that included a caring person acting consistently in a manner that was beneficial to the person cared for. That relationship was now narrowed and rigidly limited by the voluntary context within which it resided.

She like helps you. Like some kids go home and get help, I don't get any help at home, so I can get help here. It's like having someone who cares if you are learning. (11-f-19-v-10)

This illustrates how caring concepts diverge and are shaped not only by individual actors but by the context in which caring occurs.

Talking

"Talking" was an interesting variable in the research. It was frequently depicted as a means of building and maintaining a caring relationship. Participants in all three subsamples said that "talking" was an important part of how caring happened. Their comments described a communication among caring people that needed to be open, honest, spontaneous, easy to do, and frequent. The family and school subsamples offered particularly fruitful descriptions of the relationship between caring and talking. In one interview, a boy singled out talking as an activity that affected caring by drawing his family closer:

we grow very close to each other because we talk a lot, like whether it is in the car or at home or that sort of thing, so that's caring. (08-m-29-k-02)

Some identified the absence of talking as problematic:

Well, her Dad doesn't know how to express his feelings, he can't talk about them and it's been a real problem for all of us and I on the other hand can express myself without any problem, pretty much, I mean, you know, with certain people I am closed up. I've tried to teach them [her daughters] please talk, if you have something say it. (11-f-12-k-19)

With students and teachers, being able to talk frequently and easily was important to a caring relationship. A special education teacher discussed the mechanical ease she had in talking with one student who was also in her homeroom. Their frequent interactions allowed communication to be "easy and kind of nice" (05-f-01-a-008). Another teacher stressed that respect and liking must exist before students talk meaningfully with their teachers. "They tell you things as if you're their mother" when confidence and trust are established (05-f-24-b-043).

Among family participants especially, "talking" was frequently linked to sharing feelings.

I needed to discuss things with him. I just needed to know that he was interested and that he cared. Probably by telling him how I felt, by telling him that I was upset, by telling him that it was a very difficult period for me and he responded. (11-f-12-k-22)

Not all talking was easy or went smoothly. A young man confronted his stepfather with his emotional withdrawal and diminished involvement with his children after the death of his wife, the participant's mother. This exchange was difficult and it could have led to further alienation or even a rupture in the relationship.

It may sound like nothing to confront about but my father has a very stone front and most people are afraid of him. I mean I was a policeman for a while and I worked in a prison before so confrontations were second nature for me. But this was one of the confrontations that took a lot out of me actually, very hard. . . .

The confrontation resulted in a closer caring relationship. Both men had been able to share very meaningful thoughts and feelings and move on to a closer and more satisfying relationship between themselves and other family as well. (09-m-04-k-04)

Talking could thus be either confrontational and aggressive or tender and empathetic. Both kinds of talking could be mobilized in the service of fostering a close caring relationship. Talking in caring relationships was therefore both a sign that all was well and a process used to generate and maintain caring relations. Talking could be both a means and an end.

The quality of the attention to and descriptions of talking and caring were noticeably different in the voluntary setting. With few exceptions, the descriptions were brief, not well detailed, and with a superficial and casual nature. A young client said of the two volunteers who cared about her:

Even if we are not talking about basketball, we can talk about anything else and they are just fun to be around. (11-f-19-v-09)

The idea of a relaxed, comfortable, nondefensive, or cautious attitude also permeates the next description and was representative of comments made by both the caring person and the person cared for.

because I got very comfortable with her and we talked. We walk and talk about all sorts of things and nothing in particular. We just really enjoy each other's company. And it is more like taking a friend out and we just really enjoy each other's company. (11-f-19-v-05)

Absent from or faintly echoed in the voluntary interviews was any discussion about important or intense feelings, future or long-term concerns and attention to the best interests of the clients. This was in contrast to "talking" in the family and school subsamples where conversational exchanges were frequently tied to intense, personal, intimate, and somehow vulnerable feelings. With a few prominent exceptions "talking" in the voluntary subsample appeared superficial by comparison.

I grouped together the three concepts "time," "be there" and "talking" as requirements for caring to begin. These three aspects of caring were prerequisites and constants in the process. Participants continued to need time to do the work of caring and they needed to be present to do the work of caring. Talking was the mode through which the caring activities were defined and implemented.

Sensitivity

One mother said:

I respond when there is a change in someone's behavior in the household. Either sleepy or they're talking a lot or they're not talking very much; things of this nature, really noticing what is being communicated on a number of levels. That's what that means to me and the expectation that I have is that . . . is my job as a mother to be on top of things. (08-f-29-k-01)

People who cared about each other were sensitive to each other's needs. Of participants, 74 percent (64) indicated that a sensitivity to the needs of others contributed to successful caring relations. As the comment above suggests, being sensitive to a family's needs was a complex requirement. Sensitivity required consistent attention, remembering past behavior, integrating impressions, making comparisons, weighing alternatives and then responding. This did not mean, the mother quickly qualified, that there are no limits to the noticing part of the caring process.

It doesn't mean that I have to think of them first, but I have a kind of awareness if they are needing something. And if anything is amiss or lacking, then I would drop whatever I was doing. (08-f-29-k-01)

This kind of qualification is important to note, because caring is often conceived of as a one-sided fusion with another that involves little thought and reflection. But in my research, a constant balancing and interplay of several factors was required to navigate the complex interactions of caring. Negotiations between self and other(s), and thinking about the activity of caring were a ubiquitous part of the caring process.

Many teachers similarly discussed the importance of noticing, being conscious of and attending to the mood and the focus of students. Teachers spoke about the necessity of bringing students back into the classroom each morning. Students could have been up late, had an argument with Mom and Dad. They had to be refocused, drawn into the day's activities. To bring the student into the learning experience, teachers had to pay attention to students and attend to any subtle clues that their minds might be elsewhere.

Kids come in, and last night they stayed up late, or whatever, Mom and Dad yell at them because they didn't have their shoes on right, or they didn't eat breakfast, all these concerns are there, you have to get them to focus back in again to what should be important to them. So you just have to understand that, and I think some good teachers do and they see it, they try to bring people back into the crowd, into what they're doing. (05-m-29-a-011)

Although some family participants said they noticed others' needs or wants in a direct, almost spontaneous way, the ease and spontaneity of noticing the needs of others was frequently linked to the fact that family members had a reservoir of shared experiences that gave them a great deal of knowledge about one another. A father described a particularly pleasant weekend visit he had with his adult son:

Some people try too hard to have a good time that you don't have a good time. You know, he wanted to sleep in the morning and I didn't object. I'm an earlier riser and he is not. I just went down and got the newspaper and read it and I wasn't about to haul him out of bed or whatever. And it was just a very relaxing and comfortable weekend. (11-m-06-k-15)

Years of shared family experiences allowed the father to be sensitive to his son's desires. The father's sensitivity and willingness to adjust his behavior accordingly helped make the weekend enjoyable and hassle free.

Sensitivity to the needs of others came early in the caring process and was very complex. Being sensitive required time and hard work. While variations existed, nearly all men and women, caring and cared for persons spent a significant portion of their interview detailing what sensitivity meant to them. Sensitivity to others entailed a variety of emotional and cognitive tasks that in turn depended on a person willing to care. Negotiations began early in the caring process. In the family, for example, one woman handled her obligation to "notice" and "stay on top of things" with her children within limits. She was not at her children's disposal all day. She attended to her own needs and life, turning to her family when she thought they required her attention. Thinking was an integral part of recognizing and defining the needs of others, and deciding when to intervene to satisfy those needs.

The more time people had together, the more easily people could notice the needs of others. Factors such as family history or length of the school year had a positive impact on the caring person's ability to be sensitive to the needs of the person cared for. People frequently used empathy as a tool to foster an understanding of what the other was thinking, feeling and needing. These factors, along with the concrete task of attending to the cared for person's behavior in the present context, allowed the caring person to become aware of the needs of the other.

Time was linked to the task of being sensitive to the needs of others. In the view of most participants sensitivity was not an innate talent but something people had to work at. Participants said that people needed time to get to know each other as individuals in order to be sensitive to the other person's needs. Being sensitive to the needs of others was similarly complex and required more than a response grounded in feelings alone.

In the schools, teachers deliberately attended to the work of getting to know their students as individuals in order to be sensitive to their needs. It was not enough for teachers to rely on some generic notion of what students needed. Each student cared for was known sui generis. Many teachers reported this required at least a semester, if not an entire year, of continuous interaction. This layered activity involved observing each student's behavior for consistency or for signs of change. Caring teachers attended to the act of observing students.

So the first day, for instance, they walk in, they're intimidated, they are in a building, like you they don't know where they are going or how to get from point a to point b, with teachers that they don't know, with kids they don't know. If I see a kid that's upset I can tell at this point in the year whether something's going on. Because their performance or their attitude or something is off. So it's important for me to know where the students are at when they come into the classroom. (04-m-20-a-004)

A student confirmed the teacher's ideas and made an interesting analogy:

> I think the teacher has to adjust to teaching the students, because they'll take what's given in a different manner. The teacher has to understand us. To be able to see that the needs of different students are different, so they have to teach in such a manner. Sort of like a two-way radio. The teacher has to be sensitive to that, then come back and respond. (05-m-15-b-161)

Especially prominent among the voluntary and school participants, was the relationship between being sensitive to the needs of the other and seeing the other as an individual with unique characteristics. The persons cared for reported very clearly that it was important for them to be treated as individuals, people with needs, likes and dislikes, personalities all their own. They offered several brief examples of uncaring people who neglected to treat participants as unique. The resentment participants felt about not being accorded respect for their individuality also highlighted the importance of sensitivity to the particularity of personhood.

Acting in the Best Interest of the Other

"Acting in the best interests of the other" was included as an important part of caring by 75 percent of the sample. The concept appeared initially to be complex, diffuse, and without a central core of meaning. This was perhaps because acting in the best interests of the persons cared for varied according to the site, the relationship, the time of the caring events, and countless other variables peculiar to the lives of the participants. Only in the family subsample were the caring persons willing to put the needs of others above or on a par with their own needs. The family defined acting in the best interest of others as an ongoing event, a process in which family members had been there to assist in the past, were now helping, and were expected to continue acting with beneficence to promote the health, well-being and happiness of their family members.

Teachers' and volunteers' more guarded investment reflected the organizational context in which the caring relationship existed. Teachers defined themselves as acting in the best interest of their students when they were doing things that promoted the students success at school and eventually in the work world. Volunteers said they acted in the best interests of clients when they accomplished a specific or ongoing activity with clients.

Despite this diversity, a teleological perspective seemed to govern participants' views of actions or supports considered to be beneficial. Those caring wanted to understand what needed to be done in the present in order to achieve some desired end that would assure the future well-being or happiness of the person cared about. The duration and intensity of this investment varied with the site. In families, parents said they were willing to engage in long-term efforts that could benefit their children for a lifetime. The following are the comments of a father who brought his son into his business. The father was worried about his son's general lack of direction, poor work habits, and meager work history.

Well, I feel that having him work for me, giving him a sense of responsibility and a sense of purpose. He realizes that he does have some goal in life, something to fall back on, a profession, a business when I'm not here or retired or whatever. I feel that he does have a sense of knowing that without that a business to fall back on, he really wouldn't have anything else to do . . . no means to support himself, no hope for the future. (05-m-15-b-161)

Teachers acted in the present in the hope that their actions would benefit the student in the future.

I've had two individuals come up from Florida that have been in trouble and they gave me a call and asked me if they could come up because they can't find work. I said sure. They flew up and I taught them computerized drafting here, and tried to line them up jobs here, but, of course, there isn't anything right now. I even tried to get them in somewhere down in Florida. This particular individual his wife is a teacher and he's having a tough time because he's unable to get a job and they are living off her pay. He feels very bad about it, and he's trying everything he can to get a job. So finally we've got him lined up with Boeing in Seattle, and I wrote him a letter of recommendation. (04-m-30-a-002)

A few participants used the word "empower" in the context of acting in the best interest of the cared for person. Empower nearly always meant doing something now that would foster the person's independence in the future. It frequently involved not interfering—allowing the other person the freedom to decide, act independently, and maintain control. Teaching, supporting, being a positive role model, doing things in a way that was not manipulative were all strategies used by the caring person in the service of the other.

Sometimes this process was described in terms of fostering self-esteem. One teacher, for example, spoke of building the students' self-confidence and self reliance:

I want them to be leaders and in my industry sometimes that's a lot of frustration because their desires for my students and my desires are totally different. They just want someone to "be on time everyday." I tell them, why don't you just go to a high school and pick up one of those because maybe they could find them there too. I train them to be the leaders of our industry later on. There is no doubt in my mind what perception society expects of a school at this point. I don't see that they have the same aspirations as I have as far as future to do well in school and to be able to recognize her own achievements' leaders. I did a study. Industry doesn't. No industry doesn't. Society doesn't. (05-m-29-a-011)

Teachers often explained their attempts to build students' self-esteem were not just part of how things were done, but why they were done.

"Acting in the best interest of the other" was a weak concept in the voluntary subsample. Few people spoke about it, and those that did did so obliquely. As a group, volunteers were less invested in this aspect of caring. There were exceptions. One man who identified with the under-privileged children he worked with saw his role as embracing more than coaching them:

but one thing that does bend me out of shape more than anything is that if some-body says we can't do this. We don't have the money to do this, . . . When it comes to kids, I don't think there is anything that you can't do. I've never believed that. I don't think there is anything that you cannot accomplish when it comes to a kid if you are willing to really go at it. As far as with money, if you are having trouble with moneys then I would go to the police department, I would go to the fire department, to the mayor, I'd say listen you've got the money. (11-m-20-v-11)

A nurse who taught a drug prevention class talked at length about the best interests and future well-being of the clients she worked with, as did a man teaching golf. He stressed that in working with the children, making them good golfers was a secondary objective. Most important, he wanted to provide them with a relaxed setting in which they would increase their sense of competency and self-worth. Acting in the best interest of the other carried a presumption of benevolence and would be linked to the next concept—that of feeling.

Caring Is a Feeling

Caring was frequently talked about as both an activity and a feeling. Feelings and sentiment were part of what constituted caring for 75 per-cent (63) of the participants. Caring about others meant having positive feelings of concern and/or affection about the person cared for. During several interviews the person telling me a story that had been especially meaningful to him or her experienced yet again some measure of the emotion originally felt. Two teachers, both men, cried; an older married couple interrupted their conversation in order to restrain their tears. A young volunteer poignantly described his bleak childhood as the driv-ing force behind his volunteer work.

In the school and voluntary subsamples participants frequently introduced the subject of their motivation for caring. Why people cared was nearly always tied to feelings and sentiments. By feelings I mean a subjective, emotional experience and sensitivity, often accompanied by sometimes intense physical sensations. Sentiments are different, and I use this word to mean feelings colored by thought and judgment that also reflect a shared public sensibility. This distinction is relevant because the nature of the feelings changed as the research site changed. Feelings that included intense, physical, and passionate emotions were characteristic of descriptions of family caring. The nature of the feelings discussed changed sharply in the school interviews, and yet again in the voluntary subsample where they were best understood to mean sentiments. Participants in a casual, unconscious way brought up and talked about what motivated their caring. A feature of this concept shared by nearly all participants was the difficulty people had in defining and describing caring as an emotional phenomenon. One young man struggled thusly:

Without using the word caring, that's, I don't know, pretty much acceptance and love. (09-m-10k-4)

The response above was typical. Most people seemed to use the word "care" or "caring" in a relatively casual way. This may be because people are rarely asked to be specific about what they mean when they use the word "care." When participants talked about caring, they very often interchanged the phases "I think" and "I feel caring is." This suggests that participants did not usually distinguish between what they thought and what they felt. Perhaps they responded to caring interactions on both a cognitive and emotional level and synthesized these impressions into a single qualitative phenomenon that meant caring.

Feeling was the engine that drove caring in the family sample. One husband said:

When you care for somebody you feel for them, sometimes you don't always show it, you are happy when they are happy, you're sad when they are sad, you share the highs and lows, you have a genuine feeling inside you of wanting the best for them and doing what you can to accomplish that. (11-m-13-k-23)

And his wife seemed to agree:

As I said before, it's kind of hard to live up to his standards at times, but he's got all my love and respect right now and has always, even through the rough times. . . . I know you would never have known it, but I tell him that I love him ten times a day. (11-f-13-k-24)

Family participants were the only ones to identify loving, hugging, kissing, crying, and a variety of physical affections as part of the nature of caring. In this study families who cared about each other hugged, kissed, loved, and wept. Spontaneous or unexpected physical affection was often described with special enthusiasm.

The expression of feelings had a twofold connection with caring. A caring family created an atmosphere in which feeling could be shared safely, allowing the person cared about the opportunity to gratify the expression of their emotional needs. Simultaneously, the very expression of those feelings gave to the caring person information upon which to assess the needs of the other. The display of feelings facilitated sensitivity on the part of the other family members to the emotional needs of the person cared for.

Care as a feeling dropped off quickly from the family to the school subsample; 92 percent of family participants and 62 percent of school participants described caring as feelings. Two teachers cried during an interview about what it was like for them to care about students. Teachers spoke about sentiments that generally reflected empathy and hopefulness for the future of students, their achievements in their personal and work life. For one such teacher caring was a feeling of concern:

But I do think it's important. I guess it's concern. I guess I don't look upon caring as something that you have to do, it's a feeling. I think you do things out of a sense of concern. (04-f-30-a-005)

A few of the teachers who spoke about caring as a feeling did so in the context of their motivation to teach. But most teachers did not say that caring was a feeling. Considering this, I had the impression that feelings in the school setting were best left unsaid. The socialization of professionals often mandates a "distance" and "objectivity" incompatible with the open expression of emotional responses. In addition, two teachers said peers had criticized them for "caring too much" when they openly shared a warm and satisfying experience they had with a student or did extra. For example, teachers who persisted in trying to contact a student's parents to elicit their co-operation or report on their progress were admonished for wasting time with families who did not care.

Caring described as a feeling diminished still further as a concept in the voluntary subsample. When volunteers spoke of caring as a feeling, they subordinated this to descriptions of caring as helpful activities. Interestingly, volunteers often talked about their own feelings toward their volunteering, not about feelings projected outward toward the client.

Caring Is Doing

The dominant conclusion to be drawn from this research is that caring means doing for others. Caring was defined as doing things for others by 84 percent of the participants (70). Although, what people did for others, or wanted others to do for them varied substantially, what emerged from all interviews was that the essence of caring was benevolent activity in behalf of another. In this sample, this kind of activity ranged from listening to implementing the Heimlich maneuver to save a life. Consider a young mother speaking as the one cared for:

My parents, I can't say enough about them because they certainly, they help us out a lot especially since we've had [the baby]. They provide direct care to her, my mother does, a couple days a week so that I can work. And if we need them for anything, really my parents are always there. (09-f-10-k-06)

Her mother provided an even more concrete description of caring:

And when they come, I always give them dinner and then they go home and then sometimes if they have something, I've even kept her overnight, and so that's how, and a lot of times if I bake, which I bake a lot, I always send something home. And when her due date comes closer, I will probably go there an extra day a week to stay with her and help out. (09-f-10-k-05)

School and family participants frequently cited caring as complex action. School participants overwhelmingly meant that teachers who cared about students, taught them. One woman teacher did not separate caring and work, but linked caring and teaching.

I think a lot of my job is just helping these kids to organize their work to help them track themselves. So that they see that they are making progress. Caring about the students from my standpoint, as a special education teacher, is making sure that I give them the kind of help that they need to succeed in those classrooms. I see that as my basic job and my basic job, I think, is caring about them. I don't know how else to expand upon that. Just helping them to be successful. (05-f-01-a-008)

So too, students identified caring with a teacher teaching:

If I asked a teacher for help, then the teacher right away responds and helps you out or says if you need any help, after school, I'm available, something like that. Gives you a little extra attention if you need it. If you are having a little trouble, sit down with you and work it out. Like we have a teacher in science, he stays after school with the kids, he has a day he put it up on the board, and asks the kids if they need any help you can come after school. (05-f-16-b-173)

Unlike more open-ended caring in families, caring teachers did some specific, predictable task. Working through material was one task caring teachers performed.

> . . . some teachers explain it, then leave. But Mr. Edward doesn't. He explains it, if it's a small problem he explains it out in this big sentence, every step that we do until the point that it's finished. He doesn't leave, he explains it so you can understand it. If you don't understand it, then while he's explaining you can tell him and he'll explain it in another way. (05-m-03-a-014)

Students often cited teachers who spent extra time with them, or helped in some unusual way. "They aren't getting paid to go to these shows or to do these meetings; they spend months practicing" (05-m-03-a-013), and "There isn't a teacher there that isn't willing to give you extra help, if you need it" (05-f-21-a-020). In occasional instances teachers seemed to place no limits on what students could ask. One teacher offered his home phone number to a group of students and invited them to call whenever they had trouble, day or night. This carte blanche opportunity to call for help was surely the exception.

Caring volunteers, like the following, recounted stories primarily about the particular activity they engaged in with clients. This exemplified caring.

> They love basketball, and if I can teach them the basics of basketball, then I consider myself helping them out. If I can teach a girl to dribble a basketball and she wants to go out for a school team, I think that's great. Well, I think what I'm doing right is that I'm showing them the basics of basketball and they like it. (11-m-19-v-08)

In addition to the concrete work of coaching a sport or supervising a recreational activity, volunteers working with children at a boy's and girl's club offered encouragement, praise, or intervention when it seemed the children would benefit.

Some volunteers, most often women, added that their caring was expressed in their willingness to listen, talk, and be supportive to clients. But this was always in addition to doing something with the clients—driving, teaching, or shopping. A typical example was the woman who volunteered with visually impaired clients. She led a craft group, but she thought that the real benefit of the group was offering them an opportunity to get out and socialize. Few volunteers defined their caring for clients exclusively or primarily as being emotionally or socially supportive.

Essential to the success of initiating some helpful activity on behalf of the person cared for was the caring person's ability to understand the unique characteristics of the person cared for and to be sensitive to the context of the interaction. Initiating caring activity meant that the caring person assessed what the other person needed and then instituted action on the person's behalf. The person caring assumed the responsibility for recognizing that something needed doing and did it. Initiating some helpful or supportive behavior frequently meant acting assertively, without being asked. A mother thus described how she recognized and dealt with her son's tension:

. . . he said I am worried about how I am going to do in this class. . . . It is very unusual for him . . . so I reminded him of some ways to relax himself that we had learned to use physically in the house. And he just immediately felt better and, you know, getting it out of yourself and talking about it makes things get smaller immediately and he had a great time at his class. I didn't just let him know that I was aware that he was tense, but I helped him to be aware that he was tense and to give him the tools to relax. (08-f-29-k-01)

The importance of initiating caring, based on knowledge of a unique other, was also a strong concept in the school sample. In this sample especially, it was clear that much energy was expended in people getting to know each other. Unlike family members with their long history of knowing each other, students and teachers needed to accomplish this preliminary task before getting on with a caring relationship that worked. Similarly, in the voluntary setting, where relationships were often neither sustained nor frequent, most participants recognized the importance of understanding people as unique persons in order to do the right thing. School and voluntary participants felt cared about when the caring person moved beyond generalizations and saw them as individuals. As if to underscore the importance of individualizing caring, a significant number of school and voluntary participants specifically said that those who failed to treat them as individuals were not caring people.

In contrast, teachers assumed responsibility for initiating action in their relationships with students based on anticipation of what students needed generally. The teacher needed to build up a store of information about a student in order to recognize and interpret behavioral change. As one teacher explained, a lot of cognitive work is involved in such caring activity. Sometimes one makes a decision *not* to intervene:

Sometimes I'll decide, then I'll sit for a day or two. I'll watch. Because we have them all day, every day. It gives you lots of time to . . . if I only had them for forty minutes everyday, your time is much more limited. See what happens is if you jump in on everything then you are taking on all their baggage and you just get buried with it all. Plus they never learn how to solve anything themselves either, or how to deal with things themselves or how to use their peers or their family. (04-f-30-a-005)

Caring was a process, and it was work. Caring could be routine, ordered, and predictable, or it could require creativity and innovation, spontaneity, and assertion. People constantly reassess needs, make decisions, and institute new ways and means of caring. Several examples of caring experiences included people who took innovative, forceful actions to resolve an unexpected dilemma. In some instances the action taken was not asked for. The caring person, uninvited, assumed responsibility for diagnosing and remedying a problem on behalf of the person cared for.

All this explains why acting in the best interest of the person cared for was such a complex part of caring. Caring participants devoted serious attention to thinking about, negotiating and carrying out what was best for the other. In the context of the caring relationships I studied, a presumption of benevolent intent existed. Trusting the motivation of the other provided secure ground for the negotiations and balancing of needs. The caring relationships studied were all a part of larger networks and multiple networks of others. Moreover, the work of caring had a contingent quality; all participants had needs, including the person caring, and people recognized that circumstances can and do change. This sometimes generates unanticipated needs that are best addressed with creativity, assertiveness and spontaneity. The caring person, without being asked, assumed responsibility for diagnosing and remedying a problem.

Reciprocity

Caring is sometimes interpreted as self-effacing behavior, as discussed by Nel Noddings in her discussion of caring asymmetries and conflicts (1984, pp. 48–58). Caring is embedded in reciprocal relationships. Although caring is far too often interpreted as self-effacing behavior, a fusion between the one caring and the one cared for, as Noddings and others have pointed out, caring is embedded in reciprocal relationships. This was documented by the fact that 85 percent (71) of my participants identified reciprocal relations as an essential part of caring relationships. Participants described reciprocity as a mutual interchange, a give and take, most often of unequal or unlike things and activities across time. Reciprocal relations assumed and/or implied a mutual sense of obligation and responsibility. Reciprocity was the most comprehensive of the caring concepts. Understanding it required understanding all those aspects of the caring process that preceded it.

Integral to the sense of mutual obligation were the concrete negotiations involved in balancing needs. Participants often conducted this complicated activity with the tacit acknowledgment that temporal parameters would affect the process. In families needs could vary by the hour. In school the process of balancing needs was bound by the school day and year. Students and teachers had to negotiate the specifics of their caring relationships. While students might have to wait for individual attention, teachers might adjust or create a teaching approach specific to a student who was having difficulty.

In the voluntary setting, caring relationships were prearranged and negotiating space for alternative accommodations between volunteer and client often meant that a volunteer stayed longer than expected and the client made the task of volunteering easier. The range and character of reciprocal activities varied by setting. In families reciprocity was continually evolving and included a panoply of concrete supports and actions that often spanned decades. The range and character of reciprocity was more narrow in the school and voluntary settings. Slightly more caring persons discussed reciprocity than did those cared for. I believe this finding is tied to the reality of the hard work often required of the caring person. The people doing the work of caring tend to be more conscious of the demands on their time and energy.

A unique finding in the analysis of reciprocity was the many negative examples participants brought up. This was not true of other concepts. It was not unusual for participants to describe a short example of an uncaring person or interaction in order to contrast and further explain what they meant by a caring person or experience. More than for all other concepts, participants offered many negative examples to illustrate what reciprocity was *not*. The example often included lengthy and well-detailed descriptions of reciprocal relations that had not worked well—a relevant finding in a research project that was seeking positive examples. It appeared that when caring did not work well, this was often because of a failure of reciprocity. As one student put it:

I know there are some teachers that are upset with the way some of the kids care about education, because some kids don't really have enough consideration for the way the teachers try. So the teachers basically give out the work and they don't really get involved with any of the students. They don't feel that there is probably that many students out there that want to get involved. (05-m-15-b-160)

Or as another said:

They don't feel good if they've helped you and then you cut them down. Kids do that all the time. That's why I don't really blame the teachers that say they don't care about you and "don't cry to me about that." Because, the fact is that most kids are making them feel that way. I guess that's why I don't hold a grudge against any of them. . . . Yuh, it's just like everything, what comes around goes around. (05-m-03-a-015)

If a student lacked the ability to respond, teachers might in turn, give up.

The larger context in which caring occurred also could inhibit the generation of reciprocal relationships. When administration neglected to honor the extraordinary efforts of teachers, some withdrew. Theodore Sizer's work also reveals the importance of a supportive and nurturing academic environment to sustain and foster the caring activities of teachers. "My employers lack the political courage to reward the exceptionally good work that I do. Obviously, they don't value the quality that is the source of my self-esteem, my effectiveness in helping young people to learn" (Sizer 1984, p. 182).

One teacher spoke of reciprocity as a sense of mutual respect. Using a negative example, he described how he handled the disciplining of students who were getting upset, loud or rude. He was quite ready to treat them with respect and in return expected the same from his students.

I respect the fact that, number one, you came out in the hall to talk to me, because if you started to embarrass me in front of the class, I would have to come back and embarrass you in front of the class and I know how much you hate that, so let's talk. I make it a point to let them know that you should never do this. If you respect me, I'll respect you. I will never tear you up in front of the class, but I expect the same respect from you. (04-m-30-a-002)

Yet, despite many negative examples, caring relationships seemed to be resilient, able to tolerate and absorb a certain amount of error and lapses in caring. Similarly, embedded in successful caring relationships was a flexible, adaptable definition of reciprocity, involving exchanges that varied enormously in content. In his article "The Norm of Reciprocity: A Preliminary Statement" Alvin Gouldner explains this phenomenon. Making a useful distinction between complementarity and reciprocity, Gouldner argues that reciprocity is rarely an equal exchange, that "Complementarity connotes that one's rights are another's obligations, and vice versa. Reciprocity, however, connotes that each part has rights and duties." The analytic distinction has its empirical counterpart: "[W]ere there only rights on the one side and duties on the other, there need be no exchange whatsoever . . . there can be stable patterns of reciprocity qua exchange only in so far as each party has both rights and duties" (Gouldner 1960, p. 169).

With this understanding of reciprocity, Gouldner then builds on the

"Principles of Reciprocity" explicated by Bronislaw Malinowski. Three essential elements of reciprocity are

- sentiment or existential beliefs about reciprocity
- the practical exchange of benefits
- the existence of a value element, a moral norm.

The existence of the value element is Gouldner's contribution, which he claims is a norm mandating that

"You should give benefits to those who give you benefits. . . . In sum beyond reciprocity as a pattern of exchange and beyond folk beliefs about reciprocity as a fact of life, there is another element; a generalized moral norm of reciprocity which defines certain actions and obligations as repayments for benefits received." (1960, p. 170)

More simply he said that we owe others because of what they have previously done for us, because of a shared history of previous interaction with others. He claims this norm is universal, and entails two minimal demands, that people should not injure those who have helped them and that they should help those who have helped them. Further Gouldner insists that relativity is important in any analysis of reciprocal relations. One person is obliged to reciprocate only contingently, only in response to the benefits conferred by others. In addition the obligations of repayment are contingent on the imputed value of the benefit received. The actors work out problems of symmetry or equivalency in reciprocity themselves in their immediate circumstances and in accordance with other cultural norms. Conformity to role expectations (status duties), although seen as a vehicle for reciprocity, is not an adequate explanation for reciprocity.

The last integral feature of reciprocity, according to Gouldner, is time. Reciprocity is often accomplished over time. Time to reciprocate allows the actor who owes something to another time to recoup resources of whatever kind. The intervening time is a period during which the beneficiary must appear to be grateful or at least not injurious to the other.

The concept of reciprocity contains an important attribute, indeterminacy. The actors are free to work out what an equal reciprocation means and can assign a time frame that makes sense for their relationship. This give and take provides the norm of reciprocity with a generous amount of freedom and flexibility to facilitate social interaction in countless ways. The elements of reciprocity identified by Gouldner seemed everywhere extant in the caring relationships I researched. A presumption of something owed was apparent in many of the interviews.

But obvious was the indeterminate character of exactly what was needed and when.

Reciprocity lay at the end of a chain of caring events. Depending on the context, caring acts were traded back and forth over a short period of time or over a lifetime. Reciprocity sometimes involved equivalent exchanges. But, contrary to popular belief, it certainly did not demand them. Indeed, most often what the one who cared appreciated most was simply the fact that the cared for noticed and responded positively to the act of caring. The entire school sample was a singular and dramatic example of this. What teachers appreciated most was not end-of-the-year gifts but the responsiveness of students engaging in the learning process. As a nurse I have frequently observed that those patients nurses feel committed to are those who have shown some responsiveness to the nurses' caring efforts. What seems important is to heed the call to human connection—it does not matter how frail or disproportionate.

This aspect of caregiving must be widely understood if we are to counter the common assumption that those who are cared for, particularly if they are sick, dying, or otherwise handicapped or "dependent" can never sufficiently reciprocate and thus establish that they are worthy human beings. In our tit for tat, instrumental culture that values an independence grounded in material exchange, it is difficult to visualize and conceptualize a concept of interdependence in which mutuality exists. The realities of caring belie arguments of traditional exchange theory. The efforts of the caring person must be perceived and interpreted as valued by the person cared for. Caring must be understood as ongoing and mutual, a process requiring effort on the part of both persons. Successful caring relationships are relationships in which two people do not join as one, but balance closeness and solitary, giving and taking, accepting and reciprocating.

Conclusions

The purpose of the research was to understand caring when it worked well. What were people doing right in a relationship when caring could be judged to be abundant, vigorous and satisfying? What my analysis of these different people and settings suggests is that caring is an ongoing process, a phenomenon with a past, present, and future. Eight distinct caring concepts emerge as parts of this process. To begin caring, there must be people present, time to do the tasks of caring and a vehicle for facilitating the process, talking. Next the actual work of caring begins. The caring person has to attend to and be sensitive to the needs of the other, act in the best interest of the other, be emotionally invested, and most important, do helpful things for the person cared for.

The caring process then confronts the person cared for, calling out to him or her to reciprocate. The person cared for must respond in a way that perpetuates the caring process. This last period is a critical time in the caring process and is often associated with tension and conflict. If reciprocity fails, the person caring can withdraw and feel demoralized. The other is no longer cared for. To the participants in this study caring meant an ongoing process of supportive, affective and instrumental interchanges embedded in reciprocal relationships.

Caring, as I have studied it, has characteristics in common with Marcel Mauss's notion of gift exchange (see Mauss 1967), Alvin Gouldner's reciprocity, and compassion as explored by Robert Wuthnow (1991). The essence of gift exchange, reciprocity, compassion and caring is that they all connect human beings. To be caring of one another provides witness to the sense of community, and of one's identity as a part of it. Caring demonstrated, is yet one more instance of an acknowledgment of and respect for the meaning of the group. Caring can and does spread throughout the community, perhaps stopping here, but passing on to another there. Caring can be a real and a symbolic counter to self-interest, a sterile or violent social world. Robert Wuthnow writes:

What I am suggesting is that we all benefit from a better understanding of the social significance of compassion. We benefit as its meaning is amplified. We see that the compassionate person is not merely doing something that contributes to his or her self-esteem as an individual, but that compassion has meaning for us all. It enriches us and ennobles us, even those of us who are neither the care givers nor the recipients, because it holds forth a vision of what a good society can be, provides us with concrete examples of caring that we can emulate, and locates us as members of the diffuse networks of which our society is woven. (1991, pp. 308–9)

References

Aronson, Jane. 1990. "Women's Perspectives on Informal Care of the Elderly: Public Ideology and Personal Experience of Giving and Receiving Care." *Aging and Society* 10: 61–84.

Belenky, Mary Field, Blythe McVicker Clinchy, Nancy Rule Goldberger, and Jill Mattuck Tarule. 1986. *Women's Ways of Knowing: The Development of Self, Voice, and Mind.* New York: Basic Books.

Blumer, Herbert. 1969. *Symbolic Interactionism: Perspectives on Method.* Englewood Cliffs, NJ: Prentice Hall.

Boswell, John. 1984. "Expositio and Oblatio: The Abandonment of Children and the Ancient and Medieval Family." *American Historical Review* 89, 1: 10–33.

Di Leonardo, Micaela. 1987. "The Female World of Cards and Holidays: Women, Families, and the Work of Kinship." *Signs: Journal of Women in Culture and Society* 12, 3:441–53.

Finch, Janet. 1989. *Family Obligations and Social Change.* Cambridge: Polity Press.

Fox, Renée and Judith Swazey. 1992. *Spare Parts: Organ Replacement in American Society.* Oxford: Oxford University Press.

Gilligan, Carol, Nona Lyons, and Trudy Hanmer. 1990. *Making Connections: The Relational World of Girls at Emma Willard School.* Cambridge, MA: Harvard University Press.

Glaser, Barney G. and Anselm L. Strauss. 1967. *The Discovery of Grounded Theory: Strategies for Qualitative Research.* Chicago: Aldine.

Gordon, Suzanne. 1991. *Prisoners of Men's Dreams: Striking Out for a New Feminine Future.* Boston: Little, Brown.

Gouldner, Alvin. 1960. "The Norm of Reciprocity: A Preliminary Statement." *American Sociology Review* 25, 2: 161–78.

Hochschild, Arlie Russell. 1989. *The Second Shift: Working Parents and the Revolution at Home.* New York: Viking Press.

Lightfoot, Sara Lawrence. 1983. *The Good High School: Portraits of Character and Culture.* New York: Basic Books.

Mauss, Marcel. 1967. *The Gift: Forms and Functions of Exchange in Archaic Societies,* trans. Ian Cunnison. New York: Norton.

Miller, Jean Baker. 1986. *Toward a New Psychology of Women.* Boston: Beacon Press.

Noddings, Nel. 1984. *Caring: A Feminine Approach to Ethics and Moral Education.* Berkeley: University of California Press.

Popenoe, David. 1988. *Disturbing the Nest: Family Change and Decline in Modern Societies.* New York: Aldine de Gruyter.

Reinharz, Shulamit. 1992. *Feminist Methods in Social Research.* New York: Oxford University Press.

Sizer, Theodore. 1984. *Horace's Compromise: The Dilemma of the American High School.* Boston: Houghton Mifflin.

Thorne, Barrie and Marilyn Yalom, eds. 1982. *Rethinking the Family: Some Feminist Questions.* New York: Longman.

Wuthnow, Robert. 1991. *Acts of Compassion: Caring for Others and Helping Ourselves.* Princeton, NJ: Princeton University Press.

Chapter 5
Facing Up to Moral Perils: The Virtues of Care in Bioethics

Alisa L. Carse

When Carol Gilligan published *In a Different Voice* in 1982, she claimed to discern a "distinct moral voice" in the reflections of the women subjects she interviewed for her research on moral development. Gilligan dubbed this "voice" the "voice of care" and contrasted it with the "voice of justice," expressed in standard ethical theories rooted in Kant and the contractarians. Gilligan's research was designed in part as a corrective to that of Piaget (1932) and Kohlberg (1981, 1984), whose studies of moral development initially excluded women, and later found women to be "less developed" morally than men and who, in their research, equated morality with the "justice" approach simpliciter. Gilligan's research and the work it has inspired in psychology and philosophy have given rise to a set of challenges, both to "orthodox" theories of moral development and to dominant strains in ethical theory. I want to examine and motivate a number of those challenges to ethical theory and to identify their implications for bioethics.[1] I will in the end consider how we might, in light of this recent turn in ethics, conceptualize the moral goods at stake and moral skills needed in health care practice.

An early version of parts of this essay was presented in the Intensive Bioethics Course at the Kennedy Institute of Ethics, Georgetown University, June 1989. Subsequent versions of parts of the essay appeared in Carse, "The 'Voice of Care': Implications for Bioethical Education," *Journal of Medicine and Philosophy* 15 (1991): 5–28, copyright © Journal of Medicine and Philosophy, Inc.; and "Qualified Particularism and Affiliative Virtue: Emphases of a Recent Turn in Ethics," *Revista Médica de Chile* 123 (1995): 241–49. Reprinted by permission.

"Justice," "Care," and Gender

It is most helpful to understand the two moral voices as distinct *orientations* within morality. These orientations are distinguished by differences in reasoning strategies employed and moral themes emphasized in the interpretation and resolution of moral problems; they represent distinct moral sensibilities and "different moral concerns" (Gilligan 1987, pp. 22–23; Gilligan et al., 1988, p. 82).

On Gilligan's account, the "justice" orientation construes the moral point of view as an impartial point of view, understands moral judgments as derived from general, universal principles, sees moral judgment as essentially dispassionate rather than passionate, and emphasizes individual rights and norms of formal equality and reciprocity in modeling our moral relationships. The "care" orientation, by contrast, rejects impartiality as an essential mark of the moral, understands moral judgments as situation-attuned perceptions sensitive to others' needs and to the dynamics of particular relationships, construes moral reasoning to involve empathy and concern, and emphasizes norms of responsiveness and responsibility in our relationships with others. Whereas we are, on the justice orientation, viewed morally as individuals first, and in relationship to each other only secondarily, through choice, we are, on the care orientation, understood as *essentially in relationship,* though no single kind of relationship is endorsed as alone morally paradigmatic.[2]

Now it is important to note, first, that Gilligan herself denies that the justice and care orientations correlate strictly with gender. She reports that recent studies show both women and men capable of shifting easily from one orientation to the other when asked to do so, though it is women—who are most likely to exhibit a dominant care orientation—a tendency, that is, for the terms of care to take precedence over those of justice in their approach to moral problems (Gilligan et al. 1988).

Second, Gilligan claims that the justice and care orientations are not mutually exclusive:

Like the figure-ground shift in ambiguous figure perception, the perspectives of justice and care are not "opposites or mirror-images of one another, with justice uncaring and care unjust. Instead, these perspectives denote different ways of organizing the basic elements of moral judgment: self, others, and the relationship between them." (1987, pp. 22–23)

I will examine this claim critically later, because it appears to underestimate the degree of tension between the two orientations as Gilligan describes them.

My concern in this discussion is with the implications for ethical theory generally, and for bioethics in particular, of Gilligan's characterization of these two moral orientations. It is not on the empirical status of the differences Gilligan claims to have found between male and female moral reasoners that I will focus, but on the different modes of moral judgment her work has highlighted. As Marilyn Friedman has aptly put it, "the different voice hypothesis has a significance for moral psychology and moral philosophy which would survive the demise of the gender difference hypothesis. At least part of its significance lies in revealing the lopsided obsession of contemporary theories of morality in both disciplines with universal and impartial conceptions of justice and rights" (1987, p. 92).

Along these lines, I want to emphasize that we must steadfastly reject any suggestion that women speak in one moral voice; such a claim would be preposterous at best. And we must be wary of the tendency toward gender essentialism that the language of gender difference can, even unwillingly, invite.[3] Moreover, we ought not deny the crucial importance of justice and rights in affirming the wisdom and value of the voice of care. We ought, that is, defend a sturdy commitment to rights within ethics while at the same time affirming the need for an ethic more demanding than the ethic of justice—one that gives an essential place to "care" through norms of character and citizenship *for all people* traditionally thought more appropriate for women than for men.

The Care-Based Challenge

Most deeply at stake in the care-based challenge is the conception of the moral subject, of the capacities and skills constitutive of moral maturity. I want to suggest that in the narrower domain of bioethics this challenge invites us to refine and articulate a distinctive understanding of the moral objectives of care in the medical context and the conditions and skills most needed in realizing those objectives. My aim is first to set out the broad contours of the challenge. I will then explore a number of implications the challenge has for bioethics.

Impartiality as the Mark of the Moral

Recall that a first feature of the justice perspective is its commitment to impartiality as the hallmark of the moral point of view (the point of view from which moral judgment is rendered, moral choice is made). Broadly understood, the impartiality constraint on moral judgment and justification has, as it has traditionally been conceived, required that when we are deciding what morality permits, forbids, or enjoins of us, we are to refrain from giving privilege to our own (or any one else's) particular preferences, affections, attachments, or relationships as such.

So construed, the impartiality constraint ensures that what is morally required of one person is morally required of any person (at least, on some views, any person *relevantly similarly situated*) for this is to be determined in abstraction from all particularity and idiosyncrasy. On the impartialist moral paradigm, what emerges as of foremost moral significance is not what distinguishes one particular individual or relationship from another—the contingent narrative details of individuals' lives and situations—but those features we share in common, in virtue of which we are claimed to have intrinsic moral status and rights as equals. We can see the relationship between the impartiality requirement, so understood, and the conception of moral principles as abstract and universal in scope (Rawls 1971; Kohlberg 1981; Hill 1987).

Seyla Benhabib has called the impartial moral standpoint the standpoint of the "generalized other" (1987, p. 163). From this standpoint we view every individual as an independent, rational agent entitled to the very same rights to which we ourselves are entitled as independent, rational agents. In taking this standpoint, I might acknowledge *that* the other has a unique life history, particular affections, attachments, commitments, and aspirations; however, what grounds the other's moral claim on me is not any of these particular identifying features, but the fact of his or her personhood itself. Thus, from the impartial point of view, I can acknowledge the other's *personhood*, in an abstract sense, but not his or her distinctive identity as a person.

The impartiality requirement is seen by care-based critics as morally problematic precisely because it requires abstraction from the concrete identity of others and our relationships to them. Carol Gilligan writes: "As a framework for moral decision, care is grounded in the assumption that . . . detachment, whether from self or from others is morally problematic, since it breeds moral blindness or indifference—a failure to discern or respond to need" (1987, p. 24). The worry is that in taking an impartial standpoint, I become unable to see into the other's position, to imagine myself in the other's place, and thus adequately to understand the other's perspective or needs; "the other as different from the self disappears" (Benhabib 1987, p. 165). The care orientation emphasizes a close attunement to particularities of identity and relationship as a crucial feature of moral understanding. Without this attunement we are, it is argued, often unable to make good moral judgments or to act in morally responsible ways (cf. Benhabib 1987; Friedman 1987; Gilligan 1984, 1987; Held 1987; Murdoch 1970; Ruddick 1989).

One might attempt to defend the traditional commitment to impartiality by arguing that it is properly to be understood as a *justificational* constraint, not a constraint on all moral deliberation. We might, that is, hold that impartiality is crucial to the evaluation and justification of moral requirements (or recommendations), without thereby holding that impartially justified moral requirements (or recommendations) always enjoin moral agents to take an impartial point of view in going about their lives (Hill 1987). Both deontologists and consequentialists have standardly required that moral prescriptions be justified from an impartial standpoint. But nothing prohibits prescriptions so justified from acknowledging partial duties and special obligations, pertaining, for example, to people in virtue of the roles they inhabit (e.g., physician, nurse, teacher, or governor) or the specific relationships in which they stand to others (e.g., spouse, parent, friend, or neighbor).

Indeed, sophisticated attempts have been made recently to accommodate the particularist emphasis on identity and relationship within impartialist justificational frameworks (Herman 1991; Sher 1987). Some defenders of impartialism claim, for example, that if, after all, the constraint of impartiality is no more than a consistency constraint—the requirement that similar cases be treated similarly—little more follows from it than the demand that in treating different cases differently, we be able to demonstrate that the differences between the cases correlate in morally relevant ways with the different treatment the cases receive. A commitment to impartiality does not, it is maintained, in and of itself rule out the possibility of justifying special obligations and duties rooted in our specific roles and relationships, nor need it rule out as morally irrelevant facts about our attachments, identities, interests, or special needs.

An adequate response to this line of thought is impossible here. Let me say, first, that the feminist criticism of impartiality is best understood as the claim that there is no single or privileged justificational standpoint in morality. If one is contemplating what responsibilities one has generally as a teacher to one's students or as a physician to one's patients, appeal to impartially justified principles may be illuminating and appropriate. If one is trying to decide how to respond to a particular student's truancy, or to a particular patient's refusal of treatment, attunement to the peculiarities of individual need and to the vagaries of circumstance may be essential to sound moral judgment. The suggestion, then, is that impartial prescriptions cannot always inform us about how to respond to others, and morally relevant features of particular situations will sometimes be obscured through an overzealous reliance on impartial prescriptions, even those that recognize special obligations and duties (Blum 1991, pp. 720–21; also see Nussbaum 1985, 1990). To be committed to the importance of particularity in ethics means, as Lawrence Blum writes, to be "alive to the ways that a given situation might differ from others (to which it might be superficially similar), not to be quick to assume that a noted feature of a situation correlates with others with which it has been correlated in the past . . . [or] to which we might otherwise assimilate it" (Blum 1991, pp. 720–22). Most broadly, the rejection of impartiality as the mark of the moral is a rejection of the prevailing tendency in ethical theory to construe, as *morally paradigmatic,* forms of judgment that abstract away from concrete identity and relational context, and to view moral maturity and skill as residing essentially in the capacity for abstract judgment so construed. The focus on impartiality as the hallmark of moral judgment has had the effect of ascribing a derivative, secondary status to forms of epistemic skill— involving attention to nuance and peculiarity—that are, from the perspective of care, often of the first importance.

Moral Principlism

Closely tied to the traditional commitment to impartiality is a conception of moral judgment as *essentially principled.* To act on principles is to act on the basis of reasons (stated in general terms as rules or prescriptions for action) that are taken to hold with the same force for all agents relevantly similarly situated. Moral conclusions about what to do in particular cases are, on this conception, ultimately to be justified not by appeal to intuitions, stories, or paradigm cases that have emerged in local practice, but by appeal to general and abstract principles or rules of conduct that are to be brought to bear on particular cases through processes of deductive or inductive reasoning, or "specification" (Beauchamp and Childress 1989; Richardson 1990).

The care orientation is characterized by a general aversion to moral principles. Gilligan, for example, characterizes moral judgment as "contextual judgment, bound to the particulars of time and place . . . and thus resisting all categorical formulation" (1982, pp. 58–59). The resistance to principles coincides with the rejection of impartiality as a (necessary) mark of moral judgment; to act on principles is just to act for reasons that are taken to hold with the same force for all others who are similarly situated. But there is some confusion about the nature of principles and the role principles can (and cannot) play in moral judgment. Thus I want to try to motivate the movement away from a conception of moral judgment as essentially principle driven, while in the end acknowledging a reduced, but important, role for moral principles, properly understood.

An extreme conception of principled judgment asserts, with Kant, that principles admit of no exceptions. Let us consider, however, a less extreme conception of principles according to which they have prima facie status, for this is the conception generally used in bioethics (Cf. Ross 1930; Beauchamp and Childress 1989). On this conception, no single principle is granted absolute priority in cases of conflict. Rather, the weight of principles must be assessed as cases arise, and any principle can on some conditions be overridden. On this construal of principled reasoning, an apprehension of contextual detail and a willingness to tailor moral judgments to the particulars of context are deemed practically necessary to bringing principles to bear on particular situations.

The question thus arises, Why not maintain a conception of moral judgment as principle-driven, even within a care orientation? The answer lies, among other things, in the *limited usefulness* of principles in informing and guiding a caring moral response. The claim is that in emphasizing principled reasoning in our moral theories we have seriously attenuated our models of moral skill, leaving hidden and unaddressed many crucial moral capacities on which, among other things, the wise and skillful appeal to principle depends. This can be seen in several ways.

Consider the apparently straightforward injunction, central to much of bioethics, to respect the autonomy of the patient. What does meeting this injunction amount to? "Respect for autonomy" expressed in keeping "respectful distance" can help protect against physician–patient relationships that are invasive, exploitative, or imposing, and thus subversive of the patient's sense of self-ownership and self-determination. But "keeping distance"—even intended respectfully—can also be received as morally problematic abandonment or disengagement; it may, in some situations, even help undermine a patient's capacity for autonomous agency, insofar as that capacity needs to be fostered and supported in order to be realized. Consider, for example, the demands of achieving informed consent, a requirement that has in the United States been an attempt to codify the principle of respect for autonomy in the medical setting. Clearly, physicians and nurses must often play an engaged and supportive, even pedagogical or therapeutic role in facilitating patients' understanding of their medical conditions. Bringing a patient (or his or her loved ones) to an informed understanding of the medical facts and treatment options available can be a complex and difficult process, requiring an attunement not only to a patient's particular level of knowledge, his or her ability to absorb, synthesize, and retain information, but also to the fears, anxieties, or special vulnerabilities that may be interfering with the patient's reflective decision-making process. An account of moral judgment according to which it consists in the invocation of general principles such as "respect the autonomy of your patients" (even if such principles are understood to have prima facie status), leaves important pieces of the picture out. Recognizing that a general principle of respect for autonomy is relevant to a situation at hand, and understanding that principle's practical implications for action in the situation requires a capacity for perceptual sensitivity and judgment that is *presupposed by* the application of the principle itself (Murdoch 1970; Blum 1991; Nussbaum 1990; Sherman 1990).

This is an important point. Apprehending the morally salient features of a situation is not a simple or mechanical matter. As Margaret Little writes, "The morally aware person . . . is not someone who approaches each situation with some conscious grocery list of things to check *for.* The required attentiveness is a background disposition for relevant details to come to . . . the forefront of your attention" (Little 1995, p. 122). That is, this "disposition" or capacity must be in play prior to the appeal to principle; moreover, the sort of judgment at stake is one needed for the grasp of details and constellations of details that no set of principles could possibly spell out in advance (Nussbaum 1985; Blum 1991; Sherman 1996).

Furthermore, within the care orientation, it is not just a sensitivity to the particular morally implicated features of context that is integral to moral judgment, but more specifically, a sensitivity to *other people,* a capacity to perceive (as best we can) how others feel, what they fear or hope for, and how they understand themselves and their circumstances (Blum 1988). Attention is to be given to the complex, and often quite idiosyncratic conditions of others. The claim is that this attention, and the discernment of particulars it involves, is itself a *moral capacity* which can be developed and exercised with greater or lesser success.[4]

This is not to deny that impartial rules and principles can play a useful, even indispensible, *heuristic* role, as guides to our interpretation of situations and the moral demands they pose. But it is to insist that an appeal to principle can not alone establish the moral validity of particular judgments, for the appeal to principle is itself valid only insofar as decisions based on the principle are good ones. Establishing this will require a discernment of the particulars (Nussbaum 1985; Aristotle 1941 *Nichomachean Ethics* 11137b13ff). And properly discerning the particulars will require the exercise of specific forms of affective and cognitive skill—of emotional attunement and sympathetic insight which are not themselves principle-directed.

This brings us to another, related point. When we "see" that the child crouched in the corner wants to be approached and touched rather than called to or left alone, when we speak more softly to quell someone's fear or comfort someone in pain, or look away from someone who has just been humiliated, our response to the other may be direct and dispositional rather than indirect and deliberative. Though I may come to avert my eyes from someone through a process of principled deliberation I might also avert my eyes spontaneously, in direct (nondeliberative) response to that person's distress. Similarly, I might approach and touch someone or modulate my voice "without even thinking." Practically attuned responses to situations are not always grounded in forms of explicit awareness or undertaken as a result of principled deliberation. They can be the result of practical insight that is dispositional and non-inferential, a *sympathetic attunement* to others' needs or concerns which directly informs our response to them.

This suggests that it is not only the case that principled moral deliberation involves the exercise of discernment that is not itself principle directed, but also that principled deliberation is not itself always integral to generating a caring moral response to others.

Moral Intellectualism

This brings us to a third broad challenge of the care-based approach, namely, to the intellectualism of the justice orientation and the correlative assertion of the centrality to the moral personality of well-cultivated emotion. Within the broad ethical framework committed to impartial principlism, our emotions (and particularly our affections) have been seen largely to bias and distort judgment, to introduce messy partiality and inconsistency into moral deliberation. Though some will grant that our emotions, when properly cultivated, can play a supportive role, making it more likely that we will act morally by supplying psychological motivation to do so, the emotions have been seen to be largely disruptive rather than facilitative of moral understanding and response. Impartial and principled judgment has been introduced in part in an effort to protect us from the vicissitudes and biases of our emotions. The general challenge to moral dispassion raises complex and highly controversial issues, which I can only touch on here. It is useful to understand the challenge as having two dimensions: the first concerns the importance of the emotions to *moral discernment* and moral understanding; the second concerns the importance of emotion, and in particular, the *expression of emotion*, to moral response (Nussbaum 1985, esp. 183–93; Sherman 1990; 1996).

How are the emotions important to moral discernment or understanding? The claim is that the agent's patterns of emotional attunement and sensibility, as well as her or his deeper interests and commitments, are crucial to the capacity to "see," or "apprehend" the moral contours of another's situation. Our own capacity for shame can, for example, tune us in to the fact that someone else is ashamed rather than merely embarrassed or uncomfortable. Through empathy or compassion we may apprehend another's suffering, even when its manifestations are subtle or hidden. Similarly, indignation, grief, joy, anguish, fear, humiliation, hope, and *empathetic versions of these* are ways of being attuned to situations, *modes of attending*, in virtue of which certain features of the situation stand out for us as salient while other features recede from our attention. The care orientation, in focusing in particular on the conditions of others in the situations we confront, emphasizes the importance of cultivating an active concern for the good of others, an openness of heart, and a sympathetic and engaged imagination if we are effectively to understand others, or to understand the way others see and experience their own situations and to incorporate this in our moral interpretation of the situation at hand. As Iris Murdoch puts it, "The characteristic and proper mark of the active moral agent" is the "just and loving gaze directed upon an individual reality," the "patient and just discernment and exploration" of another individual that makes possible seeing her, among other things, in her own terms (Murdoch 1970, esp. pp. 34, 38, 40).

To emphasize the facilitative role emotion and affection can play in moral apprehension is not to suggest that there are no dangers in relying on our affections: we must be on the alert against the partiality, over-selectivity, unreliability, and inconsistency our affections can introduce, the sometimes stormy and fickle character of affections, or the way they can captivate and control us. There is no question that the power and partiality of affections can pose dangers that must be corrected for in the moral arena in which so much is at stake. But to view the affections, as they are often viewed in ethical theory, merely as forces that come upon us, that cloud and distort our judgments, is to overlook the crucial role they can play, *when properly cultivated*, in informing and illuminating judgment, by alerting us to morally salient dimensions of situations.[5]

In addition to their role in moral perception and discernment, the emotions play an important expressive role in moral response. As the example of respect illustrates, it is not just *what* we do, but also *how* we do what we do, that can make a moral difference in giving care. This is reflected in our gestures, the quality of our touch, our tone of voice, where and how we stand or move, how we listen—crucially, the emotions we do (or don't) express through our demeanor. Expressing the right emotions at the right time in the right way is, on this view, an integral feature of moral agency (Aristotle, *Nichomachean Ethics* 1106b21–23 in McKeon 1941). It is important to distinguish this point from the claim that we ought to act *out of* good motivation, out of interest for or loyalty to the other. What is at stake is not just the motivation from which we act, but also the *expressive quality* of our action. This is an important distinction, for the treatment of affection and emotion in ethics is standardly confined to an assessment of the motivations of action. Yet it can be morally significant not just that one acts, for example, *out of* respect, sympathy, or kindness but that one acts in a *respectful, sympathetic,* or *kind way*, that is, in such a way as to *express* respect, sympathy, or kindness through one's action. The emotional expression and manner of communication is important to the way our acts are received and interpreted by others, and thus often to their impact and effectiveness (Sherman 1996).

It appears, then, that we are not simply in need of an enriched normative vocabulary in terms of which to address those skills and capacities agents require in order effectively to *apply* general principles or rules of conduct to particular cases. We are also in need of an account of those skills and capacities agents need in order effectively to *discern* what morality demands, encourages, or recommends and, having done so, to conduct themselves in the proper *manner*, to express themselves effectively and appropriately.

Thus it is clear that the emphasis on impartial, principled, and dispassionate judgment that marks the traditional justice orientation will fall short of providing adequate guidance within an ethic of care. A key element of the care orientation in ethics, as the philosophical analysis of care is further developed, will need to be an account of the skills and character traits—the virtues—which constitute the caring person. Among the virtues will be certain cultivated emotional capacities.

Modeling Our Relationships

Let us turn now to a fourth feature of the justice orientation to which the challenge of care theory has been directed, namely, the emphasis within this orientation on norms of formal equality and reciprocity in treating the morality of human relationships. Annette Baier writes,

It is a typical feature of the dominant moral theories and traditions, since Kant, or perhaps since Hobbes, that relationships between equals or those who are deemed equal in some important sense, have been the relationships that morality is concerned primarily to regulate. Relationships between those who are clearly unequal in power, such as parents and children, earlier and later generations in relation to one another, states and citizens, doctors and patients, the well and the ill, large states and small states, have had to be shunted to the bottom of the agenda, and then dealt with by some sort of "promotion" of the weaker so that an appearance of virtual equality is achieved. Citizens collectively become equal to states, children are treated as adults-to-be, the ill and dying are treated as continuers of their earlier more potent selves, so that their "rights" could be seen as the rights of equals. (1987a, p. 53)

The commitment to equality can sometimes be indispensable in ensuring that those more vulnerable and less powerful are protected against forms of harm, for example, exploitation or neglect. But as Baier notes, this commitment also dangerously obscures the nuances of those relationships between people of unequal power or one-sided dependence, and the special moral demands weakness or dependency can introduce into a relationship:

> A more realistic acceptance of the fact that we begin as helpless children, that at almost every point of our lives we deal with both the more and the less helpless, that equality of power and interdependency, between two persons or groups, is rare and hard to recognize when it does occur, might lead us to a more direct approach to questions concerning the design of institutions structuring these relationships between unequals (families, schools, hospitals, armies) and of the morality of our dealings with the more and the less powerful." (1987a, p. 53)

The relative weight given to relations among "equals" has led to *silence* in moral theory about good and bad kinds of engagement in relationships characterized by material inequality—of power, of knowledge, of vulnerability (as with the sick or young or dependent).

This criticism is related to the second, directed to the rights-based model of moral relationship and the individualistic conception of the self. In particular, the centrality of the right to noninterference in many justice models is based on a commitment to the value of autonomy, and thus of social frameworks within which individuals are ensured the liberty to pursue their (autonomously affirmed) conceptions of the good, consistent with the equal liberty of others. On this view, if you have a right to something, then I have the duty not to impede your pursuit of it. In meeting this requirement, I respect your right to noninterference and I have a right to demand that you will respect mine. Our interactions are thus marked by a norm of mutual noninterference. What does the emphasis on individual autonomy and the right to noninterference have to do with the individualistic conception of the self? What objections have been raised against these features of the justice orientation?

One worry is that a moral model of our relationships that construes them as paradigmatically structured by rights to mutual noninterference, except when a more robust association has been voluntarily assumed, can address very few of our relationships. Just as detachment was seen, from the perspective of care, to threaten us with moral blindness, so noninterference is seen, from the perspective of care, to threaten us with neglect and isolation, especially if we are dependent or relatively powerless, like the very young, the very old, or the sick.

This brings us back to the individualism of the self on the justice perspective. On this perspective, it isn't assumed that we are in relationship, or that human relationship per se has value. The existence and value of particular relationships and of human relationship more generally are treated as resting in individual choice. Relationships are construed as among the autonomously affirmed goods we are, as individuals, to be at liberty to pursue.

Now we do, as individuals, choose *some* of our relationships. We tend, for example, to choose whom (if anyone) we will marry or divorce; we sometimes choose friends and often choose the clubs we join. But many of our relationships, our caring relationships in particular, are not undertaken through choice. We don't choose our parents or siblings, nor do they choose us; and though we might choose to have children, we don't choose the children we have (Baier 1987b, p. 45). This holds true of many of our students and patients as well. And though we can reflect critically on the *terms* of our relationships—*how* we relate to others or they to us—we can not, as individuals, independently choose or dictate these terms. Relationships require flexibility and responsiveness on the part of those in the relationship.

Gilligan writes: "As a framework for moral decision, care is grounded in the assumption that the other and self are interdependent" (1982, p. 24); that a good life is one which involves a "progress of affiliative relationship" (p. 170); that "the concept of identity . . . includes the experience of interconnection" (p. 173; cf. Baier 1987a, 1987b; Bishop 1987; Ruddick 1984, 1989). A more adequate moral model of us as individuals would more realistically recognize the full extent of our mutual *interdependence*; it would attend more actively to modes of relating to and being with others that help to sustain good relationships among individuals who are not equal in knowledge, power and relative dependence and vulnerability (May 1977, 1983; Pellegrino and Thomasma 1988). This is not to deny the demand for respect in relationships, but to affirm that addressing this demand adequately will require a nuanced and realistic view of the material inequalities that characterize many of our relationships.

The Ethic of Care

Where do these criticisms, if taken seriously, point us? The care critique has both methodological implications, for the *process* of moral reasoning and judgment by which we are to come to understand what morality demands of us, and substantive normative implications, for what it is that morality demands of us.

On the methodological front we have seen that "care" reasoning is concrete and contextual rather than abstract; it is sometimes principle-guided, rather than always principle-derived; and it involves sympathy and compassion rather than dispassion. This introduces a conception of moral psychology much thicker and richer in its skills and capacities than the conception needed on the justice perspective and suggests a movement in a more virtue-theoretic direction, in which not only our actions, but also our characters, are a principal focus of moral attention.

On the normative front, we have seen that the ethic of care asserts the importance of community with others and a concern for others' good, of a capacity for imaginative projection into the position of others, and of situation-attuned responses to others' needs. We've also seen moral importance extended from *what* we do, to *how* we do what we do—the manner in which we act, where this includes the emotional quality or tone of our actions as integral to moral response. Finally, we have seen a call for more moral acknowledgment of our mutual interdependence, for the actual limitations of material equality, and for the special responsibilities vulnerability and dependence can introduce into our relationships.

Both the methodological and normative implications of the care critique suggest that the differences dividing the two perspectives concern much more than emphasis; they concern our conception of the most fundamental elements of moral life: moral judgment, the nature of the moral self, and our responsibilities as individuals to each other.

There are strong theoretical precedents for the care perspective, so understood. A historical alternative to the deductive, principle-driven account of moral judgement is found in Aristotle, for example, for whom moral deliberation involves practical wisdom, which is understood to outrun any general rules or principles one might possibly devise (1941, *Nichomachean Ethics* 1104a1–9). Moreover, Aristotelian virtue consists in dispositions to passion as well as action, feeling the right emotions "at the right times, with reference to the right objects, towards the right people, with the right motive, and in the right way" (1941, *Nichomachean Ethics* 1106b21–23, 1109b30). The care orientation also finds a kindred spirit in David Hume, who criticizes Hobbes and Locke for what he calls their "selfish systems of morals" and who views corrected sympathy, not principled reason, as our basic moral capacity (Baier 1987b).

The Ethic of Care: Implications for Bioethics

I want, in this section, to identify some implications for bioethics of the preceding challenges to the justice-orientation in ethical theory. There are clear affinities between standard approaches taken in bioethics and the justice orientation that care theorists characterize. Bioethical theories tend to take a principle-based approach on which moral judgments are construed to be directed paradigmatically to the question "What ought morally to be done?" and thus to be concerned primarily with right action, rather than good character or virtue. Bioethical theories tend largely to emphasize, as fundamental, the impartial principles of respect for autonomy, justice, and beneficence. Much current debate in bioethics is between deontologists and utilitarians and concerns how we are to understand and rank the importance of these principles.

It is true that the importance placed on beneficence in some bio-ethical theories may seem to make these theories morally richer than the justice orientation challenged by care theorists. For the principle of beneficence requires us to do more than recognize others' rights to noninterference; it requires us actively to promote the welfare of others. Nonetheless, there is a notable difference: the care orientation empha-sizes sympathy and compassion as modes of concerned attention to con-crete and particular others, whereas the principle of beneficence urges a "love of humanity," an abstract concern for others in virtue of our common humanity (Blum 1980, esp. chap. 3).[6]

The fact that case studies are a central focus of bioethical discus-sion, that discussions of standard bioethical issues such as euthanasia, confidentiality, informed consent, or resource allocation often involve paying attention to the concrete details of particular contexts in which those issues arise, may reinforce in a second way a sense that there are strong similarities between standard bioethical approaches and the ethic of care. It is important to emphasize, therefore, that while bio-ethics discussions tend to be more concrete than some discussions in theoretical ethics, many standard bioethical approaches continue to be abstract in a crucial sense: they rely on a language of abstract rights and principles and on conceptions of obligation formulated independently of particular contexts. Details of context are consulted only insofar as they are needed in bringing abstract, general principles to bear on par-ticular cases.

The care-oriented challenge thus has implications for the ethical theory taught, the issues addressed, and the skills and sensitivities en-couraged through bioethical education and practice. Let me set out several implications here, raising related questions for further reflection and inquiry.

The Inadequacy of Rights-Based Ethics Codes

The care orientation in ethics challenges us to ask, in general, whether a bioethical approach that pictures moral judgment as essentially im-partial, principle-driven, and dispassionate might tend to overempha-size institutionally developed rights-based codes and procedures and to underemphasize the personal skills and capacities that go into good caretaking. Too much rule dependency may risk discouraging the de-velopment and exercise of the personal virtue and wisdom necessary to fostering a patient's dignity and hope and ensuring that his or her good is served.

An example of a change in bioethics which is a change in the direc-tion of an ethic of care, is found in more recent treatments of the issue of informed consent—in particular, the shift away from an emphasis on institutional rules of information disclosure toward greater attention to the quality of the patient's understanding and of the communicative exchange. What this shift in emphasis demonstrates is that in a properly caring context, respect for autonomy—the principle that grounds informed consent—will involve not only negative prohibitions against coercion, manipulation, and the like but also positive duties, to nurture and sustain the patient's capacity to exercise autonomous choices. This process demands procedurally correct forms of information disclosure, but it also requires sensitivity to the individual patient—to his or her fears, hopes, values, and capacities in the decision-making process (cf. Faden and Beauchamp 1986, esp. chap. 7; Beauchamp and Childress 1989, esp. chap. 3; Pellegrino and Thomasma 1988).

Healing Versus Curing

Illness can wreak havoc in our lives, introducing confusion and despair. Through its disruption of our projects, our sense of independence, wholeness, competency, and control, we may suffer disorientation and loss—of life as we knew it, of our confidence in the future, of our sense of self. We may come to feel helpless, isolated and alone, cut off from others and confronted with a body (our own) that now feels foreign, even alien to us, a source of pain and anxiety, even shame (Pellegrino 1979, p. 44; Sharpe 1992, p. 308).

Within a care orientation, the "good" or end to be realized through medical care includes but extends beyond medical intervention or treatment, beyond the exercise of the technical crafts of medicine, beyond curing—to *healing*. In this context "care" consists, in Patricia Benner's words, in "the promotion of growth and health; the facilitation of comfort, dignity, or a good and peaceful death . . . and the preservation and extension of human possibilities," within the bounds set, of course, by the extenuating circumstances of illness (Benner 1991, p. 2). It requires that one see the person who is ill as more than an object of treatment, monitoring, or ministration. As Virginia Sharpe writes: "a care oriented medical ethic will make demands on the character of the physician to develop not only self understanding but to cultivate emotional and interpersonal skills that go beyond 'patient management' to genuine 'patient care'" (Sharpe 1992, p. 309). This is not to deny that the commitment to cure—to the medical identification of causes and the promotion of patient survival—is, when possible, an intrinsic objective of medical endeavors. It is rather to assert that the care of patients finds a broader *ultimate* purpose or end in "healing," in responding to the suffering of patients and their loved ones and in helping to empower them in coping constructively with the *human dimensions* and assault of the illness (Pellegrino and Thomasma 1988; Sharpe 1992; Rushton 1994).

The focus on healing moves us beyond technological heroics and medical sharpshooting, beyond the articulation of moral quandaries and the defense of decision procedures to concerns about the resources of character needed by health professionals if they are to be capable of being present to their patients in an empowering way. It also raises concern about the culture and climate of the hospital and clinic environments in which physicians and nurses work. What conditions foster the responsiveness and attunement to patient well-being that a healing orientation demands? Do the systems of financial reward and professional honor reflect a focus on technological procedure and intervention? Does the way in which medical care is covered (e.g., a fee-for-payment system) encourage physicians to perform operations, administer tests, or undertake other medical procedures *in place of* committing more time to longterm patient education and effective communication?

Trust

The ethic of care, as we have seen, represents a call to attend to the distinct psychological reality and condition of the other, a call for more moral acknowledgment of the actual relationships we are in, including the actual limitations of the material equality of those in relationship. It thus highlights special responsibilities that unequal vulnerability and dependency can introduce into relationships between patients and those caring for them. The vulnerability illness brings is enhanced by the fact that in seeking help when we are ill or in need of care, we must submit to others who have knowledge and skill we do not have. This often entails that we must, as Edmund Pellegrino writes, "open the most private domains of our bodies, minds, social and family relationships to the physician's probing gaze. Our vices, foibles, and weaknesses will be exposed to a stranger. Even our living and dying will engage her attention and invite her counsel" (Pellegrino 1991, p. 73). Though as patients or patients' families we can retain broad rights of refusal and request, contract models of patient care are inherently limited given the material realities of illness and limited expertise; we are often not in a position to negotiate the terms of our treatment as equal partners. As Virginia Sharpe writes, "on the care model, moral requirements are not . . . generated exclusively by agreement between individuals who can fully articulate their needs. In fact, the care perspective insists that moral requirements frequently emerge within a relationship precisely *because* a vulnerable member of that relationship is *not* in a position to spell out his or her needs" (Sharpe 1992, p. 312). Discretionary leeway and authority must be given to health professionals to make judgments and undertake courses of action that the patient may not know to ask for and that simply cannot be fully specified or anticipated in advance (Pellegrino 1988, 1991).

Patients but also patients' families and loved ones are often forced suddenly to trust strangers to act in their best interests, in circumstances that are unfamiliar and even terrifying and in conditions providing little or no opportunity to develop more than a thin familiarity with the professionals who are to be so entrusted (Rushton 1994, p. 1). Relationships with those professionals who care for one or one's loved one must therefore of necessity be what Pellegrino and Thomasma have called "fiduciary relationships"—relationships bound by trust that is merited. In trusting we rely on the fidelity to our trust of those in whom we have placed our trust; we have faith that those entrusted with our care will not exploit our vulnerability or the power we have given them, whatever the promises of professional or personal gain might be (Pellegrino 1991, pp. 69, 71, 82; Baier 1986; 1994, chaps. 6, 7, 8, and 9). Thus we are urged to ask what features of hospital and clinic culture contribute to the erosion of trust between health professionals and their patients? How might trusting relationships be sustained, even in the extenuating circumstances of medical care? What are the virtues necessary to maintaining trusting relationships with patients?

The Significance of Communication

As we have seen, the care orientation highlights the importance of sensitivity to patients' suffering, of responding in such a way as to protect patients and their loved ones, as much as possible, from the sense of isolation, abandonment, and disablement that illness often brings. It suggests that we must pay attention in our models of moral response to those virtues needed if we are to be able to "hear" others in their own terms, and be present to them in their pain. It asks that we attune ourselves to the conditions of fear, anger, and confusion, and to the values, capacities, commitments, and felt needs that come to the center or are placed under threat through illness or crisis in a particular patient's life. Central to the conception of moral skill on the care orientation will be an account of those capacities and dispositions that enable us to be present to others, to express ourselves effectively, to interpret what others say or do with sensitivity and insight, and to remain open in principle to transformations in our conceptions of the issues and goods at stake for others in the situations they face (Walker 1989, p. 21). This suggests that more effort should be made to be attuned to our own and others' values, fears, capacities, and commitments, and to encourage the consideration of such factors in the interpretation and resolution of ethical conflicts. Thus the care-based challenge raises the question how we can widen and expand emotional knowledge and imaginative power and encourage our capacity to enter into the feelings and perspectives of others, while remaining sober about our own limitations of empathy and imagination (Walker 1989). We are called on to explore and develop the abilities that are prerequisite to good communication and to attend more explicitly to the implications of manner, tone, touch, and other forms of demeanor to the expressive quality of action—the ways in which, in Benner's words, "thoughts and feelings [fuse] with physical presence and action" (Benner 1991, p. 2).

Virtue and Character

The care orientation suggests that bioethical discussions should be addressed not only to the principled solution of moral quandaries or to the question "What is the moral status of this action (or policy for action)?," but also the questions of affiliative virtue and character—"What traits and capacities ought I to develop and express as a physician, nurse, bioethicist, or teacher who must engage with and care for others?" These questions introduce the need for a rich moral vocabulary, for the ability to address issues of character and virtue as well as right action. They also suggest that bioethical education and focus would, at its best, be aimed at developing and exploring not only intellectual skills and moral theoretical knowledge but the whole character of the health professional. It would itself be a kind of "fitness program" (Solomon 1988, p. 437) intended to sharpen analytical tools and interpretive skill useful in the deliberation about cases, *but also* to foster those affiliative virtues crucial to sustaining morally healthy relationships with others.

Moral Narrative

Of course, virtue is not fostered simply through learning theories of virtue, nor even through the presence of virtuous practitioners on whom one can model oneself. It requires practice, activity, through which one develops *habits* of sensitivity, discernment, and response. Thus, in addition to theories and role models, we need heuristic devices and guides that are capable of triggering the imagination, eliciting insight, and directing attention to matters of moral significance in the clinical situations confronted day to day.

How might this guidance of practice be institutionally affected? Many writers in the ethics of care have supported the importance of moral narrative as a heuristic supplement to abstract principles and ethical codes. Patricia Benner writes of nursing, for example, that "a historically developed set of stories that demonstrate concerns, know-how, and caring practices for preserving dignity, mobilizing hope, and preserving illusions of control and autonomy" can serve to "evoke perceptual or sensory memories that enhance pattern recognition" and "set . . . human skill in motion" (Benner 1991, pp. 10, 7–8, 11, 3). Accounts of "healing and transcendence . . . heroism . . . fostering care and connection . . . being present to and not abandoning patients," stories of "fidelity in the midst of suffering," of "disillusionment," of "confronting unavoidable suffering and death," and of learning spur recognition "uncover meanings and feelings in ways that shed light on the contextual, relational, and configurational knowledge lived out in the practice." These stories, Benner claims, are crucial supplements to the "typical codified, cryptic, efficient exchanges of professional assessment" (Benner 1991, p. 9).

Narrative accounts, stories, and paradigm cases can become embodiments of institutional moral wisdom, examples of moral excellence (or failure), and resource points or anchors to discussion and practice. They can serve to express moral aspiration and convey moral commitments within a domain of practice (such as medicine or nursing); they can in so doing inspire and guide the interpretation given to new and troubling cases as they arise. They are thus important additions to codes of ethics and virtuous practitioner-role models in health care institutions.

Acknowledging Labor Divisions and Material Conditions of Caregiving

A broad implication of the care-oriented challenge—particularly the worries voiced about impartiality and the emphasis on material inequality—is that bioethical issues ought not to be addressed in a social and political vacuum. More attention must be paid to the nature and dynamics of both particular relationships and relationship types as a significant feature of ethical analysis. The interpretation of cases must involve an acknowledgment of the inequalities of dependency, vulnerability, and knowledge within the relationships that actually structure our lives. Recognition of the inequalities and articulation of the positive duties of care and empowerment they introduce can be an important dimension of bioethical analysis.[7]

We might within bioethics also engage in critical reflection on the gender patterned occupational roles among health care providers, on the way in which the roles of physician and nurse, for example, have historically been construed as male and female roles, respectively, and on the effect this has had on the division of labor and authority in health care practice (cf. Warren 1989, pp. 77–80; Sherwin 1992). Bioethical reflection would extend to an examination of the broad social and economic implications of particular medical practices and technologies, such as reproductive technologies, and address the implications both for our access to health care and for our health care needs of factors such as age, gender, class, religion, and sexual orientation (Overall 1987, 1989, p. 182; Sherwin 1987, 1989). Finally, it would address those institutional and cultural conditions needed to support care-oriented caregivers, if we are to protect against their exploitation, particularly insofar as doing so would require institutional reform. How, that is, are we to understand the care orientation such that it has the moral resources with which to sustain itself and ensure that conditions of adequate care are met? How do those who do the principal caring work remain complicit in systems that offer inadequate care, and what conditions support such complicity? What political skills and tactics do care-takers need to defend good care-giving practices and to activate a care ethic in their work?

Some Worries

There are, of course, many worries that might be raised for the care orientation in the context of bioethics. Let me look at three that are particularly germane to the present discussion.

It might, first, be objected that there are important moral issues which fall outside the reach of an ethic of care, even if it is caring that leads us to be concerned about them. The worry is that an ethic of care will have nothing to say about certain forms of injustice, that we may, as Virginia Held has put it, "decide that the rich will care for the rich and the poor for the poor, with the gap between them, however unjustifiably wide, remaining what it is" (1987, p. 120). It is important to stress, first, that what is in question in the feminist challenge we have reviewed is not the importance of justice but the sufficiency of justice and the primacy that has been granted the justice orientation in moral theory. An adequate moral theoretical approach may well involve an integration of the justice and care orientations so as to retain their respective strengths through rehabilitated notions of "justice" and "care."[8]

Second, there might be a perceived need for detachment on the part of good physicians and nurses that is deemed incompatible with the emphasis on compassion and sympathy on the care orientation. As Beauchamp and Childress write, "A physician who lacked compassion would generally be viewed as deficient; yet compassion also may cloud judgment and preclude rational and effective responses. Constant contact with suffering can overwhelm and even paralyze a compassionate physician" (1989, p. 383). The important point to make in response to this worry is that there is nothing intrinsic to the care perspective which excludes appropriately detached forms of concern and compassion. An empathetic health care professional should be able to summon the appropriate degree of emotional detachment, or equanimity, when this is crucial to serving the well-being of the patient. This capacity would be a central feature of affiliative virtue in the health care context. Articulating or making explicit what degree of distance is appropriate is difficult, to say the least. This difficulty can help highlight the usefulness of moral stories and narratives as ethical resources. As Benner writes: "Narratives are essential to convey and preserve knowledge about the skill of involvement (getting the right kind of involvement and interpersonal distance to fit the situation), because relational skills always involve the concrete other and are always context-dependent" (1991, p. 9). Stories and narratives can help convey the subtleties of appropriate involvement with patients and their families, but this remains a difficult skill to put into practice, whatever one's moral orientation.

The third difficulty concerns the possible tendency of an ethic of care to allow, on the one hand, too much self-sacrifice on the part of the health care professional, and on the other, over-zealous caretaking, leading to too much involvement with patients, or to paternalism. In response, let me note first that a full account of the virtues of caretaking would need to spell out conceptions of proper self-regard—or care of oneself—as protection against self-effacement, problematic self-denial, or loss of identity and as a precondition of sound caring for others. Being present to another's suffering need not and *ought not* to introduce overinvolvement and overidentification with the other, or vicarious experience of the other's pain. Indeed, this would likely compromise care by bringing the focus onto oneself. A firm sense of one's own boundaries is a precondition of sound caring for others (cf. Ruddick 1984, pp. 217–18; Gilligan 1982, p. 149); it is also crucial for the self-respect of the caretaker. Secondly, it is important, in light of worries about paternalism, to build into our very conception of caretaking the requirement that the caretaker respect the person cared for.[9] A principal aim of a bioethics informed by an ethic of care would be to address how our institutions and practices of health care can further empower patients and in general encourage more active participation on the part of nonexperts in their own health care. This would involve a critical exploration of traditional construals of medical authority and reflection on the effects of power dynamics within "healing" relationships and health care institutions (cf. Warren 1989, p. 81; May 1983).

There is no question that we need, in making moral judgments or undertaking moral action, to be consistent and fair, that we must correct for our human tendencies to yield to our own biases, prejudices, affections, and attachments. We need recourse against the view that the presence in us of affection or the existence of an attachment can alone serve to determine the contours of what is morally demanded of us. It is important to emphasize that in pursuing judgment sensitive to individual need and relational context, we can and must have a way to determine which *expressed* needs or *apparent* interests are legitimate, which have a moral claim. Thus, one challenge that remains in the development of the ethic of care within bioethics is the articulation and defense of norms, guidelines, and considerations that can help direct our judgment in these ways, providing a critical vantage point from which to evaluate the cases we confront. What I want here to emphasize is that the interpretation of cases in light of these standards can and should involve an acknowledgment of the inequalities of dependency, vulnerability, and knowledge of the relationships that actually structure the cases at issue. Recognition of the inequalities and articulation of the positive duties of care and empowerment they introduce should be an important dimension of bioethical analysis.

Conclusion

The ethic of care highlights the moral perils of relying too singlemindedly on abstract judgment — the risks of blindness and incomprehension that render judgment poor and ultimately unhelpful to those whose lives or well-being is at stake. The facts of our interdependence bring to the center moral concerns about suffering and aloneness, threats of abandonment, neglect, and isolation, especially if we are in special states of vulnerability, as are those who are ill and in need of care from health professionals. I have suggested that the turn toward care-based ethics calls us to focus on community and communication, on healing rather than curing, on the importance of trust in clinical relationships, and on virtue and narrative as institutional resources.

A central question for bioethical theory concerns how we can widen and expand our emotional knowledge and imaginative power and encourage in ourselves and others the ability to enter into the feelings and perspectives of others without taking possession of others' suffering, or exploiting others' vulnerability to serve our own psychological or material ends. This is no easy task, given the pressures of hospital and clinic environments, or our weaknesses and susceptibilities as humans, capable of being fearful, self-protective, and limited in our sympathy, imagination, and emotional energy. The message of the ethic of care is that this task is a necessary one in the trustworthy and compassionate care of others.

In conclusion, we are still in need of a clear and systematic account of standards by which we can distinguish morally good from morally troubling (even morally debased) forms of "care." We also have a need for boundaries which exclude conceptions of care that serve to justify relations of domination and subordination or which threaten to bolster, rather than to challenge, existing forms of gender division and stratification (Flanagan and Jackson 1987).

But the strength of the care-oriented approach lies in its most basic recommendation: that we reflect upon the moral voices employed in moral thought and practice—the values and ideals highlighted, the forms of discourse used, and the models and paradigms central to our attempts to make sense of moral questions that arise. That challenge urges that we become self-conscious about how the dominant models shape our conception of what morality demands; it suggests that part of our job in coming to understand our moral world will involve coming to be reflective about the voices in which we ourselves speak and to listen to and learn from the voices of others. These challenges can be made an integral part of bioethical theory and health care practice.

I am grateful to those present in the audience at the original presentation of these ideas for their challenging questions, and I am especially indebted to Tom Beauchamp for helpful comments and suggestions on an earlier draft of this essay.

Notes

1. A complex and important question that I cannot pursue here is whether and to what extent Kantian and contractarian theories, generally constituting the target of attack in this feminist movement, can accommodate the care orientation. My own position is that they can do so to some extent, but not fully. Whatever position one takes on this issue, however, one thing remains true: the focus of traditional theories rooted in Kant and the contractarians is quite different from that of the care orientation. I hope that my discussion suggests some ways in which the difference is not one of focus alone.

2. This is not to say that all de facto relationships are morally acceptable on the care orientation; the care orientation can be understood as striving, among other things, to articulate norms of relationship that more adequately acknowledge the broad facts of human interdependency.

3. Though we must reject the suggestion that there is a distinctive voice that is *woman's as such*, we might understand this recent project in feminist ethics as unveiling—making visible and explicit—in our ethical theories and ethical practices *one* of the important moral orientations emerging out of women's distinctive experiences in our society, given the sexual division of labor and the social significance of gender generally as it affects identity-formation. This project does *not*, however, affirm the care orientation as most appropriate for women; quite the contrary, it affirms its importance in general—for women and men—and thus highlights forms of moral skill and moral maturity that have been overlooked or granted only secondary status in many of our preeminent ethical theories.

4. For discussions of Aristotle along these lines, see Nussbaum 1985, esp. pp. 171–93.

5. For discussions of moral salience, see Murdoch 1970: McDowell 1979; Blum 1980, 1991.

6. A notable exception is found in the treatment given the principle of beneficence by Pellegrino and Thomasma 1988.

7. William May 1977, 1983 recommends that the relationship between the health care provider and the patient be viewed as a covenant rather than a contract, because it lacks a specific *quid pro quo*. Warren Reich 1987 argues that contract models and rights language are "too adversarial" and fail adequately to capture the need for "acceptance, trust, affection, and care" which can in effect constitute the moral status of others within relationships. He emphasizes the need to encourage bonding and loyalty to those in need of care, not just respect for rights. Pellegrino and Thomasma 1988 explore the limitations of contractual models of relationship in medical ethics, stressing the unequal power and vulnerability introduced through illness. Annette Baier 1986 recommends that a language of trust be introduced into our ethical reflections to supplement if not supplant contract models. All of these proposals and others might be critically evaluated and contrasted with standard contractual models.

8. For excellent suggestions about how such rehabilitated notions might look, see Friedman 1987.

9. Pellegrino and Thomasma 1988 develop an account of beneficence which invokes, as an integral part, respect for the autonomy of the one whose good is served.

References

Aristotle. 1941. *Basic Works of Aristotle*, ed. Richard P. McKeon. New York: Random House.

Baier, Annette. 1985. *Postures of the Mind: Essays on Mind and Morals*. Minneapolis: University of Minnesota Press.

———. 1986. "Trust and Antitrust." *Ethics* 96 (January): 231–60.

———. 1987a. "The Need for More Than Justice." In Hanen and Nielsen 1987, 41–56.

———. 1987b. "Hume, the Women's Moral Theorist?" In Kittay and Meyers 1987, 37–55.

———. 1991. "Whom Can Women Trust?" In Card 1991, 233–45.

———. 1994. *Moral Prejudices: Essays on Ethics*. Cambridge, MA: Harvard University Press.

Bartky, Sandra Lee. 1990. *Femininity and Domination: Studies in the Phenomenology of Oppression*. New York: Routledge.

Beauchamp, Tom L. and James F. Childress. 1989. *Principles of Biomedical Ethics*. Oxford: Oxford University Press.

Beauchamp, Tom L. and Laurence B. McCullough. 1984. *Medical Ethics: The Moral Responsibilities of Physicians*. Englewood Cliffs, NJ: Prentice Hall.

Benhabib, Seyla. 1987. "The Generalized and the Concrete Other: The Kohlberg-Gilligan Controversy and Moral Theory." In Kittay and Meyers 1987, 154–77.

Benner, Patricia. 1991. "The Role of Experience, Narrative, and Community in Skilled Ethical Comportment." *Advances in Nursing Science* 14, 2: 1–21.

Benner, Patricia and Judith Wrubel. 1989. *The Primacy of Caring: Stress and Coping in Health and Illness.* Menlo Park, CA: Addison-Wesley.

Bishop, Sharon. 1987. "Connections and Guilt." *Hypatia* 2 (December): 7–23.

Blum, Lawrence A. 1980. *Friendship, Altruism, and Morality.* Boston: Routledge and Kegan Paul.

———. 1988. "Gilligan and Kohlberg: Implications for Moral Theory." *Ethics* 98 (April): 473–91.

———. 1991. "Moral Perception and Particularity." *Ethics* 101 (July): 701–25.

Calhoun, Cheshire. 1988. "Justice, Care, Gender Bias." *Journal of Philosophy* 85, 9 (September): 451–63.

Caplan, Arthur L. 1980. "Ethical Engineers Need Not Apply: The State of Applied Ethics Today." *Science, Technology, and Human Values* 6, 33: 24–32.

Card, Claudia, ed. 1991. *Feminist Ethics.* Lawrence: University Press of Kansas.

Christie, Ronald J. and C. Barry Hoffmaster. 1986. *Ethical Issues in Family Medicine.* New York: Oxford University Press.

Dancy, Jonathan. 1992. "Caring About Justice." *Philosophy* 67: 447–66.

———. 1993. *Moral Reasons.* Oxford: Blackwell.

Dillon, Robin S. 1992. "Respect and Care: Toward Moral Integration." *Canadian Journal of Philosophy* 22 (March): 105–32.

Faden, Ruth R. and Tom L. Beauchamp, with Nancy M. P. King. 1986. *A History and Theory of Informed Consent.* New York: Oxford University Press.

Flanagan, Owen J. and Kathryn Jackson. 1987. "Justice, Care, and Gender: The Kohlberg-Gilligan Debate Revisited." *Ethics* 97 (April): 622–37.

Friedman, Marilyn. 1987. "Beyond Caring: The De-Moralization of Gender." In Hanen and Nielsen 1987, 87–110.

Gilligan, Carol. 1982. *In a Different Voice: Psychological Theory and Women's Development.* Cambridge, MA: Harvard University Press.

———. 1984. "The Conquistador and the Dark Continent: Reflections on the Psychology of Love." *Daedalus* 113: 75–95.

———. 1987. "Moral Orientation and Moral Development." In Kittay and Meyers 1987, 19–33.

Gilligan, Carol, Janie Victoria Ward, and Jill McLean Taylor, eds., with Betty Bardige. 1988. *Mapping the Moral Domain: A Contribution of Women's Thinking to Psychology and Education.* Cambridge, MA: Harvard University Press.

Hanen, Marsha P. and Kai Nielsen, eds. 1987. *Science, Morality, and Feminist Theory.* Supplementary volume 13, *Canadian Journal of Philosophy.*

Held, Virginia. 1987. "Feminism and Moral Theory." In Kittay and Meyers 1987, 111–28.

Herman, Barbara. 1991. "Agency, Attachment, and Difference." *Ethics* 101 (July): 775–97.

Hill, Thomas E., Jr. 1987. "The Importance of Autonomy." In Kittay and Meyers 1987, 129–38.

Hoagland, Sarah Lucia. 1990. "Some Concerns About Nel Noddings' *Caring.*" *Hypatia* 5 (March): 107–14.

Holmes, Helen Bequaert and Laura M. Purdy, eds. 1992. *Feminist Perspectives in Medical Ethics.* Bloomington: Indiana University Press.

Houston, Barbara. 1990. "Caring and Exploitation." *Hypatia* 5 (March): 115–19.

Jecker, Nancy S. and J. S. Donnie. 1991. "Separating Care and Cure: An Analysis of Historical and Contemporary Images of Nursing and Medicine." *Journal of Medicine and Philosophy* 16 (June): 285–306.

Kittay, Eva Feder and Diana T. Meyers, eds. 1987. *Women and Moral Theory.* Totowa, NJ: Rowman and Littlefield.

Kohlberg, Lawrence. 1981. *The Philosophy of Moral Development: Moral Stages and the Idea of Justice.* Essays on Moral Development 1. San Francisco: Harper and Row.

———. 1984. *The Psychology of Moral Development.* Essays on Moral Development 2. San Francisco: Harper and Row.

Little, Margaret. 1995. "Seeing and Caring: The Role of Affect in Feminist Moral Epistemology." *Hypatia* 10 (Summer): 117–37.

May, William F. 1977. "Code and Covenant on Philanthropy and Contract." In *Ethics in Medicine: Historical Perspectives and Contemporary Concerns,* ed. Stanley Joel Reiser, Arthur J. Dick, and William J. Curran, 65–76. Cambridge, MA: MIT Press.

———. 1983. *The Physician's Covenant: Images of the Healer in Medical Ethics.* Philadelphia: Westminster Press.

McDowell, John. 1979. "Virtue and Reason." *Monist* 62: 331–51.

Moody-Adams, Michelle. 1991. "Gender and the Complexity of Moral Voices." In Card 1991, 197–212.

Murdoch, Iris. 1970. *The Sovereignty of Good.* London: Routledge and Kegan Paul.

Nelson, Hilde. 1992. "Against Caring." *Journal of Clinical Ethics* 3 (March): 15–18.

Noddings, Nel. 1984. *Caring: A Feminine Approach to Ethics and Moral Education.* Berkeley: University of California Press.

———. 1992. "In Defense of Caring." *Journal of Clinical Ethics* 3 (March): 15–18.

Nussbaum, Martha C. 1985. "The Discernment of Perception: An Aristotelian Conception of Private and Public Rationality." *Proceedings of the Boston Area Colloquium in Ancient Philosophy* 1: 151–207.

———. 1990. *Love's Knowledge: Essays on Philosophy and Literature.* New York: Oxford University Press.

Okin, Susan Moller. 1989. "Reason and Feeling in Thinking About Justice." *Ethics* 99 (January): 229–49.

Overall, Christine. 1989. "The Politics of Communities." *Hypatia* 4, 2 (Summer): 179–85.

Pellegrino, Edmund D. 1989. "Character, Virtue, and Self-Interest in the Ethics of Professions." *Journal of Contemporary Health Law and Policy* 5: 53–73.

———. 1991. "Trust and Distrust in Professional Ethics." In *Ethics, Trust, and the Professions: Philosophical and Cultural Aspects,* ed. Edmund D. Pellegrino, Robert M. Veatch, and John P. Langan, 69–89. Washington, DC: Georgetown University Press.

Pellegrino, Edmund D. and David C. Thomasma. 1988. *For the Patient's Good: The Restoration of Beneficence in Health Care.* New York: Oxford University Press.

Piaget, Jean. 1932. *The Moral Judgment of the Child.* New York: Free Press.

Rawls, John. 1971. *A Theory of Justice.* Cambridge, MA: Harvard University Press.

Reich, Warren T. 1987. "Caring for Life in the First of It: Moral Paradigms for Perinatal and Neonatal Ethics." *Seminars in Perinatology* 11 (July): 279–87.

———. 1991. "The Case: Denny's Story and Commentary: Caring as Extraordinary Means." *Second Opinion* 17 (July): 41–56.

Richardson, Henry S. 1990. "Specifying Norms as a Way to Resolve Concrete Ethical Problems." *Philosophy and Public Affairs* 19: 279–310.

Ross, W. D. 1930. *The Right and the Good.* Oxford: Clarendon Press.

Ruddick, Sara. 1984. "Maternal Thinking." In *Mothering: Essays in Feminist Theory,* ed. Joyce Trebilcot, 213–30. Totowa, NJ: Rowman and Littlefield.

————. 1989. *Maternal Thinking: Toward a Politics of Peace*. Boston: Beacon Press.

Rushton, Cindy. 1994. "Bridging the Tensions Between Care and Cure." In *Pediatric Ethics: Putting Principles into Practice*, ed. A. Fleischman and R. Cassidy. New York: Hardwood Academic Press.

Sharpe, Virginia A. 1992. "Justice and Care: The Implications of the Kohlberg-Gilligan Debate for Medical Ethics." *Theoretical Medicine* 13 (December): 295–318.

Sher, George. 1987. "Other Voices, Other Rooms? Women's Psychology and Moral Theory." In Kittay and Meyers 1987, 178–89.

Sherman, Nancy. 1990. "The Place of Emotions in Kantian Morality." In *Identity, Character, and Morality: Essays in Moral Psychology*, ed. Owen Flanagan and Amelie Oksenberg Rorty. Cambridge, MA: MIT Press.

————. 1996. "The Passional Underpinning of Kantian Virtue." In *Making a Necessity of Virtue: Aristotle and Kant on Virtue*. New York & Cambridge: Cambridge University Press.

Sherwin, Susan. 1987. "Feminist Ethics and In Vitro Fertilization." In Hanen and Nielsen 1987, 265–84.

————. 1989. "Feminist and Medical Ethics: Two Different Approaches to Contextual Ethics." *Hypatia* 4, 2 (Summer): 57–72.

————. 1992. *No Longer Patient: Feminist Ethics and Health Care*. Philadelphia: Temple University Press.

Solomon, David. 1988. "Internal Objections to Virtue Ethics." In *Ethical Theory: Character and Virtue*, ed. Peter A. French, Theodore E. Uehling, Jr., and Howard K. Wettstein, 428–41. Midwest Studies in Philosophy 13. Notre Dame, IN: Notre Dame University Press.

Spelman, Elizabeth. 1991. "The Virtue of Feeling and the Feeling of Virtue." In Card 1991, 213–22.

Walker, Margaret. 1989. "Moral Understandings: Alternative 'Epistemology' for a Feminist Ethic." *Hypatia* 4, 2 (Summer): 15–28.

Warren, Virginia L. 1989. "Feminist Directions in Medical Ethics." *Hypatia* 4, 2 (Summer): 73–87.

Watson, Jean. 1985/1988. *Nursing: Human Science and Human Care*. Norwalk, CT: Appleton-Century-Crofts; New York: National League for Nursing Press.

————. 1990. "Caring Knowledge and Informed Moral Passion." *Advances in Nursing Science* 13 (September): 15–24.

Wolf, Susan. 1991. "Ethics Committees and Due Process: Nesting Rights in a Community of Caring." *Maryland Law Review* 50: 798–858.

Part II
Family Caregiving

Traditional and nontraditional families and communities are societal units of care and the source of learning basic cultural caring practices and traditions. Daily rituals and routines, nourishment, care of the body, and recognition practices established in families constitute our understanding of what it means to care for and about one another. Failures and inabilities to care as well as patterns of domination and submission, control, and violence are also dramatically exhibited in family caregiving. The essays in this section describe the practices family caregivers have refined and dilemmas they face.

Colm Toibin's moving chapter from his novel *The Heather Blazing* introduces this section. This chapter follows the book's hero, Eamon Redmond, a judge in the Republic of Ireland's high court. Redmond learns about caregiving very directly when his wife of many years suffers a serious stroke. The selection captures a frequent dilemma of family caregivers of adult loved ones. Suddenly the caregiver finds that he or she must violate the borders of privacy that adults erect as they maintain their sense of competence and autonomy. They must do this if they are to deliver the most intimate bodily care.

This literary evocation perfectly conveys the wrenching moral and personal questions that so many caregivers of the sick and vulnerable encounter and the sense of loss and shame of those they care for. In this case, the one who is cared for, the wife, feels terrible shame because she is so needy and vulnerable and no longer has the bodily skills she has honed throughout her adult life. To care for her successfully, her husband must attempt to maintain her dignity while at the same time giving the most basic bodily assistance. This is a difficult balance to strike, and the risk is the kind of anger, invasion, rejection, and resentment the wife so palpably feels.

In "Mothering as a Practice," nurse Victoria Wynn Leonard applies the philosopher's and analyst's eye to mothering. Moving beyond Sara Ruddick's initial argument that mothering—parenting—in fact requires thinking, not simply "woman's intuition," Leonard explores one of the reasons we as a culture cannot truly value and understand the content of maternal work. Mothering is either sentimentalized or trivialized, and mothers are certainly not given the social support they need to help advance their important work. This is especially true, Leonard argues, today, when more mothers work both inside and outside the home.

Leonard comes to her conclusions after studying women who are moving from a full-time career commitment to motherhood. She followed these women while they were pregnant and then continued to interview them after they had their children. Included in her analysis are a number of variables including the power of family and other social institutions and the women's attempts to integrate parenting and professional life. The intricate tapestry Leonard assembles helps us to move beyond rhetoric to public policy, from trite messages on Mother's Day cards to a textured and fully nuanced discourse on maternal thought and action.

Nurse Richard MacIntyre's very personal account of caring for his friends and a lover who died of AIDS delves further into the subject of non traditional family caregiving. This intimate look at two specific caregiving relationships shows what happens to a professional caregiver when he must suddenly apply his expertise to caring for a loved one. In this case, the primary family caregiver is a gay man, who is a professional nurse and either friend or partner of the one cared for. An investigation of the shifting boundaries of these relationships highlights another of this book's themes: that caregiving can never be abstracted from the relational context in which it is practiced.

Thus professional caregivers are not simply paid *surrogates* for family caregivers, but are also *family caregivers* themselves. Their knowledge of professional caregiving may help them negotiate the universe of professional caregiving, but it is not a magic shield that protects them from the intricate dilemmas triggered when one cares for the vulnerable and dying. MacIntyre's essay points out the difference between caring and controlling, establishes a model of a community of care that will resonate in other chapters of this book, and underscores yet again the fact that in our modern urban world family caregiving comes in very different packages.

accustomed to their new lives; her slow recovery now seemed part of the everyday. He turned and walked back in the direction of the town. It was brightening up now. He wondered if he should try to keep swimming everyday even though the days were often cold. He thought that he should go down to the strand in the afternoon and see how cold the water was. He walked up one of the side streets towards the main street and then up towards White's Hotel. He sat in the lounge and took *The Irish Times* from his pocket.

He looked through the newspaper. Since Carmel's stroke they had the telephone connected at Cush and had bought a television for the house. The most important item of news for them now was the television schedule for the evening. It was the first thing he looked at in the paper. After that he checked through the news and the opinions, but he found it difficult to read many pieces from the beginning to end. He looked at his watch: another hour before she finished. He drank up his coffee and paid. Maybe in the future, he thought, he could take his bathing-togs and have a swim in the hotel pool. It would make the time less heavy.

He walked along the main street until he came to the book shop. He hardly ever bought anything more than an English newspaper in the shop but they knew him now as a regular customer. He wandered around, browsing, picking up a book and looking at it for a while and putting it back again. The classics were in a section together, all of them in black-spined paperback, the Dickens novels and novels by George Eliot and Jane Austen. He decided to buy a few of them to see if he could read them now; maybe Carmel could read them too. He picked them out with the intention of putting some of them back, but he found himself at the cash register with seven or eight paperback novels and an English newspaper. He paid for them and left. He walked as far as the old barracks, stopping to buy some fruit at a shop, and turned down towards the car park. He could easily have done the rest of the shopping in his waiting time, but he knew that Carmel needed to feel that she was involved in the life of the house, even though the consultant had told him she would only ever be able to do light housework.

As he walked along he noticed a three-story house covered in slate; he examined the narrow street leading down to the silted-up harbour, and he wondered at how it looked like nowhere else in the world. Wexford on a midweek morning in September, the light-filled sky over the harbour, the blue-black of the slate, the grey buildings all around.

At times Carmel's slow recovery reminded him of his father in the years after his operation. His father's slow limp and impaired voice, and the pretence that, despite the damage which had been done to his system, he was well. He dreaded his father telling a story in the classroom. He would start off so confidently, but some of the words would be mere blurs. There was a story he always told about the gravedigger's son who could not get his father's job as he could not read or write. All the students knew it, knew how the son had gone to America and struck oil and became one of the wealthiest men in the United States. Eamon remembered his father before he was ill using an American accent for the part of the story about the day when the gravedigger's son had to sign a contract there and then, but had to confess that he couldn't sign as he couldn't write his name.

"Here you are one of the richest men in America and you can't sign your name. Where would you be if you could read and write?" he was asked.

"A gravedigger in Ireland," was the reply.

But there was a day when his father got stuck in the story, when nothing came from him except vague sounds, and his whole face seemed drawn and twisted, but he still wouldn't stop, even when some of the students began to laugh and others looked away, uncomfortable and embarrassed. He stood there, as he always did, looking at each face in the class, acting out the story. Eamon wanted to shout out to him to stop, please stop, could he not understand that the sounds he was making made no sense? He watched as his father turned away, before the story was finished, and went to the window and stood with his back to them looking out. The boys in the class began to talk among themselves as though the teacher was not there.

He waited outside the hospital until she came out. He did not try to help her into the car. She needed to feel that she was becoming more capable. When she came out of the hospital first, she and Niamh had gone into the city and bought new clothes for her and new make-up. She was careful how she looked. A few times in Wexford he had to wait another hour for her while she went to get her hair done, but he understood her need. It was what had made her survive.

"I'm walking better, aren't I?" she asked. "There's a woman in there, and she was much worse than I was, and she was just saying that keeping your chin up is the main thing."

Her speech was slurred, but as the days went by he found her easier to understand. He believed that sometimes she said things that would require no response, thus leaving him free to pretend that he understood. But he felt that she was recovering. Her sister drove down to Cush a few afternoons a week and he left them to talk or to go for a drive in her sister's car. All her life Carmel had loved people calling, and each time her sister left he thought that she was better. He wondered if they were right to stay at Cush, now that the weather was getting cooler and the place seemed more windswept and remote.

Carmel liked the television and enjoyed the fire lit in the evening.

Eamon fetched the coal and the blocks from the small, damp shed at the side of the house. She placed the coals carefully on the fire with tongs, using all of her energy and concentration. He peeled the potatoes, but she prepared the other vegetables and salads, sitting at a table in the living room with a basin of water in front of her. She made brown bread, even though she found it hard to knead the dough; it took time, and she worked at it, patient and determined.

"Did I rave a lot when I was in Vincent's, or did I sleep?"

"You tried to talk to me, but the nurse said it wasn't good for you."

"What did I say?"

"I couldn't make it out."

"I wonder what it was."

She prayed during the day. He would find her sitting in an armchair with her eyes closed and her lips moving. She talked about God's will to him, but she knew that he did not believe.

"God knows," she said, "that you're doing your best in your own way. Everybody can only do so much."

They stopped in the village on the way home from Wexford and she got out of the car, laboriously turning so she could stand on her good leg, and went into the butcher's. He sat in the car waiting for her, realizing that each time she went into a shop, or into the hospital, he expected a face to come out and tell him that she had taken another turn.

They had lunch at the table beside the window. He put a record on, some quiet music, and they ate without speaking. The day was brightening and the sun was strong through the glass. He told her about the paperbacks he had bought, which he had left in the car.

"We should read more," she said, "instead of watching television."

A wind had blown up outside, which cleared the sky of clouds. He told her that he would take his togs and towel down to the strand to see if the water was warm enough for swimming, although he doubted it.

"Be careful down there, you could be swept out on a day like this." She was making a real effort with her speech, working on each vowel sound.

"I probably won't go in for a swim," he said. "I'll probably just go for a walk."

He cleared the dishes from the table and put them in the sink. Her sister was coming that afternoon to clean up the house and do some washing. Carmel remained at the table, looking out. She asked him to change the record before he left. She still was not able to handle the record player.

The lane was muddy with the previous week's rain. He had to walk on the verge to avoid the mud, and even then he was afraid of slipping. It was cold as well as windy and he knew now that taking his towel and his togs had been a mistake. He put the togs into his jacket pocket and the towel around his shoulders. When he came to the turn in the lane he looked over the cliff: the sea was rough, each wave as it broke released huge choppy sheets of foam. It was the beginning of the winter sea. He walked down to the strand.

He wondered if the tide was turning. He picked up a flat stone and tried to skim it along the water but it was too rough. He searched for another flat stone but he could not find one. As he walked along he listened to the sound of the stones knocking against each other on the shore each time a wave swept in over them. It was a harder sound now, more brittle and hollow than on calmer days in the summer.

As he went toward Ballyconnigar he watched the waves twenty yards out pouring over each other as though boiling. He began picking up stones and throwing them into the rushing water and listening to the shrill sounds of the gulls heading out to sea. He was enjoying the day, regretting that he had not come down earlier, but knowing that he could not leave Carmel too long by herself.

He wondered what would happen if he swam out now into the sea, how strong the currents were and how hard it might be to fight against the receding tide. The cliffs along here had taken a battering, he noticed. Huge boulders made of hard mud and stone were lying on the strand. Small clumps of clay and a tight film of sand were being blown down the cliff face as well, even now, as he walked along.

When he came to Keating's he saw that the sheds had fallen down the cliff. This must have happened, he thought, during the previous week. The last time he was here they had been in place, but now the red galvanized material was hanging down over the edge, and bits of the walls were lying on the shore where they would not last long. Two sides of the old shed had been left standing, waiting to be toppled over in a night of strong wind. He realized that this was the first building to go since Mike's house.

He turned back. The wind was still strong and a light drizzle was starting up. He put the towel over his head. The sea was the colour of slate under the grey sky. He walked as fast as he could against the wind. The drizzle turned to rain as he moved along, and then eased off again, but he knew that it would be a wet evening, and was glad of the fire at home and the television. If he were in Dublin now, he thought, he would be getting ready to brave the traffic and set off home from the courts.

He made his way up the gap, holding on to weeds and clumps of grass to keep his balance. It was raining hard and he thought that he would have to have a hot shower when he got in. When he turned into the lane he stopped for a second, startled as he saw Carmel coming towards him with a coat over her head, moving much too fast, her limp heavy and pronounced.

"It's all right," he shouted. "I'm coming."

As he drew nearer he could see that she was crying, her face distorted as she tried to shout something to him. She stopped and put the raincoat around her shoulders, letting her hair get wet. He could see that she was still crying.

"What's wrong?" he asked when he reached her, but she did not reply. They turned and walked together towards the house, his arm around her. She was almost choking with tears, desperately clinging to him.

"You're all right, love," he said. "You'll be fine when we get inside." She tried to speak again, but began to cry even harder. As they reached the gate, the rain started to pour down. He searched his pocket for the key. Once inside, he felt the house was strangely cold and uncomforting.

As soon as they stood together in the living room he knew that she had soiled herself. After her sister left, she told him slowly between gasps of tears, she had gone down to look for him, even though it was raining, and just before he came around the corner, when she was thinking of turning back she had lost control over her bowels. She started to cry again and he had to hold her.

They went into the bathroom where he let the hot water run in the bath. He emptied a bucket in the kitchen and rinsed it out. When he came back into the bathroom Carmel was standing facing away from him, resting her arms against the wall. He put Parozone into the bucket and filled it up with hot water. He held her as she continued to sniffle.

"You'll be all right," he said.

He took off her coat and hung it on the back of the door. He knelt down and took off her shoes. He tried not to smell, tried instead to concentrate on taking down her tights and her pants. He went into the kitchen with her pants and her tights and put them into the black plastic rubbish bag beside the door.

The bathroom was now filling up with steam. He put Radox in the bath in an effort to kill the smell. He felt the water to make sure it was not too hot for her. She was still standing, leaning against the wall. He opened the buttons at the back of her dress, and she slipped out of it.

"You can leave me now," she said. "I'll be okay."

"No, I'll stay," he said.

He helped her out of her slip and then opened her brassiere at the back so that she was completely naked. Her breasts hung down white and heavy. He helped her into the bath which was now filled up with suds. He took his watch off and then his jacket and shirt, and he switched on the heater.

"Lie down and relax," he said. "I'm going into the bedroom to put on the electric blanket for you."

When he came back to the bathroom the smell was still there. He did everything he could to resist a sudden urge to get sick. He closed his eyes and tried to breathe through his nose. He took a bar of soap from the wash-basin and put it under the water, letting it soften as he rubbed it along her body. He made her turn on her side and he ran it down her back and between her buttocks. He rubbed her with a cloth and with his hand until he was sure that she was clean. She was quiet now, with her eyes closed. He soaped her legs, and ran the cloth along her belly and under her breasts. The water was dirty, and he pulled the plug out to let it drain. He turned the switch to the shower and tested the water again. Carmel was still lying with her eyes closed. He ran the shower down her body, making her turn as the water drained off her and running the soap down her back and between her buttocks again and then washing it off.

He went to the hotpress and got several large towels. He put a chair for her beside the bath. There were still flecks of faeces on the floor and on her shoes, but the smell had gone. He put her dress and slip into the bucket and began to dry her. She held her hands over her breasts and shivered. He went to the bedroom and fetched her nightdress and her dressing gown.

"We'll move the television into the bedroom and watch the news," he said.

He turned the heater on in the bedroom. When he came back she was sitting on the chair with her elbows on her knees and her head in her hands.

"Do you want me to leave you alone?" he asked. "Maybe I should make tea."

She said nothing and did not move. He wondered if he should telephone her sister or the hospital.

"Are you sick?" he asked.

She said nothing. He went into the bedroom and came back with slippers for her. She stood up and let him help her put on her nightdress. He had put on his own dressing-gown and he stood there holding her, but she would not speak and soon by her shaking he knew that she was crying again.

She made no sound. They went into the bedroom together and lay down on the bed. After a while she turned away from him as though she wanted to sleep. He turned the bedside lamp on and switched off the main light. The room was becoming warm. He went out to get the pile of books he had bought. He did not know which one he would read. She was quiet now, but she was not asleep, her eyes were wide open. He thought that she was about to have another stroke, and he wondered if he should put her into the car now and take her to Wexford, or at least get a doctor. He put his hand on her waist and asked her what he should do.

"I'm all right. I'm going to sleep now," she said.

He covered her with blankets and lay on the bed beside her, flicking through the pages of one of the novels, trying to remember if he had read it before. She turned in the bed and faced him.

"I feel I don't know you at all," she said. Her speech was slurred, even more than usual, but he had no difficulty understanding what she said.

"You've always been so distant, so far away from everybody. It is so hard to know you, you let me see so little of you. I watch you sometimes and wonder if you will ever let any of us know you."

"I'm trying to help you all day," he said.

"You don't love me." She put her arms around him. "You don't love any of us."

"Carmel, I do, I do love you."

"Years ago I tried to tell you about my father and my mother and how much they fought and argued when I was a child, and how much he drank, and no matter what he did how much we preferred him to her, and how handsome I thought he was. Eamon, are you listening to me? Already you are thinking about something else."

"That's not fair," he said.

"Eamon, please pay attention to me now. We talked about this years ago, I don't know if you remember. I still feel that we are not close to each other. I am sorry that I am boring you."

"You're not boring me," he said.

"You sound bored. It is one of the things that you have learned to do over the years."

"I'm still worried about you. Should we ring the doctor?"

"Maybe I'm the one who's cold. Maybe I made you like that. Can you understand me? Maybe we looked for each other and found a match, each of us."

"Why are you talking like this?" he asked her.

"I have had this conversation in my mind so many times over the past few months. But when I imagined it, I saw you speaking too, but you won't."

"It's too sudden, and I'm not sure you're well."

"We have all night to talk," she said.

"You sound so strange," he said.

"I used to love that, how reserved you were, but I know now that it was wrong of me to want you like that. And I have long given up arguing with you. Everything I think I keep to myself now. I want this to change. I want you to listen to me."

Half the time her voice was perfect, but then it became slurred again, but she spoke slowly, making sure that he caught each word. She lay back in the bed and covered her face with her hands.

"I went down to tell you all of this earlier. I'm sorry that you had to clean up after me like that."

"Do you want anything?" he asked.

She smiled and shook her head. "We have to talk," she said.

"I'll think about what you said."

He took his book out into the living room and turned on the lamp. Slowly he set about lighting the fire. It was dark and blustery outside, but the rain had stopped. He went out to the shed to get coal. The night was pitch dark: with no moon or stars. Back inside, he sat at the window and looked out at Tuskar and the fierce beam of light which came at intervals. He watched for it, it was much slower than a heartbeat or the ticking of a clock. It came in its own time, unfolding its light clear and full against the darkness which was everywhere outside.

Chapter 7
Mothering as a Practice

Victoria Wynn Leonard

Interruption, contradiction, and ambivalence are the soul of mother-hood. It's a curious biological fact that even mothers forget the raw data of mothering as their children grow up. . . . Sooner or later, we all turn our backs on the truth of motherhood, because our culture makes it too punishing to side with it too long. Better to get a crack nanny, buy some decent clothes, and get back into the real world, the marketplace. But lingering doubts remain that those hours of pure feeling and blazing frustration, spent rocking, cleaning, feeding, and *not harming* the baby, are the real world (Jackson 1989, p. 35).

In our modern Western middle class culture we have a limited and dis-engaged way of describing mothering. We sentimentalize and trivialize it in greeting cards and television shows; we indict it as the first cause of our neuroses; we reject it as a restrictive and oppressive role for women. Government policies treat the early postpartum transition as a medical problem. Workplaces treat parenthood as a private responsibility, in-visible to corporate policies. In our modern cultural narratives mothers rarely embody the heroic and define the good in a way that shows mothering as moral, honorable and centrally important to our cultural life. In rational/empirical studies, researchers approach mothering as an aggregate of decontextualized variables (Entwisle and Doering 1981; Grossman et al. 1980; Mercer 1985). Mothers are viewed as an assem-blage of traits or variables which are viewed as context-free elements to be combined according to social science methods, the goal of which is prediction and control. These variables are abstracted from women's lives. They disembody the experience and pass over the ways mothering both gives content and meaning and a notion of the good to women's lives, and serves, through an ethic of care, to nurture and preserve both

An original essay.

individual children and important meanings and traditions within families and in the culture. Because in research on mothering context is minimized or excluded and purpose and meaning are ignored, we gain little insight into the ways our modern cultural practices and meanings make mothering difficult and stressful and threaten to undermine its moral content.

The research findings that ground this article come from a longitudinal qualitative study of the transition to parenthood of first-time mothers with career commitments. In the study, eighteen middle and upper middle class women and their families were followed from the last trimester of pregnancy until their babies were fifteen to eighteen months old. My particular concern in this study was to highlight the ways in which career women are marginalized and undermined in their attempts to meaningfully include both mothering and careers in their lives by this limited understanding of mothering. As the study participants negotiated the demands and pleasures of early motherhood, I was struck by the power of familial and institutional meanings, decisions and practices to both subvert and to strengthen a woman's commitment to her child. While ego strength and a woman's own early experiences of being parented also shaped early mothering in the study sample, I have focused more substantively in this article on bureaucratic and cultural influences because they are more appropriately addressed by a cultural-level discourse on the policies and attitudes that shape family life.

I will use MacIntyre's (1984) notion of a practice as an interpretive framework for understanding how mothering gets taken up in our culture. Understood as a practice, mothering is revealed as potentially rich in moral content and essential for the preservation of cultural traditions of nurture and care that are mothering's purpose. Mothering as a practice will then be contrasted with the increasingly evident understanding in our culture of mothering as rational technique and children as raw material to be developed. A paradigm case, from the study sample, of mothering as a practice supported by a cohesive family tradition of care and a workplace sympathetic to family concerns, will then be described. Finally, to conclude, I will turn to a cultural-level analysis of the difficulties created by the cultural context in which modern women practice mothering, and an analysis of the resources available to recover mothering as a practice and bring it to the center of our culture.

MacIntyre defines a practice as

any coherent and complex form of socially established cooperative human activity through which goods internal to that form of activity are realized in the course of trying to achieve those standards of excellence which are appropriate to, and particularly definitive of, that form of activity, with the result that human powers to achieve excellence, and human conceptions of the ends and goods involved, are systematically extended. (1984, p. 187)

Practice is here distinguished from technical skills. The goods internal to a practice can only be specified in terms of the practice and by means of examples from the practice. They cannot be enumerated in a set of rules, abstracted from the context and relationship in which they unfold. In this view, the emotional content of mothering is taken seriously because it reveals how the mother grasps her situation and what matters to her, which in turn makes her mothering activities intelligible.

MacIntyre notes that in the ancient and medieval worlds the creation and maintenance of human communities was a practice (1984, pp. 188–89). Borgmann's (1984) discussion of practice substantiates the position that practices embody a notion of the good in our culture, despite the fact that they are no longer prominent in our technological world in which the products of our labors are increasingly understood as commodities. Borgmann argues that a commodity is "truly available when it can be enjoyed as a mere end, unencumbered by means" (p. 44) and contrasts commodities with "focal things" that orient our lives by virtue of the practices through which we are engaged with them.

Mothering is a morally coherent practice, the concrete expression of which affords us an opportunity to understand the content of nurture and care, although it is a practice that is marginalized (i.e., left over from an earlier cultural tradition, it exists only at the margins of our society, not as a central focus). Unless it is recognized as a moral practice and brought to a more central place in our culture, it will lose its moral coherence and will then necessarily disappear as a practice. Children will join other aspects of our environment that have become what Heidegger (1977) calls "standing reserve": commodities to be produced, their particular needs for nurture and care indiscernible to the technical procedures required to produce commodities.

This position is not to be confused with a sentimental view of mothering that obligates women to motherhood because of their biology. This sentimental and romantic view of motherhood serves both to obscure the challenges and depth of the work as a moral practice and to further marginalize it. It should also be noted that while women most often practice mothering, it is a practice that is increasingly taken up by men sharing in the care of their children.

Mothering as Practice Versus Child-Rearing Techniques

It is critical that mothering as a practice be distinguished from child-rearing techniques. Child-rearing techniques vary with cultures and families and do not have the focusing quality nor the moral content of mothering as a practice. As MacIntyre (1984) points out, practice is never just a set of technical skills. Child-rearing techniques, understood as technical skills, may, in fact, subvert the practice of mothering, creating a strategic climate in which the particular child's needs and abilities are ignored. Means and ends both count in mothering as a practice. The purpose of mothering is found as essentially in the everyday, repetitive and contingent acts which are their own ends as it is found in the final product, the child, grown to productive adult, capable of both work and love. In child-rearing techniques which are so endemic in Western middle and upper middle-class culture, means and ends may be separated. In this strategic view, child-rearing techniques are realized in a child who walks, talks, and is toilet trained according to the canons of child development, a child who develops the requisite skills and mental abilities to admit him or her to a "good" nursery school, primary school, and college.

In the strategic view, the tasks of mothering are merely technical procedures, performed by anyone with the requisite skill, much as anyone with the requisite skill can repair an automobile; no relationship with the vehicle is required in order to perform the task. The content of care and concern, by which means and ends are merged in mothering as a practice, is absent here. In strategic mothering, the child is not allowed to show up as a person but remains an object to be dealt with and manipulated. This is exemplified, for instance, in the mother who displays her one-year-old's technical skill in eating with a spoon and not spilling. She ignores the baby's developmental need to handle her food and takes the plate away when the baby begins to resort to her hands and feel the texture of the food with her fingers. In contrast, letting the child appear and make claims is evident in this mother's response to my question about expectations she has for her child:

Well, I don't know if I have expectations; I have hopes for him. You know, I try not to have expectations cause you just, you can't really count on anything in life and you know he could grow up to be, a, uh, smoking Republican, you know; or a Ku Klux Klan member or something; I don't know. So I just feel like I try not to have expectations, but I have hopes that he'll be a happy person; that he'll be gregarious and like people. I hope that he has a social conscience, and that he has a concern for the environment and tries to live a good life and be good to other people and the world, and that he's happy and he finds a happy location. (Bonnie)

This mother understands that mothering is not a technical procedure with a clear and determined outcome. Reflected in her comments is the understanding that, as a mother, one starts with notions of good that one would like to see realized in one's child, and the mothering is framed by these notions of good. But it is only in the long-term process of working out the practice with a particular person that these goods may get realized. In the ongoing, practical engagement of a mother with her child, the particular ways her practices can reflect notions of the "good" get worked out through practical deliberation and the cultivation of her ability to recognize her child as a person.

Of course, child-rearing practices may also embody a cultural tradition supportive of the practice of mothering and of the good embodied in the practice. This mother describes her appreciation for her mother's "burping" skills:

The first week was great. My Mom, I mean it was hard, but my Mom was around a lot. My Mom and her friend would come over in the evening and they would bring us dinner, and my Mom's a real good burper. It took me a while to get the burping thing down. It's like I'd feed him and then he'd be fussy afterwards and I realized finally that he needed to be burped, and I just wasn't very good at it. My Mom's a real good burper. (Brenda)

This description of a mother's helpful expertise was unusual in the study sample. More often, women would say that their mothers had little or nothing to teach them about mothering (as one mother put it, it was like "apples and oranges") and that their mothering practices were discontinuous with those of their own mothers. This lack of a coherent tradition on which to draw attracted many mothers to "expert" theories of baby care or to the practical knowledge of friends and acquaintances.

Paradigms of Mothering as a Practice Versus Mothering as Management by Technique

By contrasting the paradigms of mothering as practice and mothering as management by technique I hope to make maternal practices more explicit. Of course, the practice of mothering does not belong to any individual mother, but is taken up by particular mothers in ways that are shaped by their own family and cultural meanings and traditions and by their material and situational contexts and concerns.

Mothering as a Practice

In the practice of mothering, the child has a real claim on the mother. This claim is emotional and physical as well as moral. This claim is not experienced as limiting, rather it provides meaning, purpose, and identity. The baby becomes what Dreyfus and Wakefield (1988) call a "paradigmatic object," reorganizing the background against which all contents appear. The baby at once is an object in the background and sets up or constitutes what is foreground and background. The mother does not view her child as an autonomous equal deserving of care by virtue of his or her rights. Rather, the child's helplessness and need and relationship to her solicit her care. An implicit notion of the good governs her care. Meaningful family traditions (understood as practical and not cognitive knowledge) and common sense, based on the mother's own intuitive understanding of *her* child, figure as a resource more prominently than prescriptive child development manuals in guiding her care. Her practice is particular to her own infant. The practice itself provides the paramount satisfaction. Play and "nonproductive" care activities like feeding, bathing, and changing also figure prominently both as constitutive practices and as ways of being a mother to this infant.

The child is a focal point in the mother's life. She sees her mothering as a "calling" and all other concerns and commitments as relativized by her commitment to her child. Satisfaction in her child's achievements is not framed by an ultimate concern with the external goods of status and achievement but, rather, in terms of her moral obligation to help her child realize her particular talents and interests and to raise a child who is equipped to become a responsible member and participant in family and community. Within the practice, a mother develops skill and an understanding of mothering, thereby extending the practice. She measures herself against very particular paradigms of mothering which embody, for her, excellence for the practice. When she seeks substitute care for her child, she makes an ethic of care a more salient requirement than professional knowledge of child development and childrearing strategies.

Anne's Story: Motherhood as a World-Defining Commitment

To exemplify this understanding of mothering as a practice, I will present a paradigm case from the study findings. Anne, thirty-eight years old when her baby was born, was a lawyer. Her work was world-defining and she was quite passionate about her professional involvement, so much so that she had rejected motherhood during her twenties. Following fertility problems and a complicated pregnancy, she delivered a healthy baby girl. Her parents came to stay with Anne and her husband, Bill, before Anne's baby, Leah, was born. They stayed for about a month.

Anne and her baby had a long honeymoon in the postpartum period while her parents lived in the house and energetically and enthusiastically helped her. She enjoyed their company and appreciated their help. As a new mother Anne drew on a family tradition of care made palpable by her parents' involvement in caring for her and for her baby after her birth.

One of the stressful incidents Anne described in the early postpartum period occurred when she ate something that gave her baby terrible gas and caused the infant to scream for hours. During the incident, she was able to recall the family story about her own babyhood in which she would sleep only when her very patient father's hand lay on her back. This memory facilitated her acceptance of his help in this situation. Acknowledging that she was emotionally and physically unable to help her baby at a certain point in the evening, she went to bed, leaving her father to comfort her daughter as she herself had been comforted as a baby. Anne's understanding of herself as well-loved and worthy served her well in this difficult incident early in the postpartum period.

Recalling her parents' departure, she commented, "I remember having tears in my eyes when they were leaving. They were so nice and I was so grateful." Her parents didn't take over the care of the baby, but helped and coached Anne. When they left a month after Leah's birth, Anne was alone with her baby for the first time. Unlike the other mothers in the study who faced their babies alone much earlier, she had by then acquired a repertoire of caring practices. She knew what *worked* and she had a sense of knowing who Leah was as a person. The coaching, care, and nurturing she received from her own parents in the early postpartum period seemed to have given her a platform from which she was successfully "launched" as a mother at five weeks postpartum. She commented after her parents' departure,

In fact, in some ways, it's nice because I don't have to share her so much and it's also nice just because I know I can manage it and it's not that big a problem. I have a whole list of things to do under various circumstances like, you know, she's fussy and I want to do something, you know, I'll try to put her down. If she cries, then I'll either try the swing—she likes the swing a lot—and if that doesn't work, then the third thing is usually the snuggly and she's very good about the snuggly. That almost always works and if that doesn't work, draping her over my shoulder. She loves that. And then if that doesn't work and I don't even know if I've gotten to that yet. I think I guess one time. Then I just give up whatever I'm doing and I sit down and, you know, rock her and do something like that. (Anne)

By the time her parents were ready to leave, Anne had also regained her physical strength. This provided her a cushion unavailable to any other mother in the study. The downside to her parents' departure was that she could no longer accomplish what she was used to accomplishing in a day. At five weeks or so postpartum, she confronted her limits and was forced to choose between accomplishing everything on her lists and just being a mother to her baby. She commented,

At first, I was very frustrated because I always—I accomplish a million things . . . or used to accomplish a million things in a day. I still do; they're just different and I wanted to kind of keep up that level. You know, I like to cook; I like to cook nice meals. I usually have lists of things that I like to accomplish in a given day and those are changing. (Anne, first postpartum interview)

I went from a phase where I was happiest if I changed her, fed her and put her down and she went to sleep because then I had time during which I could do my things you know and then I started actually wanting her. . . . one day, I realized how much fun she was and I wanted her to stay awake more. I changed. (Anne, second postpartum interview)

Anne's notions of good can be seen to shift from those that involve accomplishment to the seemingly nonproductive, endlessly repeated practices that constitute mothering, the being-with or dwelling-with that are afforded no place in the efficiency-driven world of work. This "turn" in the early postpartum period was experienced by other study mothers, though some never seemed quite able to give up being "productive," especially those mothers who went back to work before three months. Fortunately, Anne was able to stay home long enough with her baby that she was available to enjoy these developmental changes in the baby which so solicited her to "change" her way of being a mother to Leah.

I've decided, shoot, I'm home, let's just do all this stuff that's related to her and she's fine and I just sort of gave in in a way and gave up some of the sewing, the cooking is a lot less elaborate, and I find that errands that I just thought I had to do on a particular day I really don't have to do on that day. Even if I don't go to the store, Bill or I can go to the store later. If I can't get something cooked, I can ask him to bring food home. (Anne, first postpartum interview)

Anne breast-fed Leah and talked of her pleasure in feeding her. In response to my question of what she enjoyed about breast-feeding, Anne described a practice in which the needs and goods of both mother and baby intertwined and were met in a very satisfying and symbiotic way. Her breast-feeding exemplified the merging of mother and infant that Winnicott calls "primary maternal occupation" (1988, p. 93). Watching Anne breast-feed Leah I could see for myself the obvious pleasure Anne got in breast-feeding. She talked to Leah about the feeding, about changing breasts, and so forth in a high, sing-song voice, stroking her head. For the first family observation, Anne was dressed in old clothes that had been spit up on and she was unperturbed by this evidence of her breast-feeding and mothering activities.

When she returned to work at five months post-partum, Anne hired a live-in nanny to care for Leah. Anne chose Janet because she was older and had raised her own children. Anne regarded Janet as a member of her family and was not threatened by her experience in mothering practices. Not only did Janet mother Leah with Anne's blessings, she also mothered Anne, coaching her and modeling for her, nurturing her and reassuring her. What was remarkable in this situation was how Anne responded to Janet's care. Many of the other mothers in the study had more problematic and competitive relationships with their child care providers. Anne described working at her relationship with Janet, overcoming her usual reluctance to confront problems as they developed, because she felt it was so important for Leah that she and Janet be able to communicate well. This is another example of how the kind of person one is as a mother matters deeply and may prompt new ways of being in the world.

Anne was the owner of her law firm and worked with other lawyers who also had infants. She described a workplace that cultivated practices supportive of parents. In one year her firm accommodated four parental leaves, including one for a father. While she described a certain amount of upheaval that resulted from these leaves, she ardently believed in their necessity and argued that, if her small firm could afford this degree of accommodation, then other, larger firms could too. She purchased a large electric breast pump for all the mothers in the office to use and regarded this as a worthwhile service to her employees. She described an unwritten office rule that everyone went home by five o'clock because of their parental responsibilities. To stay and break this rule was viewed as making the others feel bad about leaving on time.

Just before Anne was to return to work, at four months postpartum, her baby suddenly developed a life-threatening illness and was hospitalized. Anne coped with her fear that Leah might die by trying to be as helpful as she could to Leah and to the doctors, and by focusing on maintaining breast-feeding. Anne tried to be the most complete and up-to-date source of medical information on Leah. She was Leah's advocate and guardian; she allied herself with the health care team and actually became a member of the team. She saw herself as the one who knew the *whole* story about Leah because she had been there for everything that had happened. It was as though by knowing Leah's story she could somehow affect its denouement. When I asked her if there were any principles or rules guiding her behavior in this incident, she replied,

Probably you know trying to find a role for myself in everything that was going on that was as constructive as possible, you know, just trying to see if there was anything that I could do that would help. (Anne, second postpartum interview)

With Leah's illness, Anne's plans for returning to work were put off. When I asked her whether this was a moral issue, she seemed perplexed, and responded:

Probably. But it was just sort of the obvious, natural decision but it didn't even enter my mind that I would ever go to work while she was in the hospital. I mean it just didn't even occur to me even though maybe I could have gone for an hour or two. Never occurred. (Anne, second postpartum interview)

Anne's response reflects the taken-for-granted moral claims of mothering, which form an ethos of care that (transparently) informs every decision a woman makes in her practice as a mother.

Anne's baby survived the illness, although it was unclear whether she had been affected developmentally. Anne acknowledged that Leah's illness served to point out how profoundly her life had changed:

I think my feelings (about being a mother) are just much stronger because of the crisis . . . just much deeper, stronger feelings. I mean I thought they were deep and strong before but now . . . you know, she's just the world to me right now. (Anne, second postpartum interview)

Even when faced with her daughter's possible neurological problems, Anne had a remarkable ability to see her situation positively. While she confessed to feeling unlucky at moments, her predominant feeling was that she was *lucky* to be a mother and to have this precious baby who had been so hard to have, and Leah's health problems didn't change those feelings. Even when Leah was diagnosed as developmentally delayed and placed in a special program, Anne continued to express feelings of gratitude, love and commitment for her baby and described the things that Leah did that so delighted her: "she's just a joy." While she confessed to moments of panic, these stemmed from her anxiety over how Leah would fare in the world, rather than from any feeling of rejection because this baby was less than "perfect."

As she reflected on her feelings as a mother after her baby's illness, I asked her if she felt more vulnerable now. She responded:

Oh. That's what it is! That's the word. These feelings come up from inside and you can't believe how strong they are or where they came from or why you didn't have ones like this before. I mean I have fallen in love, I've been married, all of those things. (Anne, second postpartum interview)

Anne's vulnerability arose out of her recognition that when a person, her baby, sets up her world, she also becomes vulnerable to losing that baby: she is limited in her ability to control the situation. The baby must have the freedom in the relationship to be who she is: Leah is lovely *and* has neurological problems.

In the final interview, Anne described an incident in which her nanny made a comment that Anne (mistakenly) interpreted as a criticism of her as a mother, which devastated Anne. In the following statement describing her reaction to her nanny's comment, Anne described the extent to which being a *good* mother mattered to her:

It really got to me. It is because I care. I think the worst thing anybody could say to me right now is to say or imply that "you're not a good mother." You know, it would just send me off the deep end. I think it's the worst thing. I really do. (Anne, third postpartum interview)

It was this overarching ethos of being a *good* mother to Leah that defined Anne's maternal practice. Her delight in her daughter, notwithstanding her illness, exemplified a focal concern that organized and oriented Anne's world. Her pleasure in the everyday maternal practices, in the means of mothering were never subordinate to the end of child as product or commodity.

Mothering as Management by Technique

Contrast the story above with images of women who view the mothering role as only one among several, not as a defining way of being that organizes and defines other projects. For them the ethos for mothering involves maximizing their own and their child's potential and their capacity to be a rationally choosing agent. Her child is someone she freely chose to have, and the child does not have a central claim on her. She may focus on the external goods of mothering: for instance, how soon her child walks, talks, is toilet trained, and learns to read; what schools her child is accepted into; what sports the child plays and how well. She may use manipulative techniques to resolve discrete problems. Family and childrearing traditions and rituals are enslaving and stultifying for the manager. She rejects them for herself as well as for her child, unless she can rationally choose them as prescriptive for good family life. Child development manuals and professionals may be resources for techniques of care. Since the hallmark of this kind of mothering is technique rather than care predicated on the moral responsibility of relationship, the task can be carried out by substitute caregivers who have the right techniques, who may, in fact, be better at providing the "right" kinds of stimulation for developmental growth.

I have deliberately highlighted these two positions, but they help to reveal mothering as a practice with moral content; a practice that needs to be brought in from the margins and honored, lest the paradigm of mothering by technique take over and obliterate the *practice* of mothering.

Parenting as Technical Skill: The Rationalization of Parenting by the Experts

To exemplify the cultural tendency to rationalize parenting practices I will describe a recent example of a popular parenting manual. Dinkmeyer's and McKay's *Systematic Training for Effective Parenting (STEP): The Parent's Handbook* (1989), is a current example of the highly managerial strategies advocated by child development professionals. The STEP handbook represents current notions of parent learning in the popular literature. The views expressed in this handbook are grounded in a foundational notion of knowledge: "Our basic beliefs are often faulty. Why? Because our interpretations of our experience are often inaccurate" (p. 22). The "accuracy" of our interpretations of our experience is undermined or contaminated by our beliefs, generated from childhood, about who we are and who and what others are; and by questions of value about what is important and how we should live. In other words, we have to stand outside of our basic understandings of ourselves and the world, our social and familial practices, in order to "influence our children positively" (p. 22).

The implicit assumption of this view is that there is an ahistorical, atemporal position from which one should ideally raise children and that all past parenting was not worthy of being handed down. This is a view of parenting that can offer improvement in the parenting of those who have themselves experienced devastating parenting or abuse and have no coherent or meaningful family traditions of parental care, but it undermines those family traditions that do work to facilitate maternal practice. It also ignores the gap between acquisition of formal guidelines for parenting and the experiential learning that is required in order to know how and know when to apply the techniques.

This book advocates a program of behavioral modifications through which parents can modify the behavior of their children. Parents are drilled in the advantages of positive rather than negative reinforcement. The rules for parenting are formal and abstract. Parents are told to learn them not in relation to their child but rather through reading and study. Parents are then tested with a series of "quiz" questions to see if they have "learned" the material at the end of each chapter. Finally, the parent is given a form on which to chart his or her "Plan for Improving Relationships." The very brief narrative examples do not develop a notion of the particular child of a particular parent. No distinction is made between mothers and fathers, between male and female children, nor is age of the child ever an issue. They are universal examples assumed to be relevant to all families, regardless of gender or class distinctions. The role of culture or ethnicity is ignored.

The book is replete with reductionist statements such as, "All behavior has a social purpose. The goals of misbehavior are: attention, power, revenge, or display of inadequacy" (p. 17). The inherent ambiguity and open-endedness of the parent-child relationship are ignored. Parents are not encouraged to trust their own instincts. In fact, they are told that those basic intuitions are frequently "faulty." Learning or "training" is purely a formal process.

Moreover, the entire book deals with problems of breakdown in the parent-child relationship. The very existence and popularity of the book and other manuals like it suggests the degree to which parents' confidence in a coherent and meaningful, taken-for-granted tradition of child-rearing adopted in a particular historical period by virtue of being a member and participant of a particular culture, has been undermined. The media attention given to "experts" who offer their advice in the service of producing a better "product" increasingly marginalizes such coherent traditions. For middle-class Americans who reject the parenting traditions of their own mothers, there is no taken-for-granted everyday of child-rearing. It is a painful, deliberate, and conscious process to "learn" parenting, much as one learns how to play chess or be a nurse or an airline pilot. In a very explicit, formal, conscious way one learns certain facts and rules that are then taken up haltingly and with great anxiety in the situation. There is no acknowledgment of everyday familial and social practices as resources for learning how to mother a child. Instead, these practices become suspect and must be unlearned. Frequently, it is only with a second or third child that the skills and practices of parenting come to feel taken for granted and everyday, and then the "experts" recede into the background.

A troubling aspect of this shift from learning coherent everyday traditions of child-rearing to learning from the "experts" is the fact that the everyday practices and traditions included inherent notions of the good which fit the cultural milieu of the family. The experts, on the other hand, never make explicit the goods in the service of which they, in fact, offer their expertise, other than a more efficiently produced "quality" product. This parallels the drive in rational/empirical social science research to set aside questions of value, preferring to consider only isolated, neutral "facts," a project that has come under considerable criticism (Taylor 1985a, 1985b). What is overlooked in this view is the way in which the STEP position does establish certain values, or goods, and undermines others. In particular, it promulgates a normative view of parenting in which those who deviate from the norm because of class, ethnicity, or gender show up as deficient parents. In sum, in the view of experts such as Dinkmeyer and McKay, parenting is a set of technical skills, not a coherent social practice of experientially learned skills grounded in implicit notions of individual and social goods.

The Relationship of Cultural Institutions to the Practice of Mothering

Nowhere in our culture is mothering's status as a marginalized practice more evident than in the dearth of cultural institutions that support and encourage family life. Birth is a private and often technical affair, and modern women frequently see childbirth rituals as something they have to invent, not as something given in the community and the culture. Rituals around childbirth are largely restricted to the giving of gifts at the baby shower. Women no longer look to their own mothers for material help or for advice and support. Whitbeck (1983) describes the lack of cultural stories showing childbirth at all, let alone women in childbirth as heroes, whereas men are frequently portrayed as heroes in stories of war (and frequently as heroes in labor and delivery when they function as labor coaches). When an infant is born, the mother frequently returns home with her baby within twenty-four hours. Friends and neighbors may welcome her, but they provide little material support and rarely acknowledge the difficulties and exhaustion the new infant has engendered. Nor do they give much help reorganizing the household, to say nothing of providing meaningful rituals or traditions for facilitating mothering practices or for honoring and welcoming the new family member. One need only read descriptions of community practices around childbirth in the colonial period, where women in the community descended on a birthing woman's home and set up housekeeping for weeks while the mother recovered from childbirth (Cott 1977) to realize the vacuum of social practices into which new mothers are now thrust. Fathers are generally denied the right to any kind of parental leave, effectively denying them the possibility of providing meaningful material and emotional support to mother and infant and access to their infants for the purpose of developing a relationship.

For women who take time off from a job to have a baby, maternity leave is often equated with disability leave, as we have only limited federally mandated, universally available paid maternal leave policy in this country, and disability leave is frequently invoked as a pseudo-substitute. Childbirth is thus treated as a medical condition. When the uterus and episiotomy are "healed," the mother is expected to return to work as though everything is "back to normal."

Recent research on women's physical health during the first postpartum year suggests that recovery from childbirth commonly takes longer than the six weeks currently allotted by physicians and workplace policies (Gjerdingen, Froberg, Chaloner, and McGovern 1993). This is confirmed by the women in this study in their accounts of their postpartum recoveries. Instead of feeling physically or emotionally "back to normal," a new mother returning to work has had her world transformed. She has been newly constituted by her status as mother of her particular baby. Furthermore, on returning to work she must cope with an incoherent, disorganized, inaccessible, and expensive child care system. Often, she must also cope with feelings of guilt and sorrow at leaving her infant in the care of another person. The significance of her relationship to her infant is ignored or trivialized in modern organizational, particularly corporate, life, where any felt responsibility to worthy ends is overwhelmed by subscription to the canons of bottom-line efficiency.

As children in our culture are increasingly viewed as the private property of individual parents, the business world becomes ever less encumbered with any responsibility for facilitating mothering practices. Any overarching sense of the good which frames a working mother's ethic of care is challenged by the company's demand for her primary allegiance.

In our contemporary culture we are so imbued with the importance of productivity that it is hard to "just be" with an infant. The endless job of cleaning, feeding, changing and playing with an infant often feels unproductive, empty of meaning and importance, especially since mothers aren't paid for it: the cardinal measure of productivity in our culture. In a 1986 Harvard-Stanford alumni poll (Skelly 1986, p. 26), almost half of the respondents thought that women who stay home with families are less respected than those who work. Borgmann (1984) points out that as the family's responsibility for the material circumstances of its survival are gradually eroded, so are the coherent and meaningful traditions that shape family life and give parental responsibilities meaning and weight. The result, Borgmann maintains, is that "parental love is deprived of tangible and serious circumstances in which to realize itself" (1984, p. 226).

Our cultural self-understanding in the United States makes mothering as practice problematic. Our highly individualistic notions of agency, grounded by the values of rational choice and autonomy, are inconsistent with the experience of mothering as practice. As Ann Swidler (1987) points out, present-day adult commitments represent the demise rather than the fulfillment of the search for identity:

In contemporary literature even the sacrifice of parents for their children has been brought into question. Several modern novels portray a conflict between sacrifice for someone else, including children, and the necessary attention to the imperiled self. Novelists can now portray children as predators or enemies who demand without giving, who threaten the necessary self-nurture of their parents. . . . Self-sacrifice, which once seemed the ultimate proof of love, now seems suspect. (1987, p. 120)

Mothering as a practice seeks to reassert the moral value of commitment and connectedness, of the self who finds identity through being in relationships and finds moral significance in an ethic of care. I subscribe to feminists' contention that the ethic of care embodied in maternal practices must be drawn in from the margins where it is private and invisible and made an organizing principle for all human relationships.

References

Borgmann, Albert. 1984. *Technology and the Character of Contemporary Life*. Chicago: University of Chicago Press.

Cott, Nancy F. 1977. *The Bonds of Womanhood: "Woman's Sphere" in New England, 1780–1835*. New Haven, CT: Yale University Press.

Dinkmeyer, Don C. and Gary D. McKay. 1989. *Systematic Training for Effective Parenting: The Parent's Handbook*. Circle Pines, MN: American Guidance Service.

Dreyfus, Hubert L. and James A. Wakefield. 1988. "From Depth Psychology to Breadth Psychology: A Phenomenological Approach to Psychopathology." In *Hermeneutics and Psychological Theory: Interpersonal Perspectives on Personality, Psychotherapy and Psychopathology*, ed. Stanley B. Messer, Louis A. Sass, and Robert L. Woolfolk, 272–88. New Brunswick, NJ: Rutgers University Press.

Entwisle, Doris R and Susan G. Doering. 1981. *The First Birth: A Family Turning Point*. Baltimore: Johns Hopkins University Press.

Gjerdingen, Dwenda K., Debra G. Froberg, Kathryn M. Chaloner, and Patricia M. McGovern. 1993. Changes in Women's Physical Health During the First Postpartum Year. *Archives of Family Medicine* 2: 277–283.

Grossman, Frances Kaplan, Lois S. Eichler, and Susan A. Winickoff. 1980. *Pregnancy, Birth and Parenthood: Adaptations of Mothers, Fathers and Infants*. San Francisco: Jossey-Bass.

Heidegger, Martin. 1977. *The Question Concerning Technology and Other Essays*, trans. William Lovett. New York: Harper.

Jackson, Marnie. 1989. "Bringing Up Baby." *Saturday Night*, December, 31, p. 9.

MacIntyre, Alasdair C. 1984. *After Virtue: A Study in Moral Theory*. 2nd ed. Notre Dame, IN: Notre Dame University Press.

Mercer, Ramona Thieme. 1985. "The Process of Maternal Role Attainment over the First Year." *Nursing Research* 34, 4: 198–204.

Skelly, Florence. 1986. "To the Beat of a Different Drum." *Harvard Magazine*, March–April, pp. 20–27.

Swidler, Ann. 1987. "Love and Adulthood in American Culture." In *Individualism and Commitment in American Life: Readings on the Themes of Habits of the Heart*, ed. Robert Bellah, Richard Madsen, William Sullivan, Ann Swidler, and Steven Tipton, 2.

Taylor, Charles. 1985. *Philosophical Papers*. 2 vols. Cambridge: Cambridge University Press.

Whitbeck, Carolyn. 1983. "A Different Reality: Feminist Ontology." In *Beyond Domination: New Perspectives on Women and Philosophy*, ed. Carol C. Gould. Totowa, NJ: Rowman and Allenheld.

Winnicott, Donald W. 1988. *Babies and Their Mothers*. Menlo Park, CA: Addison-Wesley.

Chapter 8
Nursing Loved Ones with Aids: Knowledge Development for Ethical Practice

Richard MacIntyre

Caring for loved ones with AIDS has been a fascinating albeit tragic experience. For me, it has provided a lens through which are refracted reflections about the kinds of tough decisions that anyone caring for someone in a dependent or vulnerable condition is constantly forced to make. My own personal experience caring for two loved ones with AIDS has helped me better to understand that family members—whether traditional ones or nontraditional ones like myself—can construct a much-needed model of ethical decision making that combines professional and intimate knowledge, one that goes beyond the professional, autonomous Lone Ranger approach without, however, embracing the kind of tortuous, process-oriented, consensus approach where nobody seems to take responsibility for anything and nothing ever seems to get done. I tell these stories of caring for two loved ones with AIDS because they are illustrative of the delicate balance between shouldering responsibility for difficult decisions entirely by oneself, and using the web of relationships which we are all involved in as the context that helps us to arrive at complex, difficult decisions.

Even though I had been practicing nursing for almost ten years, I had never thought much about ethics before 1985. Of course I had made ethical decisions that I could easily point to. One woman in her seventies did not want to undergo another cerebral arteriogram but was concerned that her doctor needed a diagnosis. She had decided against both chemotherapy and surgery and did not care whether her last faint-

An earlier version of this essay appeared as MacIntyre, "Nursing Loved Ones with AIDS: Knowledge Development for Ethical Practice," *Journal of Home Health Care Practice* 3, 3 (1991): 1–10, copyright © 1991 by Aspen Publishers, Inc. Reprinted by permission.

ing episode was due to cancer or a transient ischemic attack. To me the situation was clear-cut: she was rational and intelligent, and my job was to advocate for the patient, to empower her to make her own decisions. I told her to think of her physician as she would a lawyer or plumber who was there to give expert recommendations and to perform work only if hired for the job. The physician has no more claim to the body than a lawyer has to a case or a plumber to a leaky pipe. But I remember being very unsure about this episode: would my intervention be supported by the hospital, or even by the nursing administration? The authority structures inherent in hospitals and other health care bureaucracies sometimes have different notions of what is "good." I did not think of my decision as an ethical one. To me it was simply clinical practice.

However, behind every nursing judgment, every clinical decision, every prioritization of patient problems, there is an ethical stance. This stance is so ubiquitous that we are usually unaware of it.

Our ethical stance in any given situation is influenced by our values about what is good—what is good about people, about nursing, about health, about harmonious relationships, about families, about patient autonomy, about expert knowledge, about social norms, about life itself. Our ethical stance is also influenced by our ability to find meaning in difficult situations—meaning in pain, suffering, anger, dying. I have learned that an inability to find the "good" in caring for people with AIDS, and an inability to discover meanings in difficult situations makes good care impossible. Indeed every decision most of us will have to make when providing care to a relative is affected by these meanings.

Knowledge Requirements for Ethical Practice

Finding meaning and promoting some notion of the "good" is what nursing practice and quality caregiving practices in any setting are all about. Finding meanings and making decisions directed toward making things better (promoting the good) require generalizable, embodied, and situational knowledge. Generalizable knowledge refers to theoretical or "scientific" knowledge—knowledge that is applicable to groups of people. It tells us what happens most of the time. It yields standards of care and, in the health care professions, research-based protocols. Examples of generalizable knowledge include theories about the effectiveness of antiviral drugs like AZT and research on how soon HIV seropositive individuals should consider beginning treatment with drugs like AZT.

Embodied knowledge includes skills, like the ability successfully to insert intravenous catheters in dehydrated and emaciated patients or the ability to calm frightened children, even when they are strangers. Examples of situational knowledge include knowing an individual person or family and understanding a person's specific concerns. When nurses and physicians modify a standard plan of care to meet the special needs of a specific individual, situation-specific knowledge is being used. This last form of knowledge is dependent on a caring relationship. (The other two are not dependent on caring, but caring surely helps even there.) Because people are not simply objects, it is impossible to "know" a person in this third sense without caring for him or her. To the extent that our health science objectifies people, and to the extent that our professional practice distances us from our patients, we are less able to know, understand, appreciate, and care for them as persons.

Ever since Aristotle, theoretical or generalizable knowledge has enjoyed a much greater status than situational knowledge. This is certainly true of health care. Early this century, Flexner (Selden 1984) made major contributions to the improvement of medical care, but he also subordinated medicine's traditional purpose of providing care to the "loftier" purpose of increasing its theoretical or generalizable knowledge base. Developing knowledge of how to render individual care took a back seat to developing scientific or professional knowledge, and the "trickle-down theory" associated with professional knowledge development in the health sciences is starting to generate as much conflict as the trickle-down theory in economics.

If we are to advance our understanding of both ethics and caregiving we need to explore how we acquire knowledge of individuals and advanced caring practices. Professional caregivers like nurses have tried to participate in this effort by analyzing or describing exchanges with patients. To this end, nurses might examine how we as professionals care for our own loved ones. Although our society tends to encourage compartmentalization of our professional and family roles, being able to combine professional and intimate knowledge has some distinct advantages.

Care by Intimates

Our society tends to frown on professionals caring for family members and to encourage detached professional relationships. But most professional nurses will provide nursing care to loved ones at some point in their lives. When a loved one needs homecare, the professional nurse may find it difficult, if not impossible, to relinquish that role to an outsider. This may not always be a disadvantage—in fact, it is most often a distinct advantage. A preexisting caring or loving relationship changes the type of knowledge brought to and generated by the caregiving relationship. The personal relationship puts flesh on general theoretical principles of caregiving and creates a context where one can explore specific meanings about sickness, life, suffering, and death. While general theories and knowledge about caregiving can make personal experiences more understandable, specific experiences make these theories come to life.

I learned this through caring for Steve and Martin, loved ones who were suffering with AIDS. In both instances I created a community of decision making that would have been much more difficult in a strictly professional relationship.

Steve

It was 1977 and I was living in the gay fast lane. Life was great. I was working almost full-time as a hospital staff nurse and had just begun studies toward my BSN when I met Steve. He was 30 and I was 25. He had been the student body vice-president at the University of Wisconsin and a Rhodes scholar at New York University, where he received his law degree. He loved plants, cats, and classical music. He was sophisticated, handsome, charming, and smart. Within weeks we had fallen head-over-heels in love; somehow I knew in my bones that I had known him for an "eternity," and somehow I also knew our time together would be short. (Somehow I just knew.) We did not always have an easy relationship. Steve had lots of problems with intimacy and trust. And I probably had problems too.

Finally, after almost six years, I moved out. It was 1982 and no time to be getting divorced in the gay community. We continued to have dinner together at least once a week. I still loved him a lot but it didn't hurt any more. A few months after that Steve started having health problems. He was exhausted much of the time and had strange gait changes, difficulty getting an erection, difficulty with urination. He had two small seizures. The doctors did not know what was wrong. He was losing weight, partially, I thought, due to his not having enough energy to prepare meals. In late summer 1985 I convened a meeting of his friends. Steve lived alone in Oakland, and we wanted to ensure that he was safe and cared for. We had been watching him deteriorate for a year and were frightened. For the first time, without knowing it, I became a homecare nurse.

It was a typical September morning in San Francisco. I was on my way to work an ideal 11:30 A.M. to 8:00 P.M. shift as a nursing supervisor at a local hospital. I stopped in a restaurant near my house. Steve was having a grand mal seizure. In those days paramedics were not allowed to give anti-seizure medications intravenously. By the time the ambulance came and we got to a hospital, Steve had been seizing for almost twenty-five minutes. I don't remember his vital signs, but his blood gases strongly suggested he might need artificial life support.

The chief of neurosurgery was called in and wanted to intubate (put him on a ventilator—a machine that would breathe for him). I explained that Steve had given me durable power of attorney for health care and asked the physician to give me his rationale for the ventilator. I told him that I was responsible for the decision and needed to understand the rationale fully before agreeing to it. I explained that I was a graduate prepared nurse who taught in a baccalaureate nursing program. I assured him that I could understand his language and reasoning. But all he could say was, "You mustn't tie the doctor's hands," and "You don't want to second-guess what Steve would want." He concluded our conversation by saying something about my not understanding the difference between life support and a code blue. "Don't try to second guess what Steve would want"—isn't that my job? I asked myself. I had known Steve for more than eight years. He had been my lover for more than five of those years. For the last twelve months he had been deteriorating neurologically. He was seropositive for HIV, but in 1985 we did not have an explanation for the neurological changes he was experiencing. Steve was an attorney. He wrote his own durable power of attorney for health care which excluded the sometimes standard section that says "if two physicians conclude . . ." When I asked why, he said that the clause could be construed to give physicians decision-making authority he did not want them to have. Steve hated physicians. His fifty-four-year old father had a cardiac history and had died during a hernia repair. Steve and I did not have long discussions about the durable power of attorney. But I remembered several things: "No respirator; no intensive care units; I trust you. You're Supernurse."

What was at stake here was Steve's life and the trust he had placed in me to make hard decisions. I knew that nobody cared more about Steve's best interest than I did. And nobody was better able to make hard decisions. I loved him. I knew about hospital physicians. They did not frighten me. My years working as a nursing supervisor taught me how to listen to clinical specialists and residents argue about treatment issues. And I had the legal authority to act. In some ways this was an ideal situation. However, the physician would not talk to me, and I needed his expertise to help me make this decision. I had not worked in critical care for a number of years and was fully aware of my own limitations. So I called Rena, a nurse-colleague. She arrived at the hospital within ten minutes. Before she arrived I called Steve's brother in New York. He said he trusted me to make the right decisions and would be on the next flight out. "Your job is to convince me to intubate," I said when Rena arrived. She did an assessment, consulted with the nurse caring for Steve in the emergency department, and made an impressive argument. When she had finished we looked at each other and I asked, "Is that it?" She shook her head and hugged me. Both of us knew it was not enough. The risks of his giving up and dying due to the insult of the intubation, together with his own expressed desire not to be intubated, ruled it out. It meant I had to be ready to let him die.

I did, however, agree to his being placed in the intensive care unit (ICU). "What the hell did Steve know about ICUs," I thought to myself. But I'd better be clear about the parameters with both the resident and the charge nurse. No heroics—no feeding tubes, no intubation, no code. If Steve was going to make it he would have to do it without these. When he woke up a few hours later, he was confused and combative, so the nurses were happy to let one of us stay with him at all times. Three days later he was transferred to a ward. He had weakness in both legs and some difficulty with his speech. We had a diagnosis: AIDS-related progressive multifocal leukoencephalopathy (PML)—a progressive degeneration of the white matter in the brain—a very serious and terminal condition.

For the next four months I arranged and supervised Steve's twenty-four-hour care at home. He was able to get up with help for the first month or so, but did not move about much in bed. I wrote a detailed nursing care plan. He was to be turned every two hours and music was to be played at all times when the television was not on. He was to get up for dinner each night. Dinner would be in the dining room with friends. I usually helped feed him, although at first he was sometimes able to eat by himself. He had developed a small bedsore in the hospital. It took me two months to heal it. We discovered the wonders of blow dryers—both for keeping the wound dry and for general skin care. I wondered why hospitals had not discovered that blow dryers worked far better than heat lamps or towels. Someday, I thought, I'll write an article about it.

We instituted a systematic program to regulate his bowels. Because Steve was too weak to gulp down eight ounces of fluid with a bulk laxative, we soaked whole psyllium seeds and fed them to him in yogurt or custard. He could not urinate on his own and required frequent catheterization. The muscles around his urethra were so constricted that he was not able to urinate without it. After several days we resorted to an indwelling foley catheter. Despite some concerns that the sun was bad for AIDS patients, we took Steve out on his patio for sun several times a week. He was a sun worshiper and retaining some of what was good in life seemed more important than doing everything possible to prolong it.

The intubation decision seemed like the biggest one until Steve's temperature went up to 105 °F and he became almost unconscious. The likely cause was infection, and infections can generally be treated with hospitalization and intravenous (IV) antibiotics. I knew that Steve was dying and that his function would never really improve. I knew that infections of the blood were one way nature works to accomplish death. I knew that it was not the worst way of accomplishing the inevitable. However, Steve had never said "no IV antibiotics." Nor should he have been expected to. He designated me to make those decisions, knowing that I was a nurse and would consider what was in his best interest.

What would Steve have decided had he had the choice? It was important that I not allow my own grief and unwillingness to say good-bye push us ever further into the world of hospital treatments. Nonetheless, a few more weeks or months like the last few would not be without value. Steve was doing something, I believed. Something was going on. He ate when we fed him. He responded when we came into the room. He was not shutting out his world. True, he was in another world for much of the time. True, he was not like the old Steve. But he wasn't withdrawing—something the old Steve was fully capable of doing when he chose to.

I needed to be certain that Steve was not in physical, psychological, or spiritual pain. So I double-checked my assessment with every person who came to see him. Their responses confirmed my conclusion. We were suffering, but Steve was really doing okay. He was fighting, holding on—something he said he never wanted to do. But I was responsible to the Steve of today. I had to discern what the Steve of today wanted. I had to act on his behalf. If he was fighting, we would fight.

We made two more trips back to the hospital to treat blood infections. I put a Christmas tree up in Steve's bedroom and one in the living room as well. January came. Steve still ate but with much less enthusiasm and involvement. He still recognized us some of the time, but the light was off more than it was on. He spent more time in a kind of fugue state, not a vegetable state, but not where he had been over Christmas. His closest friends were all saddened at his *not* dying. I was sad too, but somehow felt that there was more going on than the others saw. But even what I had been seeing was disappearing.

I reviewed his care plan. I had decided not to hospitalize Steve should he develop another blood infection. I was prepared to let him go. But why was I continuing to give him antibiotics to prevent infections? It seemed clear to me that Steve had moved into the last phase, and I had no rationale for the antibiotics. It was as if Steve was moving, with all the energy he could muster, toward a soothing pool of water. Once in the water, he would be done with sickness, debilitation, and dying. What was my rationale for the antibiotics? It seemed as if I had constructed a little fence to prevent his entering the pool. He did not have much energy to spend on dying, and it seemed I was going to make him spend a bit more. It seemed I was going to force him to crawl over my antibiotic fence, to dig under it, or somehow to find a way around it. Funny, I didn't question the appropriateness of feeding him by mouth, turning him, caring for him in a myriad other ways. True, nursing care probably did a great deal toward keeping him alive. But how could we do otherwise, I asked myself. As long as he was here, we would care for him. But the antibiotic fence? Was that care, or was it a kind of stifling parental influence that interferes with normal development?

Steve's brother Andrew disagreed with my desire to discontinue the oral antibiotics. Andrew felt that stopping the antibiotics was tantamount to pulling the plug. I convened a meeting with Andrew and all of Steve's closest friends. While Andrew is "straight" and the rest of us are lesbian or gay, we had all been good friends/family for many years. We liked each other. A culture clash was definitely not an issue. Andrew loved his brother more than anyone else in the world, and I respected that love.

Andrew understood the fence analogy but felt that a fence was indeed exactly what was called for. I argued that nature might be more severe, that dying another way might cause a great deal more suffering, that he might die of something else regardless what I did about the antibiotic. Andrew understood, but still felt that these were insufficient reasons for removing the antibiotic. I insisted that as a nurse I needed a rationale for giving a medication, and that medication to prevent a condition we had agreed not to treat seemed contradictory. Andrew had agreed with my decision to let Steve go should he get another blood infection. But he argued that he was not a nurse, and hence needed no rationale for continuing the preventative antibiotic.

I finally announced that Steve had not asked me to convene a committee to decide what to do. Consensus was desirable but not required. Everyone's concern was important to me. Steve would not have wanted me to disregard his brother's feelings. But ultimately I had agreed to decide.

Andrew was leaving that evening for New York and desperately wanted to see Steve again before I took him off the antibiotics. We all explained that it was not like pulling the plug, but he was not satisfied. I agreed to one more week on the antibiotics. Andrew would have to fly back the next weekend to see Steve before I discontinued them. After all, I thought, one more week probably wouldn't make that much difference. At the end of the week Steve had another seizure. I never had to discontinue the antibiotics. Andrew arrived Friday night and at 10:00 on Saturday morning, February 1, 1986, Steve died.

Martin

Martin and I fell in love a few months before Steve was hospitalized for the seizure. I remember the exact moment. We were eating dinner in a restaurant when he simply said, "I'm a Christian"—something not often heard on a date in the Castro area of San Francisco. What moved me even more than our shared spiritual beliefs was his simple candor. He seemed no more like Steve than the sun is like the moon—except that both were beautiful. Martin was a native Californian, a dancer turned bodybuilder who had never gone to college. He worked as a hairdresser and served as a deacon in the church.

A year and a half after Martin and I met, he was diagnosed with AIDS-related *pneumocystis carinii* pneumonia and hospitalized. He was treated with one antibiotic until his bloodwork forced a change to another one. Clinically he was improving. Martin was experiencing significant nausea but little vomiting. We discovered that giving an antiemetic 30 minutes into the infusion instead of 30 minutes before helped because the nausea typically came almost an hour into the infusion. Increasing the rate also helped. But this weekend an infectious disease specialist was on call for his regular physician (an internist). The on-call physician must have asked Martin how he was doing. Martin told him he was nauseous. He offered to discontinue the offending antibiotic and to begin a course of an experimental drug that Martin would need to be on for three more weeks.

But Martin was due to complete the regular antibiotic in two to three days. His regular physician would be back in one day. As Martin's home-care nurse, power of attorney holder, and lover, I disagreed with the treatment change. I cared about Martin's discomfort with the nausea as much as anyone. But the change did not seem appropriate. We could wait another day until his regular physician could decide. I had no *legal* authority to disagree because Martin was fully competent. But he was also weak, and did not have unlimited energy for informed consent, autonomous decision making, self-advocacy, discussions with doctors, and all those other good things our society values.

The on-call physician and I discussed the matter in Martin's room. Finally—more to end the discussion than anything else—Martin said he would sign papers to begin the experimental medication. I then did what must have appeared very manipulative. I turned to Martin, told him he was very tired, and told him I wanted to discuss it further, and wanted him to make the decision in a non-pressured atmosphere. He assented to my request and the physician left to chart that I was interfering with Martin's care. With the pressure off, Martin agreed to wait.

His regular physician was glad he did. He was discharged two days later without need for additional medication.

Sometimes it is not enough to gain consent. When we "know" our friends or loved ones, we can sometimes tell when they are acting under duress. This happened twice with Martin. As he was being admitted to the hospital for what turned out to be the last time, he made a point of asking me to bring him home to die. But a few days later, when we were told that Martin only had a few more days (he was in liver and kidney failure), Martin said he wouldn't mind staying in the hospital. Everyone heard him. But I didn't buy it. What was he doing, I thought to myself? Was he trying to protect us? Was this a bit of his codependent pattern again?

I sent everyone out of the room. After a while I asked Martin if he was worried about getting up the forty-five stairs to our flat, and he said he just couldn't do it. When I told him I could get him up on a stretcher he agreed to come home.

Under normal conditions, Martin would have died in the hospital instead of at home. He would have received experimental medication. With Steve, there would have been little or no question about antibiotics. Steve would have been put on the respirator. But normally, health care personnel do not know their patients as well as I knew Steve and Martin. The long-term loving relationships I had with them made it possible to provide individual rather than standard care.

To paraphrase Benner and Wrubel (1989), intense caring sets up intense possibility. That is, the caring relationship between nurse and patient generates knowledge, specific knowledge about a person. This caring-dependent knowledge that friends and loved ones also have is often as important as the knowledge derived from more objective measures, such as lab values and the professional clinical assessment. In fact, Benner would assert that caring is a precondition for assessment.

The knowledge generated by caring relationships creates new insights and new possibilities for intervention. But caring is not just valuable because it translates into something specific we can do. The planned intervention that came out of the family meeting I had with Steve's brother and friends was never instituted. Steve did not live for another week. But knowing and caring for someone is valuable for its own sake, because it is integral to who we are as people, part of our essential being or nature. Caring requires no measurable outcomes.

As caring relationships deepen and grow over time, rich understandings are developed and knowledge is generated. As this knowledge is generated in society, the possibility for more humane, more individually relevant, more socially meaningful, and more ethical care is increased.

Quality care is nothing more than good care, and ethical care is that which seeks the highest good.

The quality of our caring determines what we see and what we don't see. During Steve's illness, the two biggest ethical decisions involved different approaches to caring, different ideas about the "good." The physician who insisted on intubation cared about his professional autonomy and the decision-making structures that protected his professional authority. He probably cared about people too, believing that physicians were best able to decide what was good for a person with particular lab values—whether he "knew" that person or not. Even though we agreed with general goals, Steve's brother saw the prevention of infection with antibiotics as an essential element of care, while I saw them as incompatible with our goals for his care. With Martin, both the on-call physician and I saw Martin's comfort (specifically, controlling his nausea) as "good." We differed over the means of attaining it. Ethical issues are not issues for which there are no answers—our decisions *are* our answers.

How we make these decisions—in what context, and with whom—is also part of our answer. The durable power of attorney for health care is like a proxy, where one competent individual is imagined to replace another. But when I reflect on my experiences with Steve and Martin I understand that caregiving relationships can allow us to move beyond this "captain of the ship" approach. While people who want to provide the best care to others must be prepared to make unilateral decisions if necessary, the best clinical and family decisions are made not on the basis of clinical or objective indicators alone, but by viewing each person in the context of his or her relationship to his or her significant others. That is why multicultural awareness is so important to health care providers—not so they can pick appropriate and culturally sensitive interventions from a list, but so that they might appreciate both the richness of possibility in human relationships, as well as the limits of those possibilities.

I have learned that respecting this community of relationship does not, however, mean that one tries to seek consensus indefinitely. Decisions about caring for vulnerable persons are weighty, and often immediate. Inevitably, the burden of this responsibility is great. The fact that everyone involved agrees with a particular decision cannot, ultimately, relieve us of this burden. Yet, too often, one sees physicians and nurses ask patients or families whether they want this or that medication, this or that intervention, this or that treatment. Often, this "everyone has to be happy" ethic becomes an excuse for torturing to death the most vulnerable among us. This ethically unjustifiable behavior is not suddenly transformed into ethically acceptable behavior just because the patient happened to agree with the decision. The new "respect for autonomy" is too often simple abandonment and no better than the imperious "Lone Ranger" approach, supposedly out of fashion.

When I cared for Steve and Martin, I viewed them as part of a web of relationships. I could not make the decisions I had to make without fully entering that web, entangling myself in its filaments. I also knew that I had to be willing to tear parts of that web if necessary and then try to repair them later. That is, I believe, the essence of family caregiving, and it should be the essence of all caregiving—the willingness to engage in a complex exchange in which there is sharing, and risk, distance and connection, pain and reward. Everyone—not just professionals—who makes these kinds of decisions for dependent and vulnerable people must learn to engage in this process. If we are to evolve spiritually and culturally, if we are improve our ability to care for each other, we need to develop new structures and skills. We need to learn how to elaborate and enlist communities of support. And we need to learn how to tolerate alone the responsibility of caring for others.

References

Benner, Patricia and Judith Wrubel. 1989. *The Primacy of Caring: Stress and Coping in Health and Illness.* Menlo Park, CA: Addison Wesley.

Selden, D. 1984. "The Medical Model: Biomedical Science as the Basis for Medicine." In *The Nation's Health,* ed. Peter R. Lee, Carroll L. Estes, and Nancy Ramsay. San Francisco: Boyd and Fraser.

Part III
Professional Caregiving

In this section we look at the contributions, ideals, and conflicts of professional caregivers in nursing, teaching, and social work. These three occupations are sometimes referred to as "semi-professions" (Etzioni 1969) because they exhibit some of the characteristics of true professions but lack others. In all three occupations, for example, members are exhorted to establish and maintain high standards of competence in the direct care of their clients, but they do not enjoy the level of prestige and autonomy generally associated with professions like medicine or law. Indeed, caring itself is sometimes seen as an obstacle to full professionalization (Reverby 1987); its ideals draw practitioners closer to their patients, students, and clients, and the *distance* that is one mark of professionalization cannot be maintained.

The first selection, Chapter 9, is a short narrative by nurse Jeannie Chaisson. Chaisson works on a medical surgical floor at Boston's Beth Israel Hospital. Her narrative not only suggests the breadth of the kinds of work that nurses do, it provides a new perspective on the difference between those who focus on care and on cure in our health care system, Chaisson's commitment to a care perspective allows her to move from her patient's disease into her patient's life. And, in this instance as in so many, it is the patient's life that holds the relevant answers. Instead of being the end point of inquiry, disease is the point of entry that allows Chaisson to understand the meaning of illness to another human being. It is only in the act of that profound, almost literary rewriting of the objective phenomenon of disease that hope resides.

In Chapter 10, "The Caring Professional", Nel Noddings discusses the problems of professionalization for caregivers. If caring is a particular kind of relationship between two people, a carer and a cared-for, can a person be both a professional, according to conventional definitions of that term, and a carer? If occupations aspire to be full professions, can they at the same time be guided by ideals of caring? Noddings suggests that it makes sense to speak of "caring professionals" if we concentrate on internal, rather than external, characteristics of a practice.

In Chapter 11, "Ella," Suzanne Gordon tells the painful and rewarding story of her own encounter with professional caregivers who believe that distance is a necessary characteristic of the caregiving professional. As a stranger thrown into a situation by her role as journalist, Gordon finds herself *addressed*, called to care by people who are suffering. As a carer, Gordon responds. Her story reveals both the shared suffering and joy of people committed to a caring relation. It also illustrates dramatically the problems raised in Noddings' chapter and other essays in this book. Can a professional care, as Gordon, a stranger, cared? Can caregiving be freely chosen and thus abandoned if it becomes too inconvenient or problematic? Can caring be calibrated? Does it not involve judgment as well as engrossment?

Chapter 12, "Two Stories of Caring in Teaching" by James G. Henderson, brings us into the classroom, where teachers enter a dialogue with their students that endures over time. In this selection from his book Reflective Teaching, Henderson describes the work of Maura Callahan and Eugene Meyers. Neither teacher has a recipe for how to infuse teaching with caring practice. Each establishes a framework in which time can be taken to get to know each student, to see each one's particularity. From that reciprocal relationship, which forms the hub of the wheel, its spokes—decisions to encourage, affirm, guide and coach—emerge.

Neither teacher abstracts the student's learning process from that student's life. Rather than abstracting their own personal lives from their professional activities and goals, these two teachers share their life experiences with their students. It is, in fact, their ability to connect and remember their own vulnerability as students that allows them to successfully connect with the children they teach.

Chapter 13 by nurse researchers Patricia Benner, Catherine Chesla, Christine Tanner and Deborah Gordon describes some of what has been traditionally depicted as the ineffable and unknowable in nursing. Treating patients in the context of a caring relation, nurses come to know them in a way that cannot be made entirely explicit. They detect significant changes before the changes show up through so-called objective indicators, like an elevated temperature or particular physiological tests. They sometimes see a quality of life that is unexpected given the objective physical condition of the patient. And, on the opposite end of the spectrum, they come to understand the despair and desperation so often denied by those physicians who treat only the patient's disease and neglect the patient's life. Benner, Chesla, Tanner, and Gordon argue persuasively for a view of nursing that makes the caring relation between nurse and patient central. This view of nursing is particularly relevant today, when considerations of cost overshadow those of quality of care.

References

Etzioni, Amitai. 1969. *The Semi-Professions and Their Organization: Teachers, Nurses, and Social Workers.* New York: Free Press.
Reverby, Susan. 1987. *Ordered to Care: The Dilemma of American Nursing, 1850–1945.* Cambridge: Cambridge University Press.

Chapter 9
Hearing the Whole Story

Jeannie Chaisson

As an experienced nurse, I am often called on to assess a person's ability to function on a daily basis. In 1991 I received a phone call from an attorney with whom I occasionally consult, asking me to review her client's appeal of a denial of social security disability benefits. Before me was a file containing an assortment of paperwork related to the application of a woman I'll call "Mrs. A." The file presented a fragmented picture of a woman in her early sixties, an immigrant who spoke a little English and had found a job working in a cafeteria. For several years she had worked diligently, but she had been fired when a new manager refused to let her coworkers assist her with the heavy lifting inherent in the job.

In a sparsely detailed application for benefits filled out by an intake worker who had been hampered by a language barrier, it was affirmed that she did not fit into the bureaucratic pigeonholes that define disability. Letters from physicians detailing her currently stable medical condition did little to bolster her cause. Her breast cancer, for which she had undergone surgery, showed no signs of recurrence. Her arthritis seemed improved on her last visit to her doctor; he could not predict when an exacerbation might recur, so she was advised to rest and take an anti-inflammatory.

Using physicians as the lens and disease as the definition of the field, fragments of a life were examined. Yet questions and answers that had little relevance to her ability to function failed to show clear evidence of disability, although I saw hints that pain might be a problem. I asked whether it would be possible for me to meet this woman and do a brief nursing assessment.

Two days later, I met Mrs. A. and her son, who served as translator.

An earlier version of this essay appeared as Chaisson, "Asking the Right Questions," *Technology Review* 95, 7 (October 1992): 47ff. Reprinted by permission of the author.

She was small and slim, and smiled anxiously as she shook my hand. Her son, a man in his early thirties, was a graduate student at a local college and spoke English well. He carried a stack of medical records containing cryptic comments that did little to illuminate or explain the life of the woman who sat stiffly in front of me with a tired, strained cast to her face.

I explained that I was a nurse and that my questions might be different from those she had already answered. Addressing me in hesitant English, or in rapid-fire phrases to her son, she talked for more than an hour.

Her comfortable life had been blown apart by revolution. One son was killed, and she had managed to escape with the other. In the United States her lack of English had disqualified her from seeking the managerial work she had formerly done. She had been happy to take *any* job, because it was blessing enough to have escaped with her life after having lost "everything but this son." But her pain increased, and when it became intolerable she asked her fellow kitchen workers to help her with lifting. They agreed willingly, but her boss refused to allow such help.

I asked her to tell me about the pain. How severe was it? Where was it located? What made it worse? What could she do to help make it better? Mrs. A's pain, which so many others had dismissed or overlooked, was a relic of eleven operations for breast cancer she had undergone before coming to this country. One by one, each new lump and node had been removed, and each time the cancer had reappeared. Terrified to permit the doctors to cut the chest muscles out and "take everything," she had gradually, bit by bit, lost both breasts. A disfigured body and horrible pain that started in her scarified chest tissue and burned and knifed its way up through her right shoulder and arm was her reward. Any activity was difficult. Nothing banished this pain, not heat, cold, or medications. Moving the right arm, or even moving the hand to write or turn the pages of a book or newspaper, was excruciating. She couldn't lie on that side at all. She had some pain in her other arm, and sometimes her knees hurt from the arthritis, but it was the pain in her right arm and chest that cut her off from life. With a tragic stoicism, she said that she didn't blame her boss for firing her. After all, she said sadly, she had been able to do less and less of her work.

As Mrs. A. continued to recount a "typical day," I heard the story of a woman vanquished by pain. The feints and parries of a few years ago—when she got up and went to work, to English classes, and to doctors for help—had given way to total defeat. Yes, she had her life, but she was not free to live it. Under an uneasy truce, she could appease this tyrant only by giving up her job, her intellectual pursuits, and her relationships with others. And now the price asked was her self-worth.

As my questions led to this tale of overwhelming loss, she became animated, then tearful. "Nobody has ever asked her about these things before," her son explained. "Nobody has cared what it is like for her."

Three weeks later, Mrs. A.'s attorney informed me that she had been granted disability benefits, and I could only wonder at the "health" of a health care system which had provided numerous surgeries, regular scrutiny of her body for recurrent disease, and prescriptions to balance the metabolism and attempt to mute the pain, yet had utterly failed to listen to the story of her illness, to bear witness to her pain. Others had talked about her disease; I had asked about her life.

Chapter 10
The Caring Professional

Nel Noddings

In this chapter, I begin with a review of what it means to care. Next, I confess some ambivalence about the nature of professionalism—at least when it implies professionalization. Finally, I explore—given my reservations about professionalization—what it might mean for teachers to be "caring professionals." Although I concentrate here on teaching, most of what I say can be applied to all of the caregiving professions.

What It Means to Care

Caring, as I pointed out in an earlier essay in this volume, is a particular kind of relation between two people—a carer and a "cared for" (see also Noddings 1984). It may occur in a brief episode or in a relationship extended over time. In the latter case, some caring relationships are mutual; that is, the members of the relation change positions regularly, sharing the responsibilities of giving and receiving care. We usually expect that spousal relationships, friendships, and collegial (peer) relationships will be of this sort. Indeed, it disappoints and angers us when the other party in such a relationship fails to reciprocate by accepting the position of carer. But some extended relationships are unequal by their very nature: adult-child, teacher-student, nurse-patient are all examples of relationships in which the first member has almost exclusive responsibility as carer. However, even in these relationships, the second party contributes something of great value if the relation can be properly described as *caring*.

When we care—when we are in the position of carer—our conscious-

This essay is adapted from a lecture given at the Seven Oaks School District, Winnipeg, Ontario, February 1993. A portion of the essay appeared in Noddings, *The Challenge to Care in Schools* (New York: Teachers College Press, 1992), pp. 22–26. Reprinted by permission of the publisher.

ness exhibits two fundamental characteristics. First, we are in a receptive mode. We attend non-selectively to the cared-for. We are, at least momentarily, engrossed in the other's plans, pains, and hopes, not our own. Second, we feel our motive energy flowing toward the other. We want to help in furthering the plan, relieving the pain, or actualizing the hope. What we actually do to enact our part in the caring relation is contingent on many factors, but these two fundamental characteristics describe our basic consciousness.

The recipient of care, the cared-for, contributes to the relationship by responding in some positive way to the efforts of the carer. An infant may smile, coo, or cuddle. A student may look up with eyes alight. A patient may nod affirmatively—"Yes, you've got it—that's where the pain is!" These responses, as all parents, teachers, physicians, and nurses know, are non-negligible. A relation cannot properly be labeled *caring* in their absence. Not only does the response complete the relation but it also provides the material by which carers monitor the effects of their efforts at care. It is part of what the carer receives in the next round of caring.

The things I have described so far are, I think, universally true of caring relations. In the moments of care, carers attend and feel their motive energy flowing toward the cared for; the cared-for makes some form of response that completes the relation. But beyond this basic description of two consciousnesses meeting in a caring relation, what actual, concrete people do varies with the situation; further, it varies across time and cultures, even across personalities and moods. This variance is indeed part of what it means to care. If I treat everyone exactly alike in situations that seem to me to be similar, my efforts will probably not produce positive responses in many of the recipients of my care. I must look at each cared-for in a special way. Simone Weil wrote:

This way of looking is first of all attentive. The soul empties itself of all its own contents in order to receive into itself the being it is looking at, just as he is, in all his truth. Only he who is capable of attention can do this. (1977b, p. 51)

In another essay, Weil (1977a) said that we must respond to cries of pain even if they are based—as they often are with children—on misunderstanding. For in these cases, she wrote, the problem lies in the inadequacy of our explanations. Here, it seems to me, another problem arises that Weil did not explore fully. Sometimes children accept explanations and assurances from us that they should reject. Sometime they believe our message, "This is for your own good," when they should doubt and resist. The Swiss psychologist Alice Miller (1983) has written persuasively on this. Examining the lives of adults guilty of enor-

mous cruelties—members of the Nazi high command among others—
she found that virtually all were raised in strict, authoritarian families.
Their parents demanded obedience ostensibly for the good of their children. But the result was adult beings with no real sense of self. It is clear
from studies such as Miller's that we need to watch not only the immediate response of the cared-for but the long-run response reflected in how
she or he grows.

Unequal relationships like parenting and teaching require time. We
need time to develop relations of care and trust, and we need time to
monitor the effects of our efforts. A firm, no-nonsense style may provide just the structure one child needs, but it may crush the intellectual
life of another child. Because it takes time for teachers and students to
understand these differences, I have recommended that students should
stay with a teacher for three or more years rather than the one year typically allowed now (Noddings 1992a). This kind of placement should be
by mutual consent. No child should be forced to stay with a teacher he
or she dislikes, and no teacher should be pressed into such an arrange-
ment. Rather, administrators should invite teachers and students to participate in this kind of program. I will return to this discussion a bit later.

The effort to care over time reveals weaknesses in both ourselves and
those we care for. Astute carers see that, to meet the needs of a variety
of cared-fors, they must increase their own skills. For example, as parents, we may be just right for very young children and not very effective
with teenagers; we may need to be more receptive and we may need
to learn new skills. As teachers, we may have to learn new subject matter to maintain the growth of our best students, and we may have to
change our methods entirely to work effectively with students who have
great difficulty learning. In a fundamental, essential way, caring implies
a quest for competence.

We realize, too, that the ways we care directly for one child may have
repercussions on others. This does not mean that we must necessarily
alter our behavior and treat everyone alike. It may be that, as Weil said,
we need only provide a more adequate explanation to those who claim
to be hurt. But it becomes obvious that we must monitor care across the
whole network of care. Not only must we evaluate the effects of our care
on the cared for and observers, but we must also attend to how cared-
fors treat others as a result of our treatment of them. Weil reminds us of
what is sacred in our fellow beings:

At the bottom of the heart of every human being, from the earliest infancy until
the tomb, there is something that goes on indomitably expecting, in the teeth
of all experience of crimes committed, suffered, and witnessed, that good and
not evil will be done to him. It is this above all that is sacred in every human
being. (1977a, p. 315)

But that spirit may not be as indomitable as Weil thought. It may, indeed, be possible to destroy it. Perhaps the most important thing children learn from us is how to interact with people and other living things. Moral education thus becomes a high priority for all carers, as I pointed out in *The Challenge to Care in Schools*:

Moral education from the perspective of an ethic of caring has four major components: modeling, dialogue, practice, and confirmation (Noddings 1984). Modeling is important in most schemes of moral education, but in caring it is vital. In this framework we are not trying to teach students principles and ways of applying them to problems through chains of mathematical reasoning. Rather, we have to show how to care in our own relations with cared-fors. For example, professors of education and school administrators cannot be sarcastic and dictatorial with teachers in the hope that coercion will make them care for students. I have heard administrators use this excuse for "being tough" with teachers— "because I care about the kids of this state"—but, of course, the likely outcome is that teachers will then turn attention protectively to themselves rather than lovingly to their students. So we do not *tell* our students to care; we *show* them how to care by creating caring relations with them.

There is a second reason why modeling is so vital. The capacity to care may be dependent on adequate experience in being cared for. Even while a child is too young to be a carer, he or she can learn how to be a responsive cared-for. Thus our role as carer is more important than our role as model, but we fill both simultaneously. We remind ourselves when we are tempted to take short cuts in moral education that we are, inevitably, models. But otherwise, in our daily activities we simply respond as carers when the need arises. The function of modeling gets special attention when we try to explain what we are doing and why in moral education. But the primary reason for responding as carers to our students' needs is that we are called to such response by our moral orientation.

Dialogue is the second essential component of moral education. My use of the term *dialogue* is similar to that of Paulo Freire (1970). It is not just talk or conversation—certainly not an oral presentation of argument in which the second party is merely allowed to ask an occasional question. Dialogue is open-ended; that is, in a genuine dialogue, neither party knows at the outset what the outcome or decision will be. As parents and teachers, we cannot enter into dialogue with children when we know that our decision is already made. It is maddening to young people (or any people) to engage in dialogue with a sweetly reasonable adult who cannot be persuaded and who, in the end, will say, "Here's how it's going to be. I tried to reason with you . . ." We do have to talk this way at times, but we should not pretend that this is dialogue. Dialogue is a common search for understanding, empathy, or appreciation. It can be playful or serious, logical or imaginative, goal- or process-oriented, but it is always a genuine quest for something undetermined at the beginning.

Dialogue permits us to talk about what we try to show. It give learners opportunities to question "why," and it helps both parties to arrive at well-informed decisions. Although I do not believe that all wrongdoing can be equated with ignorance, I do believe that many moral errors are ill-informed decisions, particularly in the very young. Thus dialogue serves not only to inform the decision under consideration; it also contributes to a habit of mind—that of seeking adequate information on which to make decisions.

Dialogue serves another purpose in moral education. It connects us to each other and helps to maintain caring relations. It also provides us with the knowledge of each other that forms a foundation for the response in caring. Caring (acting as carer) requires knowledge and skill as well as characteristic attitudes. We respond most effectively as carers when we understand what the other needs and the history of this need. Dialogue is implied in the criterion of engrossment. To receive the other is to attend fully and openly. Continuing dialogue builds up a substantial knowledge of one another that serves to guide our responses.

A third component of moral education is practice. Attitudes and "mentalities" are shaped, at least in part, by experience. Most of us speak regularly of a "military mind," a "police mentality," "business thinking," and the like. Although some of this talk is a product of stereotyping, it seems clear that it also captures some truth about human behavior. All disciplines and institutional organizations have training programs designed not only to teach specific skills but also to "shape minds," that is, to induce certain attitudes and ways of looking at the world. If we want people to approach moral life prepared to care, we need to provide opportunities for them to gain skills in caregiving and, more important, to develop the characteristic attitudes described earlier.

Some schools, recognizing the needs just discussed, have instituted requirements for a form of community service. This is a move in the right direction, but reflection produces some issues to worry about. The practice provided must be with people who can demonstrate caring. We do not want our children to learn the menial (or even sophisticated) skills of caregiving without the characteristic attitude of caring. The experience of caregiving should initiate or contribute to the desired attitude, but the conditions have to be right, and people are central to the setting.

Next, practice in caring should transform schools and, eventually, the society in which we live. If the practice is assimilated to the present structures of schooling, it may lose its transformative powers. *It* may be transformed—that is, distorted. If we were to give grades for caregiving, for example, students might well begin to compete for honors in caring. Clearly, then, their attention could be diverted from cared-fors to themselves. If, on the other hand, we neither grade nor give credit for such work, it may inevitably have second-class status in our schools. So long as our schools are organized hierarchically with emphasis on rewards and penalties, it will be very difficult to provide the kind of experience envisioned.

The fourth component of moral education from the perspective of caring is confirmation. Martin Buber (1965) describes confirmation as an act of affirming and encouraging the best in others. When we confirm someone, we spot a better self and encourage its development. We can only do this if we know the other well enough to see what he or she is trying to become. Formulas and slogans have no place here. We do not set up a single ideal or set of expectations for everyone to meet, but we identify something admirable, or at least acceptable, struggling to emerge in each person we encounter. The person working toward a better self must see the attribute or goal as worthy, and we too must see it as at least morally acceptable. We do not confirm people in ways we judge to be wrong.

Confirmation requires attribution of the best possible motive consonant with reality. When someone commits an act we find reprehensible, we ask ourselves what might have motivated such an act. Often it is not hard to identify an array of possible motives ranging from the gross and grubby to some that are acceptable or even admirable. This array is not constructed in abstraction. We build it from a knowledge of this particular other and by listening carefully to what she or he tells us. The motive we attribute has to be a real, a genuine possibility. Then we can open our dialogue with something like, "I know you were trying to help your friend . . ." or "I know what you're trying to accomplish. . . ." It will be clear that we disapprove of this particular act, but it will also be clear to the other that we see a self that is better than this act. Often the other will respond with enormous relief. *Here is this significant and percipient other who sees through the smallness or meanness of my present behavior a self that is better and a real possibility.* Confirmation lifts us toward our vision of a better self.

It is worth repeating that confirmation cannot be done by formula. A relation of trust must ground it. Continuity is required, because the carer in acting to confirm must know the cared-for well enough to be able to identify motives consonant with reality. Confirmation cannot be described in terms of strategies; it is a loving act founded on a relation of some depth. When we turn to specific changes that should occur in schooling in order to meet the challenge to care, I will put great emphasis on continuity. Not all caring relations require continuity (some, as we have seen, are brief encounters), but teaching does require it.

Confirmation contrasts sharply with the standard mode of religious moral education. There we usually find a sequence of accusation, confession, penance and forgiveness. The initial step, accusation, causes or sustains separation. We stand in moral judgment and separate the other from ourselves and the moral community. In contrast, confirmation calls us to remain in connection. Further, accusation tends to produce denial or rationalization which we, then, feel compelled to overthrow. But the rationalization may in fact be an attempt on the part of the accused to find that possible motive and convey it to us, the accuser. Because we have to reject it in order to proceed with confession, penance, and forgiveness, offenders may never understand their own true motives. This sequence also depends heavily on authority, obedience, fear, and subordination. We can be harsh or magnanimous in our judgment and forgiveness. Our authority is emphasized, and the potential power of the offender's own moral struggle is overlooked.

I do not mean to suggest that there is never a place for accusation and confession in moral education. It is not always possible for us to find a motive that is morally acceptable; sometimes we have to begin by asking straight out, "Why did you do that?" or "How could you do such a thing?" But it is gratifying how often we really can see a better self if we look for one, and its identification is a first step in its realization. (Noddings 1992a, pp. 22–26)

What It Means To Be Professional

So far, I have described the basic nature of caring relations and the form of moral education that is central to such relations. Now let's examine what it means to be a professional, and then we will see if carers and professionals can co-exist in the same bodies.

Current efforts to reform education in the United States include recommendations for the professionalization of teaching (Carnegie Task Force 1986; Holmes Group 1986). Using law and medicine as exemplars of the professions, reform groups have suggested that preparation for teaching be conducted at the graduate level, that a professional teaching hierarchy be created, and that a board of professionals should oversee the testing and licensing of teaching candidates. All of these recommendations can be challenged both from within a professional framework and from perspectives that criticize the very idea of professionalization as it is now defined (Noddings 1992b).

Initial reaction from teachers to recommendations for professionalization is often positive. After all, I regarded myself as a professional when I taught high school mathematics, and most teachers no doubt also regard themselves as professionals. However, it turns out that teaching manifests only a few of the characteristics sociologists have identified with true professions. Professions, sociologists tell us, are marked by self-selection and regulation, specialized knowledge, altruism or service, privilege and status hierarchies, collegiality, and autonomy (Bledstein, 1976; Flexner 1915; Hall 1968; Larson 1977). Teaching is certainly a work of altruism and service, but it does not clearly exhibit any of the other features. The very structure of schools and the school day precludes real collegiality; supervisors and administrators often tell teachers exactly how to teach, so autonomy is warped into passive resistance; advancement to administrative work usually means no more teaching; teachers do not select and regulate members of the occupation; and, although some prominent educators insist that teachers have highly specialized knowledge (Shulman 1987), many critics doubt that this is so. Both teaching and nursing are, perhaps, better described as semiprofessions rather than professions (Etzioni 1969).

Now the question arises whether we should feel bad about this and push for full professional status. I confess to mixed feelings about the movement. On the one hand, I believe that good teachers—people who uphold the highest intellectual and ethical standards of teaching—are already "professionals." But, on this definition, members of any occupation—mechanics, plumbers, bakers, police officers—are all "real professionals" when they consistently do an admirable job. Indeed, we use the term "professional" as an accolade in all such situations. When we are pleased with the job our regular mechanic or plumber does for us, we often say appreciatively, "He is a real professional." Similarly, when we in education direct our attention to this sense of "professional," we are concerned with the internal standards of teaching. We earn the title by perfecting our skills, promoting the growth and satisfaction of our students, and gaining the recognition of peers and parents.

But the current movement does not emphasize the internal practices of teaching. Its focus is on the external marks of professional life—those I listed a few moments ago. For example, we are sometimes urged to introduce status hierarchies into teaching. Suggestions have been made that perhaps 10–20 percent of the profession should be called "career professionals" or some other honorific title. The possibility of achieving such status gives teachers something to work toward, a way of advancing in the profession. The trouble is that achieving this status might involve acquiring credentials that have little to do with one's influence on students and, that once ensconced in that higher niche of the hierarchy, a teacher would spend less time with children. Thus those people who acquire advanced degrees, those who have the time and energy to create impressive portfolios and videotapes, those who can afford testing and licensing fees are more likely to achieve high status than those who simply do a devoted and superb job year-in and year-out in the classroom. Recognizing this undesirable possibility, we could, of course, create hierarchies that do not favor those who perform tasks other than the actual teaching of students. But, as feminist theory has made so clear, hierarchies are always suspect because they introduce (or reflect) relations of domination and subordination.

As we look carefully at each recommendation to increase the professional status of teachers, we see that the connection between the professionalization of teachers and the growth and well-being of students is by no means clear. It is inferential at best. For example, if teachers take charge of admitting candidates to teaching and approving them for upper level status through national board examinations, how will this help students? One could simply argue that with higher status teachers might take more pride in their work, or that the skills demonstrated to pass such licensing procedures would ensure better teaching. But the example of medicine suggests caution. It is by no means clear that the professionalization of medicine produced better patient care. On the contrary, many would argue that the benefits we now enjoy are products of medical *science*—more effective drugs, diagnostic instruments, and the like—and that actual medical *care* has deteriorated. Alternatively, and more honestly, one could argue that the professionalization movement does not have to promise benefits for students; it is enough to show that teachers will benefit. But this argument flies in the face of what we hear regularly from people applying to teacher education programs. Overwhelmingly, these people want to "make a difference" in the lives of individual children. So I would press advocates of professionalization to tell us how *professionalization* will affect *professionalism*.

Let's consider another aspect of professionalization—possession of specialized knowledge. Most of us give glad assent to the assertion that teachers possess specialized knowledge. But specialized knowledge often implies a highly specialized language. Physicians and lawyers are notorious for their use of words and expressions that defy translation into ordinary language. Must teachers use "educationese" to impress the public? It has not worked so far! One deleterious effect of using a highly specialized language is the separation it creates between professionals and clients. (This result could, of course, be described positively if we concentrate wholly on status: separation, then, tends to elevate the party in possession of highly specialized language.) But, in the language of professional*ism*, we want to reduce, not increase, the distance between us and students and their parents. As professionals, we pride ourselves on our ability to communicate, not to obfuscate. Thus, any claim we make to specialized knowledge should not necessitate a corresponding claim to specialized language.

Besides altruism and service, which clearly mark teaching, professionalism and professionalization share one other feature—autonomy. To do the best possible job with a variety of students, teachers must be free to use their professional judgment in matters of management, curriculum, and instruction. Both the internal and external criteria of professions require appropriate levels of autonomy, and it is precisely the lack of autonomy that frustrates and humiliates teachers today. It is also one of the lacks that prevents teachers from establishing relations of care and trust. This observation sets the stage for an analysis of what it might mean to be a caring professional.

Caring in Teaching

To be caring professionals, teachers need not set aside all aspiration to higher status and salary. It is entirely appropriate to work for these things. But, if we are honest about what it means to be a professional, we see that the chief criteria are internal to the practice. To be a professional is to be highly skilled in a practice and to be dedicated to the growth and well-being of the people with whom we practice. Indeed, most people become teachers because they see teaching as a "worthy" profession or because they want to make a difference in the lives of children (Goodlad 1984). In our teacher education program at Stanford University, we hear the latter reason more than any other from our applicants.

It is not surprising, then, that people often give as their reason for leaving teaching that they cannot make the difference they intended. Something in the structure of schooling keeps teachers and students from connecting in ways satisfying to either. James Comer (1988) has commented on the complaint commonly heard from inner city students, "Nobody cares!" It echoes everywhere. High school students, especially, do not feel that their teachers care about them. But when we consult teachers we often find that most express deep concern for their students. Here we seem to have students who want to be cared for and teachers who want to care, and yet we do not have caring relations. Kids behave badly while they are in attendance, and all too often drop out of school. Teachers become frustrated and disgusted, and they, too, leave school for more rewarding work.

The problem seems to be that teachers cannot be caring professionals in today's schools. Traditionally, the greatest rewards for teachers have been the positive responses of students. When these responses disappear, teaching becomes a job, and teachers turn to the external trappings of professionalization for compensation. Is there any way for teachers to be caring professionals today?

There are probably many ways to approach this problem, but it seems to me that two issues are central. First, teachers, after their initial apprenticeship, must be allowed to exercise their professional judgment in all classroom matters; second, school structures should be redesigned with caring uppermost in mind.

Let's consider the issue of autonomy first. It is understandable that administrators should apply scientific measures to evaluate teachers when parents and politicians clamor for higher performance on test scores, and no one really knows how to produce higher scores. But, consider. Administrators do not monitor the day-to-day work of physicians and lawyers. If something goes badly wrong, physicians and lawyers are called to account for their decisions, but no one evaluates them on their adherence to specific moves or strategies with every patient or client. Yet teachers today are often evaluated on whether they have a specific learning objective for every lesson, whether they use a 5-step (or 7-step) lesson, and whether they use a particular form of classroom management or discipline.

I think this has to change. Teachers should be asked to account for every failure, to suggest what might be done for every child experiencing difficulty, and to explain what they have done for each child in their care, but they should be free to decide how to conduct their own teaching. I really believe teachers need to be adamant on this. In the best of all possible professional worlds, teachers in a given school (in a "practice") would list their qualifications and describe their methods, and parents would apply to have their children study with particular teachers. This would represent choice in the best sense. But, in the absence of family practice modes of teaching, teachers should insist on at least this modicum of autonomy: they should be in charge of how they teach and manage a classroom.

Now, because children are not adult clients, someone does have to be sure that they are not being treated cruelly, being led astray morally, or developing more slowly than they might intellectually. Thus classroom visits and tests have their place. Additionally, far more professional conversation should take place. Time should be provided for teachers who are working with a particular group of students to talk with one another about these students—their growth, problems, needs, and aspirations. Teachers should visit one another's classrooms, ask questions, and make suggestions. Real educational leadership should address itself to bringing out the best in teachers and teacher collegiality, just as we want teachers to bring out the best in students.

Professionals who want to care must also press for changes in the structure of schooling. To care adequately for students, teachers need to know them better than is possible under current conditions. In California today, it is not unusual for a mathematics teacher to be responsible for 160 to 175 students a day. Furthermore, all of these students are new to the teacher in September. By April teachers may feel that they are beginning to know their students as individuals, but the year is almost over! If finances make it impossible to reduce class size, at least half a teacher's student load should be students returning for a second, third, or fourth year. Teachers and students should, by mutual consent, stay together for several years. This is a plan that can be enormously satisfying for both students and teachers, and it costs nothing.

To reap the rewards of teaching as a caring profession, teachers need to get a positive response of some kind from students. A positive response may manifest itself in a variety of ways: Some students may respond enthusiastically to the subject matter itself; some may show greater interpersonal awareness; some may grow in self-understanding; some may come to trust the teacher and, finally, have an adult to confide in; some may simply find school a safer, happier place to spend the day. But none of this can happen if it isn't legitimate for teachers to spend time on the establishment and maintenance of caring relations. Teachers must insist on the autonomy to exercise their capacity to care.

As we look at education through the lens of caring, we see that more attention has to be given to human relationships—to continuity of place, people, and purpose. It should be understood by teachers, parents, and students that the purpose of schooling is to produce competent, caring, loving, and lovable people. Of course, we will attend to academic and intellectual matters but the purpose even of these is to contribute to the complete growth of every child. Looking this way is, as Simone Weil said, first of all attentive. We do not restrict ourselves to abstract problem solving on matters of schooling but, rather we *look at* our students. Listen to some comments from a 1992 study conducted by the Institute for Education in Transformation:

High school student: This place hurts my spirit!
Elementary teacher: Everything I like about teaching is related to students.

High school student: Teachers should get to know their students a little better, not to where they bowl together but at least to know if they have any brothers or sisters. I have found that if I know my teacher I feel more obliged to do the work so I don't disappoint them. Once my trust is gained I feel I should work for myself and also for the teacher. (1992)

This is what caring professionals know—that teaching and learning and life itself go better in an atmosphere of care and trust. Teachers should be encouraged to spend time creating such an atmosphere. It should not only be legitimate to spend time sharing and caring; the practice should be encouraged. We need to engage in dialogue with our students not only about routine issues in the prescribed curriculum but, more important, about alternative definitions of success (not just "making it" financially), about various forms of the good life, about the meaning (or lack of it) of life itself, about the possibility of immortality, and the meanings of love, friendship, and commitment. None of this should be done dogmatically; it should always be expected that students should ask how, why, and on what grounds. And, of course, teachers should not spend *all* of their time rapping or storytelling. But some time thus spent may be morally obligatory in teaching. Kids desperately need this kind of sharing. Stories told generously and judiciously invite students to participate in immortal conversations. Surely this is just the sort of work to which the caring professional is called.

References

Bledstein, Burton J. 1976. *The Culture of Professionalism: The Middle Class and the Development of Higher Education in America*. New York: W. W. Norton.

Buber, Martin. 1965. "Education." In Buber, *Between Man and Man*, trans. Ronald G. Smith, 83–103. New York: Macmillan.

Carnegie Forum on Education and the Economy, Task Force on Teaching as a Profession. 1986. *A Nation Prepared: Teachers for the Twenty-First Century*. New York: The Forum.

Comer, James P. 1988. "Is 'Parenting' Essential to Good Teaching?" *NEA Today* 6: 34–40.

Etzioni, Amitai. 1969. *The Semi-Professions and Their Organization: Teachers, Nurses, and Social Workers*. New York: Free Press.

Flexner, Abraham. 1915. "Is Social Work a Profession?" *School and Society* 1, 26: 901–11.

Freire, Paulo. 1970. *Pedagogy of the Oppressed*, trans. Myra Bergman Ramos. New York: Herder and Herder.

Goodlad, John I. 1984. *A Place Called School: Prospects for the Future*. New York: McGraw Hill.

Hall, R. H. 1968. "Professionalization and Bureaucratization." *American Sociological Review* 33, 1: 92–104.

Holmes Group. 1986. *Tomorrow's Teachers*. East Lansing, MI: Holmes Group.

Institute for Education in Transformation. 1992. *Voices from the Inside.* Claremont, CA: Claremont Graduate School.

Larson, Margali Sarfatti. 1977. *The Rise of Professionalism.* Berkeley: University of California Press.

Miller, Alice. 1983. *For Your Own Good: Hidden Cruelty in Child-Rearing and the Roots of Violence,* trans. Hildegarde Hannun and Hunter Hannun. New York: Farrar-Strauss-Giroux.

Noddings, Nel. 1984. *Caring: A Feminine Approach to Ethics and Moral Education.* Berkeley: University of California Press.

———. 1992a. *The Challenge to Care in Schools.* New York: Teachers College Press.

———. 1992b. "Professionalization and Mathematics Teaching." In *Handbook of Research on Mathematics Teaching and Learning,* ed. Douglas A. Grouws, 197–208. New York: Macmillan.

Shulman, Lee S. 1987. "Knowledge and Teaching: Foundations of the New Reform." *Harvard Educational Review* 56: 1–22.

Weil, Simone. 1977a. "Human Personality." In *Simone Weil Reader,* ed. George A. Panichas, 313–39. Mt. Kisco, NY: Moyer Bell.

———. 1977b. "Reflections on the Right Use of School Studies with a View to the Love of God." In *Simone Weil Reader,* ed. George A. Panichas, 44–53. Mt. Kisco, NY: Moyer Bell.

Chapter 11
Ella

Suzanne Gordon

I met Ella in the worst possible circumstances—on the day of her admission to an oncology unit at a major American teaching hospital. She was a Russian Jew who had emigrated with her family—a husband and two children—to the United States from the former Soviet Union, only to learn that she had a particularly vicious form of cancer. Her doctor, in fact, believed the cancer was a result of the accident at the Chernobyl nuclear reactor, which had been only several hundred miles from her home. Like the other inhabitants of the former Soviet Union, she had learned of the accident two weeks or more after its occurrence, too late to take adequate precautions against exposure.

Ella and I were never conventionally introduced, but rather were plunged into the course of each other's lives. She was a patient on a hospital unit which I had entered as a journalistic observer. In researching nursing, I had come to this floor to chronicle the activities of the expert nurses who are the backbone of our medical system. On that particular day, I was following a nurse we'll call Joanne Carey and her associate nurse, Denise Sullivan. Ella was assigned to Joanne's care. She was in excruciating pain and about to start her first of five rounds of largely futile chemotherapy in one of medicine's brave but misguided lurches to defeat even the most untreatable disorders. For the five-day period she was in the hospital, her nurse fought with interns and residents who were terrified to give her enough pain medication, brought in social workers to help with her and her family's many emotional problems, and managed the side effects of the intense chemotherapy she was receiving.

As a journalist trying to learn about the meaning of caregiving in an acute care hospital, I followed not only nurses but also their patients.

An original essay.

If caregiving, as I believe, is a relationship between two people—and more—then it is crucial to grasp what caregiving means not only to those who deliver it but to those who receive it. In my capacity as anthropologist analyzing a culture of care, I talked often to patients and families.

And in this particular case I got very close to one of them.

That involvement—and the many rewards and conflicts it engendered —is at the heart of this story. It happened, like most human connections, without premeditation or reflection. Indeed, when I look back on it, there seemed to be no choice or option but to connect, help, and witness. Once I got to know Ella and her family, once I understood what was happening to them and what particular skills I could offer, I *had* to help.

When we first met, Ella lay on her bed writhing in pain, surrounded by her two sisters-in-law and her husband. The one thing that struck me about her then was her hair. On this unit, full of patients whose hair had been chemically sheared and who thus appeared in hats, turbans, or entirely bald, her long mane of thick black hair seemed a special gift. As she shifted restlessly on the hospital bed, her hair rippled across the pillow. It was, it seemed, the crown of life, and the slow shedding of follicle after follicle seemed to symbolize everything she had to lose.

Later, when her nurse Joanne had gotten her pain under control, I sat and talked with Ella. Open and receptive, eager to confide and be cared for, it soon became clear why she would become one of those patients who seem to be magnets for affection. She never talked directly about her suffering. Nor, at least to me, did she ever demand help and support. But, unlike so many others, she never resisted vulnerability, defenselessness, and connection. Quietly, without words, she told you she wanted you to be there. Silently, she seemed always to convey gratitude for your help. Everything you gave her and her family, every thought, visit, telephone call of inquiry, hand held, or bedpan emptied became a gift. It was impossible, no matter what the burden or the response of others, to stop or inhibit the flow of that exchange. The human connection was just too strong.

On the second night of her admission, as her nurse, sister-in-laws, and husband were standing outside her hospital room talking about the Chernobyl catastrophe, her husband turned to me—the writer—and asked if I would help compose a letter for him to send to his employer. He wanted to thank his boss for all his help during Ella's illness. I could hardly say no.

We sat in the solarium—a narrow room with a television and a crush of large blue imitation-leather recliners, a couple of neglected potted plants, a scattering of magazines, and a large television set—and he dictated the sentiments I was to translate into grammatical English. After the letter was satisfactorily executed, he broke down in tears as he confided his concerns for his dying wife and two surviving children—eight and eighteen respectively.

I reached out my hand and put it over his and he wept while I sat by his side in silence. There was nothing he asked for. Yet faced with the intensity of that suffering I felt the same kinds of pressures doctors and nurses encounter every day. I had to do something. I wrote my telephone number down on a piece of paper, told him to call if he needed anything, and, as we left the room, gave him a hug.

Over the next days I would visit Ella. As a journalist skilled at asking questions and getting information, I would ask her questions. But, as a human being suddenly caught up in the flood of someone else's pain, I simply could not stand there and objectively observe. Whenever I could I also tried to help. When Ella needed the nurse, I went out to call her; when she needed assistance getting to her portable commode, I let her lean on me and drew the curtain to give her some semblance of privacy. If her hair needed combing, I offered to do it. If she was thirsty, I went off in search of ginger ale, held the cup to her mouth, or cut up her food and sometimes fed it to her if she was too weak, as she often was, to do it for herself. Whenever it was possible to perform some minor act of succor, it seemed impossible, absolutely unthinkable, not to do so.

When she was not too tired, we would also talk. She told me something of her life in Russia, described her journey here and what she did when she first came. While we chatted, the meticulous former teacher would fastidiously collect any stray strands left on the bed and roll them into a tight coil she would deliberately place in the waste basket at her side. When she was too exhausted from the chemotherapy and anti-nausea antidotes she would ask me a few leading questions and encourage me to talk about my life in the United States. It became clear to me, that I was somehow her last American. She seemed to imbibe the stories of my life as if I was perhaps the American dream she was to be denied. So when she asked a question—where did you go to school? where did you live afterwards? how did you become a journalist?—how could I not answer? To refuse such personal revelation would have been an act of aggression.

The day she was discharged from the hospital, she asked if I would visit her at home. Again, it was impossible to say "no, sorry, you're the subject, I'm the objective observer, our relationship is merely instrumental and can go no further than this hospital room." Were I her nurse or her doctor, the sharing of these moments would have been far different. But I was neither and could use that freedom to follow the relationship as it developed. So, I said yes, I would call to see how she was, and visit if I could.

We met several times at her home for brief visits and when she was in the hospital for another round of chemotherapy. When I learned that her youngest child was the same age as my oldest daughter, I invited him over to play and picked him up and drove him home. When it was time for her son's birthday party, he invited my girls. The party was held at Chuck E Cheese's, a huge American pizza emporium with games for the children. Kids flowed like flood waters through the vast sanitized dining rooms when the pizza was served, only to drain away when the cake was eaten and the electronic games in an adjacent play area beckoned.

Ella was very sick by then. Her face was pallid; her long mane had been cropped short after her first round of chemotherapy and had grown sparser and sparser with each toxic treatment. She seemed able to walk only by drawing her two hands across her stomach and grasping them tight, as if constructing a girdle that would strengthen her failing musculature. This was supposed to be a joyous event, but she could barely smile. Her expressive face had suddenly become a canvas for variants of only one set of emotions—pain, suffering, and loss.

But she wanted to be there, had to be there, at what she knew, or at least suspected, would be the last birthday she would ever celebrate with her son. It was my role, I tacitly understood, to sit with her so that this event was not an unendurable exercise in loneliness. While the children raced in rambunctious oblivion through the commercial delights of Chuck E Cheese, and the fathers supervised, I kept Ella company in a deserted booth in a back room and bore witness to her pain.

Over those months I was overwhelmed by the sense that there was nothing I could *do* to help, and yet convinced that simply being with Ella was, in fact, doing a great deal. When she was in the hospital for one of her many rounds of chemotherapy, I visited each day at lunch time trying to dissuade her from ordering the overcooked fish that made even me nauseous. Order the baked potato, I encouraged, and when she did, I fed her small mouthfuls with the sour cream she so relished. Afterward she would sometimes doze off and then reawaken to ask," Is it okay that you're here? Do you have to go back to work?"

"Yes it's okay," I'd answer. Released from her anxiety her face would break into a wide, relaxed smile and she would command, "Tell me something interesting!"

"About what—the cosmos, the planet, the state, the family, politics, literature, or art?"

"Tell me about the children," she invariably answered. "How are your children?"

It was during one of those visits, on her fourth or was it fifth round of chemotherapy, one that seemed to be designed mainly to make her physician feel useful since it seemed to do no therapeutic good at all, that my role of supportive acquaintance turned into that of more active caregiver. Ella's condition had dramatically deteriorated, and with it the stress on her and her husband had escalated. I saw him and spoke with him frequently and could see how distressed he was. She was increasingly worried, too, about the fact that her sister—who was in the Soviet Union—could not seem to get a visa to visit the States and be with her during this critical period.

Because I'm a journalist and an inveterate asker of questions, I knew her story and each successive physical and emotional response to the treatments she received. I had, I was to realize afterward, become the repository of her illness narrative, a modern-day oral historian recording her needs and fears. Originally, I had no intention of putting this accumulated knowledge to use in the service of getting her the kind of care she needed. But one morning, when I came on to the unit and asked her nurse about her condition, I found I had no choice but to turn that peculiar status of scribe to work for her and her family.

When I questioned this nurse—one new to her case—about Ella's condition, the nurse willingly told me the physical details but confessed unabashedly that she had no idea how the patient was faring emotionally. Ella's primary and associate nurses were on vacation, and it was impossible to get a full account of this complicated case from the shorthand of the nursing and medical notes in her chart. "I just don't know her at all," the nurse said with regret. On further inquiry it turned out that the family had never asked the social worker on the unit to become much involved with her case, and the primary nurse on the outpatient unit, to which she had been only the most infrequent visitor, also had little intimate contact with her (this nurse was also having serious health problems of her own and was not able to reach out to Ella as she might normally have done.)

On gathering this information, I did not excuse myself, sit down, make a list of the pros and cons, and then make my decision. The decision imposed itself on me. Because I knew Ella and her family well, I quickly volunteered, "Would you like me to tell you what's troubling her and her family?" The nurse—a professional genuinely eager to gain any information that could facilitate better care—swiftly assented. I filled her in and then spoke with Ella's social worker. Over the next month, I became an informal liaison between family and professional caregivers.

My function, I soon realized, was not only narrator but translator and cultural guide. Even most Americans have difficulty navigating the turbulent waters of illness. As Russians recently immigrated to the U.S. they were doubly disadvantaged. Like the set of Russian dolls the family had brought with them to America, they found themselves enclosed in one foreign culture—America—only to discover that almost immediately they were to be entrapped in yet another—the culture of high-tech medicine. If they were only semi-literate in the language of the larger culture, they were totally illiterate in that of the subculture of medicine. Moreover, they were peculiarly ill-adapted to the demands of a how-to, voluntaristic culture where one is expected to advocate for oneself and establish an instant rapport with a shifting cast of professional caregivers.

These were people, after all, who had spent their entire adult lives in the Soviet Union mastering a stoic acceptance of whatever the system dictated. They were hardly disposed to advocate aggressively for themselves. Even had they been more confrontational or assertive, they were utterly bereft of the kind of knowledge that is the essential foundation for such confident self-assertion. How could they ask for hospice care when they didn't know what a hospice was? How inquire about DNR (Do Not Resuscitate orders) and code status, when these terms were truly a part of an indecipherable code to them?

But it was not code to me. So I helped to tutor them in this new vocabulary. My job, I knew, was not to presume to be able to answer questions, but simply to advise them about what the right questions were and to whom to address them. Ask your nurse, ask your doctor, was my constant refrain.

It also became my job to clarify murky and confusing signals that the family sent out to the professional caregivers. Near the end of Ella's life, for example, her nurse Joanne Carey worried because the family had not brought her eight-year-old son to the hospital to see his mother before she died. Aware that many families assume that a child visiting a dying parent will be so traumatized by the experience that it is better to simply let the parent die and tell the child after the fact, she wanted the family to know that a parent's disappearance can be even more traumatic than final good-byes.

She explained her concerns to me, and described the family's difficulty hearing them. The next night, when Ella's husband called me, he talked about his desperation and grief. I realized I had an opening. "Are you going to bring your son to see Ella?" I asked. He paused and one could hear the anguish infusing his silence. He expressed the concern which Joanne Carey had identified. It was a terribly difficult thing to say—one of those walking-on-eggs experiences that had come to typify each encounter—but I tried gently to tease out his fear. "You know, it's your decision, and we'll support whatever you choose. But don't assume that it will be worse for him to see his mother and say good-bye than not to see her. Sometimes it's worse for a child to have a parent simply disappear than to be able to say good-bye to her. But remember, it's your decision. Just make it soon because she may not be conscious and able to say that good-bye."

The next afternoon he brought the two kids to the hospital. Ella was conscious and they said their good-byes. That night I knew I had to say mine as well. When my father was dying of cancer years before, and a friend of lung cancer only two months earlier, I gained first-hand experience of the windows of opportunity death constructs. When someone is dying, you cannot have closure too early, or too late. A hasty revelation of one's affection and grief can make your loved one anxious—"Why is she saying this? he or she may think "Does she know something about my imminent demise that I don't know?" Nor can you wait too long, when they are too sick, perhaps even comatose, and cannot listen.

That evening I exercised this new-found skill. I knew Ella would die soon and that her death would be preceded by a period of unconsciousness. If I wanted to say good-bye, I had better say it now. So before leaving I gently tugged her back from her drug-induced sleep.

"Ella, I'm going for the night. I'll be back tomorrow," I whispered, and bending over I kissed her and said, "I love you."

She smiled one last beautiful smile and said "I love you too."

The next morning all her systems "crashed." I had come to the hospital early to see her and found her nurse outside her room worriedly reviewing her chart and checking her lab results. "Everything has shut down," she explained and then added with an almost frantic sense of urgency, "but they have her scheduled for an MRI and she's getting all this fluid." The nurse explained that moving a dying patient in and out of bed, onto gurneys, to other floors, into a huge machine and then back again, would be sheer torture—and for no reason whatsoever. After all, the patient was dying. That was obvious. What useful purpose would further information about the progress of her disease serve since there was nothing further to be done? She also explained that giving a patient too much fluid when her kidneys have shut down only causes fluid overload and greater agony.

Recognizing how easily the invasive medical machine can literally run over patients even when providers want it stopped, I caught her urgency and insisted, "That can't be allowed to happen. What can be done?" She needed to talk to the intern, she said, who then in turn could alert Ella's attending physician to her status. While she did not hesitate to do this, my presence and assurances that this is what Ella and the family would want seemed to sustain her. We walked down to the nurses' station where the intern—a tall, tired-looking man in his early thirties, sat reviewing charts. After she explained the changes in Ella's medical status, he agreed that treatment should be stopped. Moreover, he seemed relieved to hear that others shared his opinion.

But he had to consider the medical hierarchy—notably the attending physician who had ordered these tests. "I don't want to torture her either," the intern said. "We should stop and just let her go. But I'm not getting clear signals from the attending. This is always the way it is with him, one minute he tells us he wants us to let the patient go, the next he's ordering a battery of tests and hydration."

The nurse cut to the quick of his dilemma. "You need to call and tell him what's happening. He hasn't been here, he hasn't seen the labs, and doesn't know. Her kidneys have totally shut down. What's the point of all this?"

He reached for the phone and called the attending physician, who, thank goodness, concurred. Then she told the intern to tell the attending the family should be called to come in to be with Ella.

That done, he put down the phone and smiled. For them, it was not a moment of sadness but one of great triumph. I understood the real meaning of the term—almost a cliché in the health care field—of a "death with comfort and dignity." Now they had been liberated to care for Ella. That was a victory, not a defeat.

During her last two days, Ella lay in bed, sedated, as if her spirit were simply awaiting release from a body whose only mission was to end its sojourn so that her soul could move on. I came to visit several times before she died, and spent hours as her husband and sisters-in-law kept their vigil. Each time I planned to leave, something seemed to interfere. Her husband needed a break, but didn't want to leave his dying wife alone. So I stayed while he went for a much-needed walk. Ella's sister-in-law worried because the sedated patient had lain in one position for a day and a half. She asked the nurse to turn her and we stayed and watched. But this simple physical act jarred her out of her sedation. Her eyes opened with a look of agony and she screamed "niet, niet" (no, no). Horrified by the thought that she requested an act that hurt this vulnerable, dying woman, her sister-in-law collapsed in my arms and begged me, "Suzanne, please don't leave me alone." So again, I stayed.

As I sat through those almost endless hours, I was impressed with what it means to be what Patricia Benner has called the compassionate stranger. I was someone these people could talk to about their memories, their fears, their past, and their future. They told me about Ella's life in Russia, about their own struggles coming to America, the difficulties of adjustment, learning a new language, building a new life. And then this! they lamented, shifting their eyes to Ella as if, in that simple glance, conveying a universe of despair.

I was also impressed with the power of ordinary conversation in times of crisis. After we talked about Ella's life and her dying, the conversation would magically turn to the most prosaic—a recipe for herring salad, where to buy provisions, the new markets and restaurants the Soviet Jews had created in this new land. I remember, looking cautiously at

Ella while her sister-in-law and I discussed the intricacies of whitefish. Could she hear? Would she mind that we had found a moment of respite in the comforting details of daily life? Then I realized that this was my function now—to let her loved ones lead me where they needed to go so that, while Ella lay groaning so, they could both resurrect her and affirm their own lives—life itself.

Ella died on Saturday morning. Her nurse was with her, but not her family. At the family's request, I came to the hospital to see her and accompany the family to the funeral home to make their final arrangements. Again, I was the American interpreter—in this case the American Jew explaining some of the intricacies of an orthodox Jewish funeral to Soviet Jews who, despite their persecution, had been able to learn nothing about the Jewish religion.

Apart from the sustained contact I knew her family and I would have, I thought this hospital engagement with Ella and her dying was over. It appeared that there was one final complication to face—the very unexpected, but on reflection hardly surprising, response of some of the professional caregivers who seemed unable to understand or tolerate my "involvement" with this case.

I was not prepared for this because most of the professional caregivers I worked with seemed to appreciate and honor my relationship with Ella. These penultimate caregivers knew that someone like me—a person neither insider nor outsider to the medical treatment system— could be helpful to an immigrant family with little knowledge of the dizzying array of death "choices" available to the modern consumer of health care. They recognized clearly that in the last days of Ella's life, she and her husband were not going to become "educated health care consumers" who could take responsibility for their own health care outcomes. Although they were concerned about how I would react to the inevitable outcome, they were delighted to help me provide assistance in any way they could.

Moreover, they also understood that my experiences as a caregiver would help me comprehend their work and dilemmas more immediately and effectively than hours of interviews and observation sessions. Having taken the time to get to know me, they also realized that this involvement was not soul threatening but soul enhancing. As one of the nurses said to me one day, "There are some patients who just break your heart. And if they don't it's not worth working here." Thus their mission was not to save me from myself but to allow me to be myself, not to save me from pain but to allow me to learn from it.

That was not, unfortunately, the case with some physicians and even some nurses. Indeed, their responses to my involvement with this dying woman and her family were some of the most instructive and illuminating experiences I have ever had. Unlike the expert caregivers I was writing about, I believe they interpreted my concern and involvement as a disturbing and unwelcome challenge. Because of the heavy dose of sorrow nurses and physicians must tolerate, some feel they have to draw lines in the sand, boundaries neither they nor patients and families are supposed to cross. One of Ella's nurses, for example, expressed great frustration when, during the final days of her life, Ella's husband wanted the nurse's home phone number. "He wants to deal with only one person about all this. But I can't do that. He has to learn to trust the other nurses."

I could certainly understand her need to keep her private and professional lives separate in order to prevent a total fusion of the two. For nurses and physicians, this constant barrage of suffering can become intolerable, and rituals of distance are crucial to their ability to maintain their commitment to their profession. I also learned later that her nurse-manager heartily discouraged any personal "involvement" with patients. On the other hand, I could also understand the family's despair, their need to have one person they could trust. I tried to explain that in this chaotic, anguished period her family could not be expected constantly to shift the gift of their confidence from one professional to another. She listened, but in that moment, torn between her supervisor's dictates and the family's needs, she placed me in the family's camp and perceived me as a judgmental participant blaming her and finding fault.

It is thus, I realized, that conflicts arise between families and professionals. Family members feel that their world is collapsing when a loved one is sick or dying. They demand an exclusive focus on their agony, an appreciation of what they will lose or have lost. When their education and institution supports it, some professional caregivers can convey the sense of devotion that enables families to survive this kind of ordeal. In this case, however, some staff seemed to try to control rather than facilitate the delivery of care.

I was caught in the middle.

What was more alarming was the fact that these staff members extended their rules of limited emotional engagement not only to the nurses they supervised but to me as well. When it became clear to them that I would not abide by their rules, that I was breaking frame and could no longer be neatly compartmentalized as either objective journalistic observer or family caregiver, this seemed to cause them considerable discomfort.

Whenever I appeared in Ella's room, one senior nurse seemed to withdraw into purse-lipped disapproval. Sometimes she would corner me in the hallway and grill me about "how I was doing." Her concerns were always cast in the most altruistic language. Nonetheless, it soon became evident that when she said, "I'm worried about how you're doing and how you're going to handle this," she really meant she was worried about her ability to deal with my relationship to Ella.

Similarly, when I was walking outside Ella's room early one morning, another nurse came up to me and frantically began to warn me against "over-involvement" with a patient. "You just can't do this with every patient," she ordered "You'll never survive over the long term if you do." In vain, I tried to explain that I was not a nurse, that I was not going to be on her floor for the next five years, or even the next year. Nor did I have any intention of getting involved with every subject I observed. Heedless of my words, desperate to save me from myself, she sputtered on, repeating the same caveats until, fortuitously, the incessant ringing of one of her patients' buzzers extricated me from the weight of her concern.

Then there was an oncologist I had gotten to know. He, too, was worried about my long-term emotional survival. In the clinic hall one afternoon, when I burst into a brief flurry of tears, he told me that I would have a harder time with Ella's death than anyone else on the unit. "You identify with her," he announced confidently," and you don't have the professional buffers we have."

I received his concerns politely, but could not help musing on the all too common assumption that any involvement or caring for others must be governed by some deep narcissistic identification with that human being. All through Ella's illness I was struck with precisely the opposite. What Ella had, in fact, taught me were the limits of identification. There was clearly a bond between us—two dark-haired Jewish women, one a sufferer, one, at least for that moment, an observer of suffering. Two women whose families had escaped from the same country—one more than a hundred years ago, one only two years ago. Two women with children—one who would leave them soon, the other who would remain near her own as long as she could.

Yet, throughout her illness and our intermittent exchanges, I think we both recognized how little we knew of each other and how small and constricted were the places we filled in each other's lives. I remember with great immediacy the hugs we shared when we greeted each other when she was well enough to stand on her own. We held each other for a few moments as if acknowledging this peculiar bond. She knew that I knew very little about her and that she did not have the time or energy to alter that fact. I knew that she knew very little about me and that I would not, nor could not, remedy that. Nonetheless, she knew that I cared about her and her family, and I knew that fact meant a great deal to her.

In spite of my realization of the otherness of Ella, this notion that one can only care for someone else because of an intense, almost uncontained identification seemed to prevail. When I was leaving the hushed hospital one evening, I bumped into an oncology fellow, who asked me how I was doing. When I told him about Ella's condition, he cautioned, "Just remember, Suzanne, there's one rule in the House of God. The patient has the disease, you don't." Floored by this meaningless slogan, a kind of medical "Read my lips—no new feelings," I replied, "Martin, I know I don't have cancer" (unless, that is, he knew something about my body that I didn't). To which he retorted. "Well, it keeps you sane."

"So do feelings," I hurled at his departing posterior.

By the time Ella died, I realized that the concerted efforts of these well-meaning professionals to keep me from feeling any sorrow were becoming more difficult to cope with than Ella's dying itself. Sorrow, anger, loss, grief—these were all emotions I could confront and accept. But this constant need to feint and parry in what had apparently become an obstacle course of caveats and controlling concerns took more energy and was more depleting than helping Ella and her family negotiate death.

During the period when Ella was actively dying, these "professionals" managed to make me feel I was doing something wrong by visiting her on the floor and providing comfort to her family. Because of their purse-lipped disapproval, I refrained from coming to relieve her husband the morning she died, and as a result she died alone.

By the time I arrived at the hospital to say good-bye to my dead friend and share her family's grief, I thought I would throttle the next person who offered me some neatly packaged platitude about the virtues of detachment. And indeed, as I was walking off the unit with Ella's husband and sister-in-law, who had asked me to accompany them to the funeral parlor to make burial arrangements, a very well-meaning, young nurse came up to me and hugged me. As she expressed her condolences, she also shared her puzzlement. "Do you do this because it makes you feel good, because it makes you feel useful?"

Standing there, at the nurses' station, I felt like screaming. "No it does not make me feel good to see this lovely woman lying in her bed stone cold dead. No I don't enjoy trips to funeral homes, or endless discussions about hospice versus hospital care. Sometimes you do things because people need help!" But there were people around, places to go, a grieving family to deal with and a woman to bury. So I said nothing and walked out in silence.

My relationship with this dying woman and her family had clearly affected a number of "caregivers" in ways I had not predicted. Even as long as two months after Ella was dead, one of these nurses pursued me, inquiring why "this involvement" had occurred. She wondered repeatedly if "*it* would happen again" with another patient. Although we never actually addressed the issue directly, her concerns gave me a taste of the kinds of pressures professional caregivers experience. Rather than celebrating connection, she and many others had pathologized it. In their presence, this profoundly human act of gift exchange was something that had to be justified. I finally understood that this nurse might be using me as a messenger. Through my example and her response to it, she was reminding others to respect the boundaries she had erected. The very fact that she was concerned least "it" happen again, signal that for her engagement with other human beings was something one should feel guilty about, rather than proud of.

It was thus that I realized how toxic caring has become in a society bent on disengagement and autonomy. Here, in capsule form, swarming around this episode, were all the various fears and anxieties about caregiving I had been reflecting on and writing about for the past four years. Apart from the expert caregivers I worked so closely with, most people seemed to assume that any but the most circumscribed involvement with people in trouble would be engulfing and endangering. They seemed unable to recognize that professionals and even some nonprofessionals can calibrate involvement, that, as that one nurse said, if some people don't break your heart it's not worth it.

Similarly, none of these Cassandras seemed able to believe that human beings can mobilize judgment even in the midst of the most deeply felt engagements and experiences. Seduced by the logic of the rationalistic philosophies that so dominate our culture, many are convinced that you cannot let down the iron curtain of detachment once without demolishing it forever. Despite my assurances that this was to be my "one involvement," (now I marvel at the fact that I was coerced into giving such assurances in the first place) people seemed certain that I had somehow become a sponge for sorrow, someone who would forever prowl the halls of hospitals looking for lost causes and desperate cases.

And finally, of course, I kept hurtling against what clinical nurse specialist Adele Pike calls "malignant entitlement," the belief that only medical professionals can shoulder the burdens of the human condition and tolerate pain and sorrow. It is indisputably true that in our unbalanced world some have a greater share of death and disease than most others. But those outside the hospital walls are also not strangers to suffering. We have friends who die or are in trouble. We have had problems of our own and have developed the skills to cope with these dilemmas. In this peculiar perversion of the ethic of universal benevolence—this oh-so-modern desire to save others from suffering—we oddly refuse to allow others to learn that sanity does not only lie in the path of detachment, but can also abound on journeys of the most intimate personal and emotional discovery.

After two weeks of shielding myself from this kind of concern, I began to clearly understand the terrible toll of the medical education in detachment. I was 46 years old when Ella died. I'd had a death or two in my time, friends in pain, years of attempts at reflection and self analysis. I was ten or fifteen years older than most of the people counseling disengagement. I could easily insist and believe that "feelings keep you sane." But what if I were 25 or 30? How would I respond to my teachers and mentors who had only this one-note samba to sing. Would I persist in my quest to understand not only disease but illness, not only organs but the complicated reactions and experiences of the people who shelter them? Or would I begin to doubt myself, wonder if I was some sort of "care addict," afflicted by a terminal case of "burn-out," who needed to recover not explore? It is in the installation of this insidious variation of self-doubt, I believe, that the medical system constructs its greatest tragedy and imposes its greatest barrier between the world of care and cure.

I began as well to understand the inadequate explanations we often offer to explain our deepest human engagements. Ella was supposed to be my "journalistic subject." But she hardly fit into that compartment. I have never believed in the all-American myth of journalistic objectivity. If I like and connect with the people who allow me into their lives, I do not deny the pull of friendship and affection. In this particular case objectivity was impossible. I have said that I learned more about caregiving from Ella than I have ever learned in my life. That learning could not have emerged from distance. It had to come from closeness. The border between journalist and subject had to be crossed.

That did not, however, make me a "family member," as some of the nurses and doctors who were so dismayed or disturbed by our relationship seemed to believe. I was most definitely not that. Indeed, I would never have been able to help Ella and her family if I had been some kind of co-dependent, over-identifier, or even worse, a newly adopted member of her family. Had I been a family member, I would never have been able to tolerate the question-asking and information-gathering process her death demanded and calmly comfort her relatives during and after the dying process. To do this, I had to be an outsider—a compassionate stranger, or Good Samaritan, temporarily occupying the same space as the wounded traveler, but moving toward a different destination.

Finally, there was another category into which our relationship did not fit—that of "professional volunteer," a recruit ready to enlist in the service of every hard case that came along. The doctors and nurses who were so puzzled by my relationship with Ella kept flailing at this myth: if I cared with such intensity for Ella, I would inevitably fall into a deep and bottomless pit filled with grasping, drowning victims who would suffocate me in the quicksand of their suffering.

This notion denies the very essence of caregiving as many professional caregivers define it. Over and over again, some of the same nurses who complained about my relationship with Ella advised me that caring is not intuitive, not dependent on hormones, but is rather a skill, gleaned not only from books but through the process of social learning. Caring is something nurses learn about from their patients and from each other, they repeated. In its service you use judgment, set limits, and delineate boundaries. These boundaries are not fluid; these judgments are often based on skilled intuition; the limits vary according to the individuals involved. How ironic, then, that in their obsessive concerns about my relationship with a dying patient some caregivers were denying their abilities as teachers and role models.

What caring for Ella helped me understand is that caregiving creates new spaces and new categories. For me, Ella occupied a space reserved for relationships that lie outside of the comfortable geography of professional or even everyday personal exchange. Although I am not a religious person, from the very first I think I recognized that Ella occupied a spiritual space in my life. Because there was nothing material I could do to save her, my role was quite simply to help her die. Our relationship was formed around the unspoken sacredness of that trust, around my gradual understanding of it and her acceptance and need of it.

I did not want her to die and would have done anything possible to prevent it. I hoped she would have as long as she could without the agony and disgrace of that futile, final battle. It was because I was not caught in that tight circle of companionship whose destruction is always so intolerable, unthinkable to those within that I could cope with her dying, and therefore had no need to deny or delay, hasten or confront.

I could mobilize my skills to ask the questions that needed to be asked, find out to whom to address them and tell her story to whomever needed to know it. None of this was ever done dispassionately or objectively — those ridiculous words with which we burden our most human acts and impulses; everything was excruciating, a parade of clichés — "walking on eggs." Because my energy was not devoured by anger, anxiety, fear, or despair, I was available to her family and to her professional caregivers.

I did this without ever imagining that I had replaced either the latter or the former. Indeed, the fact that I was not a professional caregiver working in the institution in which Ella was treated gave me the same kind of freedom of action, negotiation, and inquiry that my status as non-family member provided. I was not responsible for the systems or strategies of professional care upon which Ella depended at the end of her life. I did not have to feel guilt because I could do so much and no more. No one ever imposed on me the kind of unrealistic demands professional caregivers in our medical system are expected to fulfill. No one ever imagined that I could save Ella, provide round-the-clock assistance to her and her family, or erase her physical and emotional pain. Because of this freedom of movement, I could utilize my intimate knowledge of the system in which professionals deliver care to hopefully help them deliver it.

Ella remains for me a living presence. She was not a friend. The imperatives of her condition made impossible the kind of reciprocity and mutual sharing of history upon which friendships are based. What I know of her life is how she lived her illness and her death. What I know of her history, I learned when she lay dying or after she was dead. She was not a subject, a family member, the object of the charity of a devoted volunteer. She inhabits the world of care—a space which can accommodate relationships that defy the conventional categories to which we assign and categorize our human encounters and connections. In her dying, for me, she lived on a vast, horizonless plain that allows one the freedom to be human for and with another. Now that she is gone, she resides in that same limitless and impossible-to-chart territory of joy, sorrow, and compassion—only this time in memory.

Chapter 12
Two Stories of Caring in Teaching

James G. Henderson

Editors' note. In the following stories, we hear the voices of caring teachers. Readers will be impressed again by the competence that accompanies genuine caring. When we care, we work hard to meet our professional and personal responsibilities. Both Ms. Callahan and Mr. Meyers are reflective problem-solvers. Indeed, the author of the book in which these stories appear emphasizes the teachers' competence as inquirers. Caring is manifested in many ways, but clearly, it always involves direct, receptive attention to the recipients of care and reflective attention to one's own attempts to meet their needs.

Introduction

Maura Callahan and Eugene Meyers exemplify the inquiring, reflective teaching model. Both teachers fit Noddings's (1984) description of the caring teacher. They take the time to dialogue with their students; they work cooperatively with them; and they help each individual discover his or her best self. Eugene Meyers's description of how he teaches the concept of point of view and Maura Callahan's technique for teaching persuasive writing are examples of applied constructivist learning theory. When problems arise in the classroom, these teachers invest the time and energy necessary to find the solution that is best for the student, not just for themselves. Finally, both teachers are questioning, challenging, probing individuals who seek personal professional growth for themselves and intellectual, emotional, and social growth for their students through the process of inquiry.

An earlier version of this essay appeared in Henderson, *Reflective Teaching* (New York: Macmillan, 1992), pp. 1–25. Reprinted by permission.

Maura Callahan: Unless It's Me in That Work, What Good Is It?

Maura Callahan has been teaching elementary school children for 6 years. She began teaching in a Catholic school on the northwest side of Chicago. Later she taught behaviorally disturbed preadolescent boys in an urban residential facility. Now she teaches in a combination learning disability/behavior disorder first-grade classroom. She also coordinates a holistic reading and language arts program for the first through fifth grades.

Building on Her Past Experiences

As a beginning teacher Maura Callahan was unsure of her six-year-old students' developmental levels and interests. She *was* sure, however, of her own basic philosophy of learning: "Unless it was me in that work, what good is it?" She explains, "Learning is not going to be any fun unless it's about me. And if it's not any fun, it's not going to be worth anything."

Ms. Callahan's philosophy grew out of her own learning experiences. She recalls her elementary school education as dreadful, bleak, and boring. Her teachers were impersonal and distant. "Nobody taught *children*, they taught *subjects* to children," she observes. When Ms. Callahan began teaching she was determined to make a better impression on her own students. From the start she felt a strong sense of identification with them:

I could have been that child sitting in that classroom. I really wanted to let them know that I was a human being, and I was a kid once too. It's hard to be a kid, and I always told them that.

As a college art student Callahan had realized that she achieved her best results when she saw a connection between herself and her work. When her work was not tied to her own experiences in some way, she was not motivated to learn. "It would have no meaning for me," she recalls. Today all her teaching decisions are guided by that one premise: that no matter how old students are or what their abilities, each student must find something of "me"—something of that student's self—in the curriculum.

Confirmation and Dialogue

Ms. Callahan's recollections of her own early school experiences made her sensitive to her students' needs. For example, she remembered that she had difficulty each morning getting focused on school. "I remember myself," she says, "coming from a rather stormy home, the lack of concentration, thinking about what went on at home. I couldn't have cared less about capitalizing the pronoun 'I.'"

To ease students' transition from home to school, Ms. Callahan invites them to discuss, privately and in confidence, anything they want to talk about during a daily session she calls "talk time." She knows that addressing students' concerns early in the day enables them to turn their attention more quickly to the tasks at hand. The ritual of talk time sets the stage each day for meaningful student learning. Callahan's caring approach toward her students is a reaction to negative experiences in her own childhood, when teachers talked to her in an intrusive, contrived manner. Today she consciously strives for a positive, supportive, and genuine relationship with her students.

Ms. Callahan believes that focusing on each individual's talents helps students find their own best selves. She and her students often discuss their talents:

"I think I have talent in art," and, "I did such and such at home," or, "I enjoyed these types of pictures that you showed me." We go at it from that angle. Because they know that's the angle I am stressing in the classroom. Apparently it clicks with them then. They look within themselves to see what their talents are, what they like to do, and what they need to do to get some help to do some more. Budding artists come to talk to me because they know that I was in art before teaching. They think that is really neat, that a teacher who isn't in the art room can draw.

Ms. Callahan tries to help each student in her classroom "to find himself or herself in terms of what they're about, what they're good at, what they can do, and what's important to them." She has never had a set formula for helping students find their best selves. Rather, she encourages them to follow their dreams. She tells them that they can do and have things in life that they may think are not possible.

While helping her students to find their best selves, Ms. Callahan shares her own self with them. She tells them about her experiences as a child and as a commercial artist, about her talents and interests, and about the people who helped her during various stages of her life. By confiding in her students, Ms. Callahan encourages them to confide in her. She hopes her students perceive her as a person whom they can talk to and a person who will really listen.

Constructivist Teaching

In her first year of teaching Ms. Callahan considered various established methods of teaching young children to write, such as rote learning, copying, dictation, and sounding out letters. Guided by her philosophy of "unless it's me in that work, what good is it?" she rejected all these methods. She chose instead to have first-grade students write about the babyish things they used to do.

The students generated their own ideas following her examples. Each student gathered ideas, and she helped them with writing and spelling. They learned how to write a rough draft and proofread one another's papers. Using samples from the library, Ms. Callahan showed them different ways to make a book containing their own texts and illustrations.

They had a vehicle for structure in which they could start to write, plus they could bring in their own experience. Because I felt if we were not talking about ourselves, who would care to write?

Ms. Callahan recalls some of her students' writings: "I used to think babies fell out of the air. I used to think that God was sneezing when there was thunder. I used to think there was a little man in the radio talking." The class delighted in the fact that one idea was funnier than the other. The students were excited about their initial writing experiences because "these were all things that came out of their lives." Ms. Callahan had found a connection between the school's curriculum and each student's self.

Maura Callahan has often had to choose between teaching in a "bookish format" and teaching "within the realm of the world that they know." She steadfastly has chosen the latter.

Anything that I ever taught, I've always tried to see what it would mean in terms of their day-to-day life. Because I really don't believe that it would mean anything to them unless it was connected.

The way she accomplishes this is "totally my own way" and never through prepackaged materials. When she teaches rhyming couplets, for example, "there I am with the kids, a hunk of paper, and a bag of markers." Together they create couplets using the students' suggestions. "A lot of it is from their day-to-day lives," Ms. Callahan notes, "and that's that."

As a reflective teacher Ms. Callahan relates subject matter to her student's experiences, needs, and interests. In her fifth-grade language arts class she draws on her students' familiarity with commercial advertising to teach persuasive writing techniques. First she asks students to list their favorite television commercials. She selects a few examples to analyze with the class. Ms. Callahan describes their reaction:

It's a very interesting experience, because they are extremely enthusiastic about this. We talk about what it actually means to persuade somebody to do something. I have them bring in the ads because this is one of the most obvious forms of persuasion. I have them think about how you explain to your mother why you need to buy a certain thing, or why she should drive you to a baseball game. What you're trying to do is to change somebody's mind. They actually analyze their own kind of strategies in conversations that way. Then I say, "how would you like to make your own commercial?" They get very excited, because this is one thing they've never done.

Ms. Callahan encourages her students to create an innovative product of their own. Students analyze and carry out all the steps of a presentation to make people want the product. They write scripts and work out illustrations. Then Ms. Callahan guides them in putting it all together. They deliver the presentation themselves, on tape, so that they learn about voice, inflection, and how to address a group. "We end up with the most wonderful back-to-back ads show that you would ever want to see," declares Ms. Callahan.

To judge the effectiveness of her methods, Ms. Callahan observes students' reactions in class. Her class is always noisy, filled with laughter and fun. It is loud "with a purpose," she explains. "I'm always looking for something I can make their own."

I used to see in our reading lab situations with teachers who are very much by the book and for the book. The kids used to sit there like bumps on a log. Get somebody with a more creative bent, who connects the learning experience to the kids' real lives, and you'd have the same kids literally jumping on desks — much to the chagrin of those other teachers, who would complain about the noise. But that's how I've always judged it.

Ms. Callahan makes a distinction between teaching methods that are both fun and meaningful and those that involve "pulling a rabbit out of a hat," or fun that does not sustain any meaningful learning. Examples of the latter include such activities as work sheets or games that keep kids busy but don't help them learn.

I've seen children dance, clap, and jump up and down with teachers who pull rabbits out of hats. Those are the types of lessons and experiences in school that may be fun for awhile, but it's nothing that continues on, or really reaches anything in a meaningful way.

Ms. Callahan notes that many new teachers have learned plenty of "rabbit-out-of-the-hat techniques" in their methods classes. She suggests that teachers need to evaluate the purpose of such activities before using them.

Artistic Problem-Solving

Her 6 years of teaching have not been without challenges. Ms. Callahan recalls Mark, her first learning disabled student to be mainstreamed for reading. Even though he did well in the reading group, he would return to class emotionally drained, and he sometimes became violent. Ms. Callahan spoke to the reading teacher and to Mark, but was unable to identify the problem. She then contacted Mark's mother, who described Mark's unusual behavior at home. Every morning Mark would stare at himself in the bathroom mirror and say he hated school. His appetite was decreasing and his temper tantrums at home were growing more frequent.

On the basis of what she had learned, Ms. Callahan decided to take a low-key approach at school. One day when she found Mark hitting another student during recess, Ms. Callahan embraced him and said, "I know that you're really hurting inside, Mark. Something is bothering you, and I'm not sure what it is." She continued this supportive, nonjudgmental approach and consulted frequently with Mark's mother. Eventually they discovered that Mark was upset because students in the mainstream class had ridiculed him for his weight and his clumsiness in gym class. Mark feared he would never have any friends in the new classroom.

Relieved that students were not stigmatizing him because of his learning disabilities, Ms. Callahan continued to offer Mark her support. She helped him realize that his violent reactions would not make students like him better. In time, Mark was able to make friends in the new class. Once he knew that his classmates really did care about him, his aggressive behaviors ceased.

A less caring teacher might have handled this situation quite differently. Instead of looking for the cause of Mark's problem, she might have punished him for the symptom—aggressive behavior—and ostracized him even further. Perhaps this situation would have culminated in Mark's removal from the mainstream class. Such disciplinary action would have been easy and convenient for the teacher, but it would have been a serious disservice to Mark. Instead Ms. Callahan gathered information, reflected on the situation, and made the decision to support her student in overcoming his problem and moving one step closer to his own best self.

Cooperative Practice

Ms. Callahan encourages strong parent-teacher relationships, a practice she established during her early years in the Catholic school. "Having the interaction with parents, and trying to look at children holistically, was second nature to me, because this is what happens in a private school." The parents wanted their children to be there, and many made financial sacrifices to enable them to attend that school. Teachers and parents shared the common goal of educating the children. In the public school, some colleagues found Ms. Callahan's focus on parent-teacher relationships unusual.

But looking at the children and their needs, I realized immediately that I couldn't do this job without the help of all of those parents. Most of the kids came from single-parent homes. I got to know a lot about what went on out of school. I knew there was no way that school could mean anything unless we were all in this together.

Keeping in touch with students' parents is not easy. Ms. Callahan often stays at school until 6:00 p.m. and invites parents for informal meetings. She is convinced that the extra effort is worth it. With parents' cooperation, she believes, any problem can be resolved.

I tell the parents, "You're here and I'm here, we can work this out. We can do it." It requires getting to know the parents and building a trusting relationship with them.

Ms. Callahan noted that parents' eagerness to provide the best for their children sometimes seems to backfire. Numerous parents hold second jobs to help pay for music lessons, sports equipment, fashionable clothes, and the like. With all the activities and jobs, however, some families never have the time to eat a meal together. Families are physically and emotionally fragmented, and some kids have no one they feel they can really confide in. In addition, Ms. Callahan worries that constant shuttling among organized activities stifles students' natural creativity.

Sure, they might be learning how to dance or swim, but I think they are learning how *not* to have one imaginative bone in their bodies, or to dream, or to just sit and watch a cloud go by like I used to do. I think the shuttling kind of dulls their ability to get in touch with that creative part of themselves.

Students are so accustomed to structure and organization that they are unable to respond creatively when no structure is provided. Instead they express boredom and a desire to be entertained. Fortunately, Ms. Callahan was surprised to discover, it is not difficult to stimulate their imaginations.

I think everything I do and the way I do it is so different from anything they have seen in a schoolroom that I am very appealing to them. With young children, if they like the teacher, they'll go along with you. Once they're in your power you can turn them on to the power within themselves.

Eventually students carry their excitement about classroom learning to their out-of-school lives. They begin to talk about school with enthusiasm and share their schoolwork with their parents. In turn, parents visit the classroom to see why their children are so excited about school.

Setting and Achieving Personal-Professional Goals

How did Ms. Callahan develop the agility to meet administrative criteria without sacrificing her own teaching values and philosophy? She feels that confidence in herself and her goals was the key.

I know I am a good teacher, and I'm confident about what I'm doing. If the principal walks to my room, I am able to explain the rationale for what I am doing. I'm not fearful. I'm not fearful because I believe in my teaching, and I believe that I can provide a rationale that in some way will be compatible with the objectives of the district.

She admits that this confidence is not handed out along with your degree. It requires hard work, careful self-evaluation, and a willingness to adapt. Unfortunately many pre-service teacher education programs fail to provide students an opportunity for reflection. She advocates a more diversified approach.

We may have to throw out the teacher manual and look for each person's "raw material." We need to recognize the people involved are the primary source, not some book. A strong sense of reflection within one's own experiences, within one's own curriculum, is what brings a person to the realization that "unless I am in this, it's not going to have any significant value to me at all." If anything is really going to stick or take place or have an effect, then it has to come from within. That's a belief a teacher must have. And unless that belief is conscious, there will be no evidence of it in practice.

The structure of many educational institutions does not encourage reflection. Instead, Ms. Callahan notes, the institutions require people to play games—"games within classrooms at school, games to obtain credentials, and games to satisfy the expectations of the district." Having to play such games clouds a person's own philosophy.

We waltz around in this cloud of denial, in this cloud of artificiality that is not as passive a thing as we think it is. It's destroying the chance to really speak the truth, and to identify the problem, as we pretend that it doesn't exist.

Ms. Callahan strives for a return to reality. "I think that more kids can be reached by getting down to the nuts and bolts . . . to what really is going to matter, what really is going to last when we learn anything in life." In many school districts, however, teachers are expected to simply follow the philosophy imposed from above rather than their own. In Harry Wolcott's (1973) book *The Man in the Principal's Office* he states, "There are no individual philosophies in a school district, there is only one [top-down] philosophy, the rest are merely attitudes."

When a teacher's own philosophy, which I believe should be the guiding force, is reduced to a mere attitude, we have a very serious problem. I've seen many good teachers put to death by an attitude. When I read that statement, it occurred to me that our organized learning attempt has been, in a sense, our own death warrant. (290)

When teachers who know what students are interested in and would like to pursue or teach something else instead, both teachers and students end up leading a double life. Ms. Callahan adamantly refuses to do this. She attributes her success as a teacher to her philosophy of "always striving for the reality to come through" in her classroom.

Eugene Meyers: Celebrating Students, Friends for Life

Eugene Meyers is a veteran of 21 years of teaching. He taught for 10 years in primarily black schools in Chicago. Eleven years ago he was reassigned to his current location, a racially balanced school in an integrated area. Mr. Meyers teaches English to academically talented seventh- and eighth-grade students. He also teaches independent studies in literature and creative writing to juniors and seniors.

Constructing Personal-Professional Knowledge

Unlike Maura Callahan, who conscientiously applied her insights about her own learning to her teaching, Eugene Meyers began teaching without a clear idea of the type of teacher he wanted to become. At first, he recalls, his greatest concern was maintaining control of the class.

I always used to think my options were either to have everyone sitting behind a desk or to have Cuisenaire rods flying all over the place. Later I learned there was a way for me to have sufficient control over the dynamics to be able to go where I wanted to go and teach my students in a much more real way.

He was inspired by visions of caring teaching portrayed in movies and books from the 1960s, such as Sidney Poitier's character in *To Sir with*

Love. But he quickly discovered that it was impossible to emulate some-one else's style of teaching. "You can't be somebody else," he says. What you can do, however, is work on developing your own personal teaching qualities, values, and beliefs.

Eugene Meyers struggled with the same issues you are most likely to struggle with, such as developing successful problem-solving, cur-riculum, and classroom management strategies. He began his teaching career with the standard knowledge of educational theory and meth-ods, as well as his own romanticized images of teaching. Through his classroom experiences and interactions with other teachers, Mr. Meyers began to develop approaches that worked well for him. He constructed his own personal-professional knowledge as he went; this developmen-tal process was slow and difficult. Looking back he observes, "Teaching is a wonderful profession, but no way is it easy. You have to decide what kind of teacher you want to be, and then you have to work at it."

Mr. Meyers's teaching strategies evolved over a 20-year period. For example, in his early teaching years Mr. Meyers randomly gave vari-ous kinds of assignments. Some of them worked, and some did not. He began to notice that certain kinds of assignments were more effective than others. He also noticed that his observations about effective assign-ments could help him find better ways to achieve academic goals.

It struck me that, just as I liked to talk about myself, students get most involved when they're talking about themselves. Writing makes one feel very vulnerable. The more involved the writer is in the writing, the more willing he or she is to tolerate that vulnerability.

Constructivist Teaching

Although Mr. Meyers sets traditional academic goals for his students, he achieves those goals by integrating his students' life experiences into the classroom. He concluded long ago that if school is separated from a child's life, it is pointless.

I think the reason schooling is sometimes irrelevant to students is no one shows them its integration. The more we can integrate school and the real world, the more learning will actually get inside them. Through subject matter we're help-ing them actualize themselves. If drawing on these other aspects of their lives helps them get the skills they need, then they should bring those aspects into the classroom. We have to provide them with avenues to bring them into the classroom.

For example, he teaches grammar in a practical, problem-solving way. Students bring in what they perceive as awkward sentences or grammati-cal errors from newspapers, television, or radio. They then justify their perceptions using examples from their own writing or outside sources.

Such integration must take place within academic areas, as well. Rather than teach the traditional components of English as separate strands, Mr. Meyers combines them to show the interrelationships among grammar, writing, and literature. For example, he uses a writing assignment to help students grasp the literary concept of point of view. Then students rewrite it as an autobiographical story from a first-person point of view. Students experience first-hand the strengths and limitations of narrative perspective. They also begin to develop an appreciation of psychological elements such as emotional distance. Knowing how language works in certain situations allows students to read in a more involved way. And involved readers usually become life-long readers.

Teachers' and Students' Personal Purposes

Reading, discussing, and writing about literature have another benefit.

English is a subject that asks us what it means to be human. If it's taught well, it's a very inviting subject. It asks us what it means to be alive, to be ourselves. It allows us to freely talk about things like our fear of death, our fear of falling in love, the confusion of being in love, in the context of *Hamlet* or *Romeo and Juliet*. In one sense it becomes very risky when you're writing about it, but in another sense it's kind of protective, because you're talking about yourself through other people.

Creative writing offers students another opportunity to talk about themselves. Mr. Meyers emphasizes to his students that they create an atmosphere out of their own experiences. "You're the god of your own story," he tells them. They write for themselves and for each other, not just to complete a classroom assignment.

Although his students may not love English, he is confident that they feel closer to it because they approach it through their own life experiences. "If you give students assignments that let them talk about themselves," he explains, "the kids feel more of a commitment to the assignment, to you, and to what you're teaching."

Encouraging students to express their ideas about what they read helps them become lifelong readers. "They talk about ideas," he says, "because I make ideas exciting to talk about." *Hamlet*, for example, is not a work most teenagers come to eagerly, but he enables them to see something of themselves in the protagonist. Mr. Meyers recalls a discussion about Hamlet believing in the idea of providence and of God. One student turned to him and asked plaintively, "Well, do you believe in them?"

I think he didn't want Hamlet to have such an easy answer, because he himself didn't believe in it. I said to him, "No, I don't. I'm not that happy a person that I think there's a future that God has planned out. I don't see life as that organized and that wonderful, but I'd be very happy if I did." I thought it was lovely that he was able to ask me that in that kind of a voice. This kid was really thinking, "Gee, I hope that there's somebody out there who's as hopelessly lost as I am." And of course I was. So it was a relief for him.

Educational Inquiry

To enrich his teaching Mr. Meyers turns to his own interests in literature, music, art, and theater for inspiration. He designed a course, for example, that focuses on how literary patterns change in different media. Students study a literary work that has been made into a movie, television program, ballet, opera, or symphony. The students themselves are a great resource as well.

This kind of energy and experiences and information that students bring is phenomenal. If you were to read the stories . . . their knowledge of material that is not taught in school, cultural things, like life in other countries, what it's like to be a dancer, what it's like to play the harp. I don't mean naturally be good at baseball and pick up a team. Their sense of commitment to activity is more extensive than most children I've taught elsewhere, because they have experienced the emotional commitment to doing something over an extended period of time. Whether it's a ballet class or swim team or choir, they're more in touch with their own emotions. I think they tend to understand literature better, and in their own writing they portray emotions more vividly.

Artistic Problem Solving

Most students like the teacher more than the subject matter, Mr. Meyers suspects. "If you knew that your teacher cared about you, you would like his class, and him." Occasionally he encounters a student who does not easily accept him or the class. A youngster in his class a few years ago was afraid to participate in class discussions, but did average work on his individual written assignments. He couldn't talk about himself aloud, but he began to do so through his writing. Mr. Meyers's acceptance and support enabled this student to express in writing his feelings about a literary work. In turn, this student had a profound influence on Mr. Meyers.

More than any student I've ever had, this was *my* child. I really seemed to have nurtured something good, something important in him. There's more to the world than just math and science, and I mean math and science as a metaphor for this sort of tight world of rules. One of my best experiences was with this kid.

Mr. Meyers continues to help those students who are more vulnerable bring something of themselves into their work. "They sometimes don't do it exactly the way you would expect them to, or the way everyone else does, but they do it, in their own way," he said.

Caring

As a veteran teacher Mr. Meyers continues to reflect on how he interacts with his students. He concludes, "I do a lot of metaphorical sort of hugging with the kinds." When students leave his class, he hopes they take away more than just an appreciation of literature.

I think they also take away the feeling that I really care about them. I really hope they learn something about English. I think they do. I think they also learn something about ideas, that ideas are exciting, and thinking about ideas is exciting.

Mr. Meyers thinks that being a friend to your students is worth the effort it takes to cultivate that friendship while maintaining mutual respect.

Through reflection I discovered how much my students mean to me, as people. I spend my entire day with them. I have an investment in believing that my students are valuable, because my closest co-workers in this process are the children. The relationship you have with your students is yours alone. The 9 months you share can be an intimate, unique, and caring experience. Sometimes children feel frustrated, there's tension, and disagreement, but my kids know that I love them. And I love them educationally, constructively, and by trying to help them become more successful learners. My students know when they leave my class that they have a friend for life.

Service

It is a mistake, Mr. Meyers believes, to reward teachers professionally and monetarily by moving them into nonteaching, administrative positions. Although he's certain he would be a good administrator, he would rather devote his life to teaching. He also believes veteran teachers should contribute to the profession by mentoring novice teachers.

Mentoring allows people who come out of the university to have somebody there to help them with the whole process of acculturation into a school. It also allows the veteran teachers to have contact with the university. They can be involved in making the study of the process of education better.

In particular, Mr. Meyers wants to help beginning teachers develop child-centered classrooms, in which children are involved in both the curriculum and the process of education.

Some teachers think it's okay to throw in some occasional student participation, just a few crumbs. What I'm saying is that the student has to be fully integrated into the process, even into the goals of the process. I teach English, and my goals are English goals. But I know that my students want to communicate effectively. Once they admit that they want to communicate effectively, I try to suggest ways in which they can do that. But they start out by believing in *their* goal, and they're involved in the process. That's the only way they're going to learn anything.

Getting more schools to practice child-centered education is difficult. Institutions want to maintain the status quo, teachers believe what they are doing is adequate, and boards of education mistakenly think educational reform must mean more money and smaller classes. "They have to think about student involvement in the classroom and in their own education," Mr. Meyers contends. Teachers must make students' education an integral part of their lives, not something that's separate from their real world.

Think about why you want to become an educator, Mr. Meyers suggests. Education is exciting, joyful, and fulfilling. Too many people enter the field of education for the wrong reasons. When they encounter the bright students who are excited, they think the students are being unruly, or talking back, or getting off task. To be a good teacher, Mr. Meyers believes, you have to be excited about education.

References

Noddings, Nel. 1984. *Caring: A Feminine Approach to Ethics and Moral Education.* Berkeley: University of California Press.

Wolcott, Harry F. 1973. *The Man in the Principal's Office: An Ethnography.* New York: Holt, Rinehart, and Winston.

Chapter 13
The Phenomenology of Knowing the Patient

Christine A. Tanner, Patricia Benner, Catherine Chesla, and Deborah Gordon

Research on clinical judgment in nursing has generally assumed that nurses acquire objective facts about their patients' well-being, as well as obtain specific information about their patients' social and family histories, ways of coping with and managing their illness, and so on (Tanner 1987; Corcoran 1986). This formalized and explicit information is used through complex reasoning processes to identify problems and issues, and/or to develop a plan of care. In our early pilot work on the role of intuition in clinical judgment (Benner and Tanner 1987), we noticed a recurring discourse among nurses about "knowing the patient"—a reference to how they understood the patient, grasped the meaning of a situation for the patient, or recognized need for a particular action. In expert nursing practice, this kind of knowing is very different from the formalized, explicit, decontextualized, data-based knowledge that constitutes formal assessments, yet it is central to skilled clinical judgment. In our current study of the development of expertise in critical care nursing practice, knowing the patient has continued to be a central theme in nurses' everyday discourse about their practice. The purpose of this article is to describe analyses related to two questions: (1) What

This essay is based on research carried out at the Oregon Health Sciences University, with data interpreted by Sheila Kodadek, Martha Haylor, Peggy Wros, Dawn Doutrich, Yoko Nakayama, and Monica Dostal. An early version of the work was presented by Peggy Wros at the Western Society for Research in Nursing Annual Scientific Meeting, May 1991. An earlier version of the essay appeared as Tanner, Bender, Chesla, and Gordon, "The Phenomenology of Knowing the Patient," *Image: Journal of Nursing Scholarship* 25, 4 (1993): 273–, supported by a grant from the Helene Fuld Health Trust. Reprinted by permission of *Image: Journal of Nursing Scholarship*.

do nurses mean by knowing the patient? and (2) What difference does knowing the patient make in nursing care?

Background

Rationalism is the doctrine that reason alone is the source of knowledge and is independent of experience. The rational tradition, represented by Descartes and Spinoza, holds that all knowledge can be expressed in self-evident propositions or their consequences. Nursing has been influenced by the rational tradition and has increasingly sought to formalize all nursing knowledge in order to legitimize it. The goal has been to make nursing knowledge explicit and eventually propositional as a means of making formal knowledge claims for nursing.

Studies of nurses (Benner 1984; Benner and Wrubel 1989; Benner and Tanner 1987) and of other practice disciplines (Schon 1983; Dreyfus and Dreyfus 1985), have demonstrated the importance of clinical knowledge—the tacit, embodied know-how that allows for the instantaneous recognition of patterns and intuitive responses that characterize expert practice. This clinical know-how, in Polanyi's (1962) terms, is ineffable—it is something these practitioners know but can describe only vaguely. This is not to say that they are completely inarticulate. They can give the best account of what can be explicitly stated.

The inability to spell out completely the operative principles of expert health care practices sometimes occurs due to immature or incomplete science, but here we are pointing to the ineffability that comes from not being able to formalize human concerns, meanings, and practices. All of these involve timing and the unfolding of indeterminate clinical situations where immediate historical understanding is essential. If health care practices were only science or technologies, then, in principle, the knowledge of expert practice could be made fully explicit. But, as Bourdieu points out, the logic of practice and the logic of science are necessarily different:

> . . . if practices had as their principle the generative principle which has to be constructed in order to account for them, that is, a set of independent and coherent axioms, then the practices produced according to perfectly conscious generative rules would be stripped of everything that defines them distinctively as practices, that is the uncertainty and "fuzziness" resulting from the fact that they have as their principle not a set of conscious, constant rules, but practice schemes, opaque to their possessors, varying according to the logic of the situation, the almost invariable partial viewpoint which it imposes, etc. Thus, the procedures of practical logic are rarely entirely coherent and rarely entirely incoherent. (Bourdieu 1980/1990, p. 12)

In recent years, nursing literature has acknowledged other legitimate ways of knowing (Carper 1978; Chinn and Kramer 1991), but on these views knowledge gained from experience is highly personal, subjective, and idiosyncratic. However, following the views of Heidegger (1962) and Dreyfus and Dreyfus (1979; 1986), Benner (1984) has argued that experience is not purely subjective, that knowledge gained from experience is shared in language and practices. Meaning is not subjectively held but is already present in shared language and everyday practices. This understanding of knowledge and experience implies a different possibility for how nurses might know patients.

The analyses reported here are part of a larger interpretive phenomenological study. The aims of that study were (1) to describe the nature of skill acquisition in nursing practice, extending the work of Benner (1984) and Dreyfus and Dreyfus (1986); and (2) to delineate the kinds of practical knowledge exhibited in expert nursing practice. Here we will describe in some detail one aspect of practical knowledge, that of knowing the patient.

Methods

Sample

The sample for the study consisted of 130 nurses who practice in the intensive care units of eight hospitals, seven of which are located in two western regions and one in the eastern region of the United States. The informants practiced in neonatal, pediatric, and adult intensive care units; those practicing in adult units were distributed evenly across surgical, medical, cardiac, and general ICUs. Because we sampled for a relatively homogeneous group, 98 percent of the nurses held a minimum of a bachelor's degree. They were selected for their expected level of practice (advanced beginner through expert) based on years of experience and peer/supervisor nomination.

Data

All informants were interviewed in groups of four to six nurses, again clustered by expected level of practice. In these interviews, the informants gave narrative accounts of their clinical practice, describing specific episodes or patient situations. Group rather than individual interviews were used to create a natural conversational setting for storytelling and to encourage participants to talk with each other as practitioners in natural practical discourse about particular clinical situations. The naturalistic small group setting made it possible for nurses at similar levels of practice to talk to each other and not "up" or "down" to the two research interviewers. Each participant was encouraged to listen actively, asking questions for clarification and understanding, and also to add similar or contrasting experiences from their own clinical practice. Discussions about generalities and ideology, while allowed intermittently, were limited by the request to "tell a story" about particular situations with as much conversation, thoughts, feelings and expectations as possible, staying within the language of the familiar everyday narrative discourse about their everyday practice (Bourdieu 1990).

In addition to these group interviews, 48 of the nurses were interviewed individually about their work history and early perceptions of nursing and nursing education. These 48 nurses were each also observed during their practice at least three times.

Analysis

Analysis of the data occurred in several phases:

(1) Transcripts of interviews were reviewed by members of the research team individually. Interpretive summaries of each clinical episode were prepared by each member and presented and discussed in group meetings. These interpretive summaries were used to develop beginning descriptions of recurring themes and issues.

(2) Observational notes were examined to reveal aspects of everyday practice that would not be apparent in the narrative accounts and to augment/dispute beginning interpretations of practice.

(3) Themes derived from background frameworks (e.g. the Dreyfus model of skill acquisition and Benner's domains of nursing practice), from pilot work (Benner and Tanner 1987), and from early interpretive summaries were labeled with short descriptive terms and broadly defined. For example, some themes relevant to this analysis were labeled KNOWPT for knowing the patient, PARTICGEN for the recognition of the particular as an instance of a general class.

(4) All text was reviewed by at least two of the project staff. Text that contained descriptions of particular clinical situations was labeled "clinical episode" to set it apart from text that contained more general discussion, not related to particular stories. In addition, the labels used to describe major themes were applied to sections of the text so that segments could be retrieved using the software program "Ethnograph" (Seidel 1987).

(5) Whole clinical episodes that contained excerpts tagged as relevant to "knowing the patient" were retrieved for in-depth interpretation

along two major lines: what nurses mean by knowing the patient and what knowing the patient means in terms of practice.

(6) Whole clinical episodes that had been tagged as practice which was "off the mark" were analyzed as contrast cases, exemplars in which nurses did not know the patient.

Results and Discussion

What do nurses mean by "knowing the patient"?

The language nurses used to describe "knowing the patient" was clear, direct and simple. In their stories of particular clinical episodes, they would often comment "I really knew him." Or "I was the only staff member who knew him." In cases of breakdown, it was not uncommon for nurses to explain as a source of breakdown, "I didn't know him." Embedded in the discourse of knowing the patient is meaning central to the nurses' practice: getting a grasp of the patient, getting situated, understanding the patient's situation in context with salience, nuances, and qualitative distinctions. The nurses frequently described knowing the patient as getting a sense of the patient as a person:

It's something, I think, that's hard to describe, but I find with most patients, I feel like I get to know them differently than when they're normal, I'm sure. There's some sense of who this person is. It's when you touch them, or when you say something to them, what happens on their monitors. Or maybe just to see that the effect of what you're doing shows up in what's happening to the patient, how they look, even when they're paralyzed, just whether their features look a little different, something looks different about them, if they seem to be comfortable when you're there.

In many exemplars, like the one above, nurses describe understanding the relationship of particulars—the effect of a nursing act on cardiac rate and rhythms, the slight change in a vasoactive agent on the patient's blood pressure. While they may describe recognition of particular responses and patterns, all that they know about the patient, how they notice subtle changes and interpret responses remains largely ineffable.

Nurses talk about getting to know the patient at the beginning of the shift. In the following dialogue, a nurse describes how a patient had extubated herself at the beginning of the shift. She describes her experience of not being situated:

I hate it when things happen right at the beginning. Not my time of day. Let me get everything organized . . . you get tuned in where all your lines are, you know, if something happens then you know exactly where you are. During the first hour, I try not to let any visitors in the room because they'll come in and say what's happening and my answer is, "I don't know yet. From the report I got they're doing OK." I cannot say myself that they're doing OK. . . . You have no idea, you don't have a feeling for that patient either, about how they're going to react when you turn down the nipride [an intravenous drug to control blood pressure] or how they're going to react when you turn up the epi [epinephrine]. You don't know that particular patient and how they react to anything.

Here the nurse has acquired from end-of-shift report the objective information about the patient, her disease, and its course. But she still doesn't know that particular patient. Knowing the patient, in short, means an immediate grasp, an involved rather than detached understanding of the patient's situation and the patient's responses, an understanding that is directly apprehended and may remain largely ineffable.

Two broad categories of knowing the patient emerged from nurses' descriptions of particular patient situations in which they felt they had a good grasp of the patient: (1) in-depth knowledge of the patient's patterns of responses and (2) knowing the patient as a person.

Knowing the Patient's Patterns of Responses

Nurses, in the context of particular clinical episodes, describe their detailed knowledge about the patient's patterns: how she moves; what positions are comfortable; how his wounds look; how she eats; how he tolerates being off a ventilator; how infants tolerate feedings and respond to comfort measures; what rituals soothe and reassure; what timing of care works best. These are all very local, specific knowledge about particular patient's responses, physical functioning, and body topology. Within this broad category are several particular aspects of knowing the patient: (1) responses to therapeutic measures; (2) routines and habits; (3) coping resources; (4) physical capacities and endurance; and (5) body topology and characteristics. Here is an example of one such description:

Nurse: I took care of a baby who was about 26 or 27 weeks who was about 900 grams who had been doing well for about 2 weeks. He had an open ductus [patent ductus arteriosus, occurring when the fetal connection between the aorta and the pulmonary artery fails to close normally after birth]. The difference between the way he looked at 9:00 and the way he looked at 11:00 was very dramatic. I was at that point really concerned about what was going to happen next. There are a lot of complications of patent ductus, not just in itself but the fact that it causes a lot of other things. I was really concerned that the baby was starting to show symptoms of all of them. You look at this kid, because you know this kid and you know what he looked like two hours ago. It is a dramatic difference to you but it is hard to describe that to someone in words. You go to the resident and say, "Look, I'm really worried about X, Y, and Z" and they go,

"OK," then you wait one half hour, 40 minutes, then you go to the fellow and you say, "You know I'm really worried about X, Y, Z." They say, "We'll talk about it on rounds.

Interviewer. What is the X, Y, Z you are worried about?

Nurse. The fact that the kid is more lethargic, paler, his stomach is bigger, he's not tolerating his feedings. His chem strip might be a little strange. All these kinds of things . . . there are clusters of things that go wrong. At this time, I had been in the unit I think a couple or three years. I was really starting to feel like I knew what was going on, but I wasn't as good at throwing my weight into a situation like that.

Here the nurse is talking about particularizing her theoretical knowledge of the complications of patent ductus to this particular child. Because she knows the child, she is able to recognize changes in the way he responds—being more lethargic, paler, not tolerating feedings—qualitative distinctions that require prior local, specific, and ineffable knowledge about how this child usually responds. This nurse describes a situation that was not at all uncommon—having a grasp on the patient situation but not being able to describe the specifics sufficiently in order to make a case with the physicians.

The nurse sought assistance from a second nurse who was more experienced. Rounds started shortly after that and she walked up to the attending very quietly, "sidled up" and said, "You know, Sara is really worried about this kid." She told him the story and said, "He reminds me of this child we had three weeks ago." Everything stopped. He got out his stethoscope and listened to the child, examind the child, and said, "Call the surgeons." The more experienced nurse "made the case" not by recourse to calculative reasoning and elemental bits of information but by pointing out the resemblance of this child's particular situation to a prior shared experience. She made the case by knowing how to approach this particular physician, one who reportedly practiced "anecdotal medicine," by having shared understanding and experiences, and by having won his respect through several years of working together.

Knowing the Patient as a Person

Two nurses from one unit participated in describing a patient, George, who became our paradigm case for knowing the patient as a person. George was in his mid-sixties. He lived in a residential care facility and was admitted to the ICU with septicemia. He had been quadriplegic for many years from injuries sustained in a motor vehicle accident. He had also had a radical neck resection 15 to 20 years prior to admission. His situation provides a dramatic example of the difficulties of getting to know a patient in extreme circumstances:

What happened with him is that people really didn't get to know him . . . he was really deformed . . . you couldn't really read his lips. You couldn't write a note. I think the bottom-line question was quality of life. If we get him off the ventilator then what is it that he's going to be going back to. I think that happens (with residents from this particular facility). That's the last ditch effort, then they come here to die. It turned out that he had an excellent quality of life and we all didn't realize that or didn't think of it as quality of life.

He was there for five months, and it took months for people to get beyond looking at him, first his face and judging him on where he came from, and also his communication was almost impossible. You had to not base any kind of care you gave him on anybody else. He didn't have a family, didn't have a support, you couldn't communicate with him, but he was really in there. I mean he wanted to watch the ball game. That is what he wanted to do, and he would get upset. He would mouth the words "Ball game!" And people would ask him, "Are you saying bowel movement?" And finally we learned what he meant.

The nurses go on to describe how expressive George was, despite his quadriplegia and significant facial deformity. The nurses learned to communicate with him. Eventually, his story was filled out through piecing together information from his friends at the residential care facility and a social worker, and through George himself during a brief period of time that he had a talking trach:

It turned out that he was a spokesperson for patients (at the residential care facility), that a lot of people there had alcohol and drug problems and he helped them out with them. He had a girlfriend there who was also wheelchair bound. They were the Valentine's King and Queen. We would get these strange calls from people at the residential facility. You would pick up the phone and nobody would speak for half a minute but you would know that someone was on the other end. People who would call would just stutter and stutter and then finally say "George!"

Before the nurses got to know George, the physicians had decided not to treat him fully,

. . . based on what he looked like, and what we thought he was. I stood up for him. I don't think some people ever go beyond just looking at him and saying, "This man is disfigured and not able to take care of himself."

When asked what was different about the way the nurse looked at George and how the doctors saw him, when they thought that he wanted to die, she responded:

I don't think they stood with him and looked at him or gave him a Pepsi or knew that he derived a lot of pleasure from living. I think they looked at him and they saw that this is as good as it gets and this is really depressing and he is really depressed, so why continue? This is torture. And it was definitely border-line whether he is ever going to get out of here, but still he was glad to see you. He wanted to watch the ball games. To me that is not someone who has given up. Somebody who is that active in planning my day really is not somebody who doesn't want to deal with living. The more we got to know him, the more we learned that quality of life for him was really very good.

Here the nurse is describing the uninvolved, detached stance that comes of not knowing the patient as a person. The outside-in view of George was of one with an impoverished quality of life, that his depression was completely understandable given all his physical disabilities and deformities, a perception supported by prior notions of what life is like for people at this particular care facility. The nurse came to understand George's concerns, his enthusiasm for life, and his importance to his friends. She got to know George in an involved, attached way.

The detached stance is a common moral position. It allows clinical decisions that are based on external interpretations, not on the meanings as constituted by the patient. But the nurse who knows the patient, as these nurses came to know George, is able to assume an advocacy position of caring, from an involved stance (Benner, Tanner, and Chesla 1992). Knowing the patient is the expression of caring as a commitment to protecting the patient's vulnerability, while enhancing that person's dignity (Gadow 1989). As one of our informants explains:

Nurse: I'm taking care of someone right now who is unresponsive. He is awake but he doesn't follow commands and he doesn't communicate. And from what the chart reads, he was out at a nursing home and that basically was his level of functioning. But he has someone who calls in every day, so there must be a little higher level of functioning. I want to know what he was like before he was sick.

Interviewer: Why?

Nurse: Because it makes me humanize the person or patient more. I treat them more as a human being. I work mostly at night so it is real easy to lose perspective. When I see a patient with glasses on, or a photograph of them, it is so much easier for me to think of them as someone's father or a businessman, or someone with a life, like mine or someone else's. You only lose that as the days go by and you keep the person totally unresponsive, hooked up to machines . . . just a body that you are turning, and cleaning, and dressing. I think it is easy to lose the human aspect.

By their very presence the family can enable the ICU nurse to establish and maintain an involved rather than detached stance with patients. In the presence of family the patient is revealed as a husband, wife, daughter, beloved grandfather rather than a clinical entity. Through the family, acutely ill patients who cannot communicate their needs, wants, or essential humanness in any way show up as persons with lives beyond the ICU. When families attend at the bedside, nurses can understand the composition of patients' everyday lives, their work, commitments, fears, and hopes. This knowledge is essential to everyday caring practices as well as to larger decisions about treatment. In the following example, a nurse's knowledge of a patient, derived almost entirely through the family, allowed her to advocate for discontinuing support measures despite strong opposition from some of the physicians involved. The patient was a middle-aged gentleman who came to the hospital with minor complaints, was taken to cardiac surgery, suffered a cerebral infarct during surgery, and never recovered.

> I had never, ever spoken to this man, but I grew to know him because of the family. Because I became real close to his wife and the son who still had a lot to resolve with his father.
>
> The day that he went into the hospital, he was planting beans and he had a little bit of pain, so he went in. That's the last time he (the son) ever got to talk to his father. But they knew that he was a very independent person and his quality of life, there would be none. He would not like to live this way, so they had to make a decision. So after the report came back that he had an infarct, he probably wouldn't have regained any kind of normalcy in this life at all, and he would be a burden to his family who weren't in the best financial situation either. Then they wanted to withdraw support at that time.

From a more distanced position, the attending physician ordered that supportive measures be maintained for an additional ten days after the cerebral infarct had been confirmed. The nurse advocated for the family, arguing that the additional time on support would not change the clinical course and yet would bring significant suffering for the family. From her engaged advocacy for the patient and family, support measures were terminated several days earlier than had been planned.

In much smaller ways, nurses learn of patients' personalities, normal modes of expressions, likes and dislikes, and personal habits and practices through the family. Nurses often meet patients when they have totally succumbed to sedatives, analgesics, and paralytics. Families have an important role in helping the nurse learn about and assess the patient as he or she recovers. Families cue nurses into the fact that the patient is typically irritable, demanding, or anxious, and that the reappearance of these behaviors is actually a sign of recovery rather than a cause for concern. Alternatively, families signal the nurse about patient behaviors and responses that fall outside the patient's familiar patterns and therefore demand closer monitoring.

Family members often have the most constant contact with the patient throughout a hospitalization. Some nurses use the family's capacity to note minute changes in the patient's condition as one of their early warning signals. Nurses also follow family members' suggestions about what comforts or distresses a patient. For example, we observed the care of an extremely anxious ventilated patient who was at grave risk of pneumothorax and whose sedative management was complicated by blood pressure instability. The patient's wife explained his fear of alarms. In the previous hospital, every alarm meant a cardiac arrhythmia. Once the nurse was cued into this particular fear, she comforted the patient and quickly explained what was going on each time a vent or IV pump alarmed, clearly easing his tension and allowing him rest.

What difference does knowing the patient make in patient care?

The narrative accounts provided by the nurses in our sample, as well as related literature supports the following assertions:

1. Knowing the patient is central to skilled clinical judgment and is broader than what is captured in formal assessments of physical systems.
2. Knowing a patient is a practical nursing discourse that points to specific nursing skills of seeing and involvement.
3. Knowing the patient creates the possibility of advocacy.
4. Knowing individual patients sets up learning about patient populations.

Knowing the Patient as Central to Skilled Judgment

Knowing the patient, as these nurses describe it, goes beyond formal assessments in several ways. First, because the nurse knows the typical patterns of responses, certain aspects of the situation stand out as salient and others recede in importance. Second, making qualitative distinctions and comparing the current picture to this patient's typical picture, are made possible. And third, prescriptions and abstract principles can be particularized. The rational model of clinical judgment holds that deciding on a course of action is simply a matter of instrumental application of scientifically based knowledge. The limitations of this model have been well described by Dreyfus and Dreyfus (1985) and Schon (1983). Nurses in their narrative accounts in this study show repeatedly how clinical judgment requires particularizing formal prescriptions and abstractions through understanding how *this* patient responds under *these* circumstances. Knowing the patient is the nurses' basis for particularizing care. The following nurse describes knowing a premature infant and how that influences her care and judgment of the infant:

> The baby I'm taking care of now is a twitty little preemie. She is the ultimate preemie. All you have to do is walk in front of her isolette and have a shadow fall across her face and she desaturates [blood oxygen level drops]. She cannot stand knowing there is anyone else in the world, but I found that I was able to suction her [clear secretions from her airway] by myself and keep her saturation in the 90s just by being slow and careful. This baby usually has terrible bradycardia [slowed heart rate] and desaturations when she is suctioned. She developed a reputation for being a real little nerd, but I haven't had any problem with her for the first couple of hours.

Knowing the preemie is personalized and particularistic even though this baby's responses are typical of premature babies: as the nurse notes, "she is the ultimate preemie." Knowing the particular baby and her responses is at the heart of clinical judgment about the source of the baby's oxygen desaturation and bradycardia and directs the nurse's care for the baby. The practical discourse about knowing a patient spans extremely deprived situations in critical care and the more communicative situations of general care as illustrated by the following negative example in the pilot study on a general medical unit:

> *Nurse:* This patient was acting weird but no one knew her baseline. I spent a lot of time with her, walking her down the hall, doing her care, because I didn't know her and couldn't figure her out. She had been confused and goofy, but now she was mellowing out, but we didn't know if that was her baseline. . . . I felt so frustrated all day long . . . I had read her chart, but I still didn't get a feel for this patient, although I was doing all these things. I went into report and gave a much more comprehensive report than on any of the other patients, because I think my anxiety level was higher, because I don't feel I know this person. It may be that I took care of a patient two weeks ago, but two weeks later, I still don't know *that* patient. It makes me feel very uncomfortable.

> *Interviewer:* What do you mean by really knowing a patient?

> *Nurse:* It is getting an idea of what they look like, how they talk, how they eat their breakfast. It is stupid stuff, it is not even medical.

This interview illustrates that, despite its centrality, the informal discourse on knowing patients is underdeveloped without the legitimacy and status of technical-procedural discourse. Nevertheless nurses describe knowing their patients as central to good clinical judgment and practice. In the above excerpt the patient is on chemotherapy and at risk for sepsis due to immunosuppression; therefore, knowing the patient is essential for early detection of changes. The excerpt also illustrates that "knowing a patient" discourse is current, situational, particularistic and contains the immediate history of the patient's condition.

Knowing the Patient and the Skill of Involvement

Learning a practice requires one to learn the culturally appropriate levels of involvement and interaction between the practitioner and client. The expected levels of involvement for family member, friend, physician, lawyer, therapist, clergyperson, and nurse are different. But the differences cannot be spelled out completely by formal instruction because they must be socially enacted in multiple contexts by actually being a nurse, physician, friend, or therapist. The practitioner's learning is social and personal. The skill of involvement and the skill of seeing salient patient changes are based upon engagement in the clinical situation, and these are central in the informal discourse about knowing a patient where they show up as present, absent, or in the process of being learned.

Learning the skill of involvement requires experience. It is not a trait or talent of the nurse, or abstract knowledge. Knowing the patient as these nurses describe it is a way of involvement. In a study of nurses in Scotland, May (1991) describes knowing patients as being of central importance to involvement. Using interview excerpts which sound strikingly similar to those produced by American nurses, May points out how involvement is viewed as an everyday, non-problematic aspect of practice that is characterized by knowing the patient, reciprocity, and investment.

Knowing the Patient as Advocacy

Nurses, in their exemplars, clearly see themselves as advocates, as persons who stand along side of and empower patients and their families to have a voice when they are weak and vulnerable. They talk about their commitment to be vigilant in ensuring that adequate care is given, that early warnings of patient change are attended to, that medical therapies are given with an understanding of the particular patient's responses:

Nurse: My first concern was my patient. I can't leave him.

Interviewer: Why not?

Nurse: Because I knew the patient the best. If anyone came to the bedside and started mucking around with things, I'd say, "No, wait a minute. If you asked me first, then I'll tell you what you can do with the patient. If you want to move the patient, etcetera. But don't try to set him up and listen to lung sounds, if you don't know the patient."

Knowing the Patient as Part of Clinical Learning

Getting to know many particular patients with similar illness situations allows the nurse to learn common issues and important qualitative distinctions within particular patient populations. For example, the following excerpt illustrates the particular issues of knowing patients with electrophysiological problems:

We have a general report and we know what drugs you can't give to certain people. Like Mr. Smith in Bed Two is refractory to Lidocaine, Pronestyl, and Bretylium [drugs used to treat dangerous cardiac rhythms]. And you do rely very much on that nurse who is taking care of that patient, but you never expect one of our electrophysiology patients to follow an algorithm [standard treatments for dangerous cardiac rhythms]. So in a crisis situation, the first question is what *can* you give instead of "Let's give this."

Knowledge of particular patient populations is built up with many instances of knowing particular patients. This way of knowing helps fill out one's understanding of common issues, common expectations, and common timetables. Thus, assessments become much more differentiated and nuanced within this range of historical, particular knowledge.

The development of particularized knowledge of specific patient populations stands out when a new patient population is formed. For example, neonatal intensive care nurses in this study were struggling over learning to recognize when babies were withdrawing from crack cocaine:

We've trained nurses to evaluate babies using scoring sheets so that there's not so much guesswork involved or so much opinion of, "Well, I think this is really a fussy baby; therefore it must be withdrawing." There are lots of fussy babies that are not withdrawing.

The distinction between fussiness associated with withdrawal and fussiness associated with other causes is learned over time by knowing the patterns of particular babies who are later confirmed actually to be withdrawing from crack cocaine and contrasting their knowledge of these "crack babies" with others who are fussy for other reasons and who have different patterns of fussiness. Thus knowing particular babies sets up the possibility of knowing a patient population by collecting instances and contrasts over time. And in turn, knowing a patient population sets up a context for knowing variations and particularity within that population.

Summary and Implications

Knowing a patient is a central aspect of nursing practice and is pervasive in the everyday practical discourse of nurses. Knowing the patient is a primary caring practice. As a moral concern, knowing the patient creates the possibility for advocacy in its most basic sense—limiting the vulnerability of persons and preserving their dignity and integrity (Gadow 1985). Knowing the patient is essential to patients feeling cared for and about. In an empirical study of patients' experiences of caring, Brown (1986) found that patients place at the top of their list of caring acts not being "just another case," but rather that care was personalized, and thus not routine. Similarly, from a series of studies, Swanson (1991) described "knowing" as one of five dimensions of caring, defining it as "striving to understand the meaning an event has in the life of another" (1991, p. 163).

It is striking that such a pervasive phenomenon has been overlooked in most research on clinical judgment, as well as in most formal systems designed to support nursing practice. Nursing care plans, nursing diagnoses, and standard protocols all derive from the rational model of practice and cover over the significance of knowing the patient. Rational models of clinical judgment also assume that what is important to know about a patient can be explicitly stated and formalized in context-free processes and rules. The practical discourse on knowing a patient and its significance to clinical judgment simply cannot show up when practice is viewed through the lens of the rational models.

The practical discourse about knowing the patient points to the private-public juncture of nursing practice. The informal practical discourse on knowing a patient illustrates an informal everyday understanding that is further developed and finely tuned in a practice such as nursing. Knowing a patient is highly specific, situated knowledge, and by it nurses never claim an inclusive, all-encompassing knowledge; "knowing a patient" is always specific to what can be known in the nurse-patient-family interaction and clinical context. Discourse about knowing a patient is bounded by the understanding of the patient that is required for what the nurse understands to be good nursing care and clinical judgment.

Knowing a patient, as these nurses describe it, is always situated by time constraints, clinical situations and the nature of the nurse-patient-family relationship. Culturally, nurses are given access to private knowledge about care of the body and maintaining a sense of integrity and selfhood in the midst of breakdown and high vulnerability. Over time, nurses have developed an informal practical discourse to describe their knowledge about these intimate regions of physical and interpersonal care. Much of this knowledge can be extended and refined by making it more public and consensually validated. However, it would be a mistake to think that this discourse could be made completely formal, explicit, general, and objective, because it is the discourse of the particular so essential to clinical knowledge. Clinical knowledge by its very nature cannot be made completely general; it must always incorporate the particular, historical understanding of the clinical situation and the concrete other. That is why narratives of actual practice must be made public because in the narrative lies the possibility of describing the knowledge embedded in the particular, historical, clinical relationship.

The informal discourse, and indeed the possibility for nurses to know their patients, is constrained by the organizational arrangements and economic constraints of the practice. When nurses work in situations where it is impossible to know their patients sufficiently to see changing relevance, recognize early warnings, or protect patients from violation of patient–family concerns so that their vulnerability isn't threatened then the very ground for safe and astute nursing care is undermined. In such situations, and if nurses lose their practical knowledge of "knowing their patients," nursing is reduced to a technology and loses its ground as a practice with notions of good internal to it (MacIntyre 1981; Benner 1994). In order to preserve the possibility of knowing patients we will have to extend and protect forms of nursing care delivery such as primary nursing that allow for it. Even in an era of cost-containment, we will have to protest views of "advanced nursing practice" as removed abstract decision making organized so that the disengaged decision maker delegates the direct physical and interpersonal care of patients to auxiliary workers. Such a view overlooks the myriad decisions embedded in providing the care. Likewise case management versions of nursing practice must be designed so nurses can know their patients.

References

Benner, Patricia. 1982. "From Novice to Expert." *American Journal of Nursing* 82, 3: 402–7.

————. 1983. "Uncovering the Knowledge Embedded in Practice." *Image: Journal of Nursing Scholarship* 15: 39–41.

————. 1984. *From Novice to Expert: Power and Excellence in Clinical Nursing Practice.* Menlo Park, CA: Addison-Wesley.

————. 1994a. "Discovering Challenges to Ethical Theory in Experience-Based Narratives of Nurses' Everyday Ethical Comportment." In *Health Care Ethics: Critical Issues,* ed. John F. Monagle and David C. Thomasma. Gaithersburg, MD: Aspen.

————. 1994b. "The Role of Articulation in Understanding Practice and Experience as Sources of Knowledge." In *Philosophy in an Age of Pluralism: The*

Philosophy of Charles Taylor in Question, ed. James Tully and Daniel M. Wein-stock. Cambridge: Cambridge University Press.

Benner, Patricia and Christine A. Tanner. 1987. "Expert Clinical Judgment: The Role of Intuition." *American Journal of Nursing*

Benner, Patricia, Christine A. Tanner, and Catherine Chesla. 1992. "From Be-ginner to Expert: Gaining a Differentiated Clinical World in Critical Care Nursing." *Advances in Nursing Science* 14, 3: 13–28.

Benner, Patricia and Judith Wrubel. 1989. *The Primacy of Caring: Stress and Coping in Health and Illness.* Menlo Park, CA: Addison-Wesley.

Bourdieu, Pierre. 1980/1990. *The Logic of Practice,* trans. Richard Nice. Stanford, CA: Stanford University Press.

Brown, L. 1986. "The Experience of Care: Patient Perspectives." *Topics in Clini-cal Nursing* 8, 2: 56–62.

Carper, B. 1978. "Fundamental Patterns of Knowledge in Nursing." *Advances in Nursing Science* 1: 13–23.

Chinn, Peggy L. and Maeona K. Kramer. 1991. *Theory and Nursing: A Systematic Approach.* St. Louis: Mosby.

Corcoran, S. 1986. "Planning by Expert and Novice Nurses in Cases of Varying Complexity." *Research in Nursing and Health* 9: 155–62.

Dreyfus, Hubert L. 1979. *What Computers Can't Do: The Limits of Artificial Intelli-gence.* Rev. ed. New York: Harper and Row.

Dreyfus, Hubert L. and Stuart E. Dreyfus, with Tom Athanasiou. 1986. *Mind over Machine: The Power of Human Intuition and Expertise in the Era of the Computer.* New York: Free Press.

Gadow, S. 1989. "Clinical Subjectivity: Advocacy with Silent Patients." *Nursing Clinics of North America* 24, 2: 535–41.

Heidegger, Martin. 1926/1962. *Being and Time,* trans. John Macquarrie and Edward Robinson. New York: Harper and Row.

MacIntyre, Alasdair C. 1981. *After Virtue: A Study in Moral Theory.* Notre Dame, IN: Notre Dame University Press.

May C. 1991. "Affective Neutrality and Involvement in Nurse-Patient Relation-ships: Perceptions of Appropriate Behaviour Among Nurses in Acute Medical and Surgical Wards." *Journal of Advanced Nursing* 16: 552–58.

Polanyi, Michael. 1962. *Personal Knowledge: Towards a Post-Critical Philosophy.* New York: Harper Torchbooks.

Schon, Donald A. *The Reflective Practitioner: How Professionals Think in Action.* New York: Basic Books.

Seidel, I. 1987. *The Ethnograph.* Boulder, CO: Qualis Research Associates.

Swanson, K. M. 1991. "Empirical Development of a Middle Range Theory of Caring." *Nursing Research* 40, 3: 161–66.

Tanner, Christine A. 1987. "Teaching Clinical Judgment." *Annual Review of Nurs-ing Research* 5: 153–73.

Part IV
The Politics of Caregiving

It has often been said that caregiving, traditionally women's work, is inherently conservative. Like the traditional stereotype of the woman in the home trying to protect her domestic haven from external invasion, caregiving has been accused of fostering a politics of accommodation or adaptation rather than one of transformation. This negative stereotype has been particularly insidious in an era when more women have tried to liberate themselves from traditional roles and stereotypes. The liberated woman has often been depicted as a female version of the successful upper class white male. She is supposed to work in an "elite" profession, master the skills of competition, careerism, and hyper-individualism and—most importantly—get as far as she can from the caregiving professions (Gordon 1991).

Caregiving has suffered immensely because of negative societal stereotypes that impede rather than advance our understanding of this important social and human activity. They have made it hard to analyze what is positive within caregiving. Because caregiving work has historically been women's work and because women's work has been devalued and degraded in our society, most analyses of caregiving work in and outside the home have focused on its exploitative qualities. Because of these historical factors, many conclude that caregiving is inevitably exploitative, particularly to women. Indeed, today, many consider those who continue to remain committed to caregiving work to lack ambition or intelligence and or to suffer from the oh-so-modern malady of "codependence."

This final section of the volume challenges this view of the politics of caregiving. The chapters in this section describe the transformative political and personal power of caregiving. They demonstrate that the care perspective can provide guidance that enables individuals to better evaluate proposals for reforms, such as reforms to our health care system; to pose challenges to hierarchical power structures like those in organized male-dominated religions; or to redefine the goals of movements for liberation, like feminism, and restructure social institutions.

Ellen D. Baer's and Suzanne Gordon's short essay (Chapter 14) on what is happening today in health care analyzes the complexity of caring work in nursing and suggests how nurses can respond to the threat to their profession. It uses an understanding of the importance of caregiving to promote concrete political action. The political activity that the authors recommend stems directly from their appreciation of the very texture and value of caregiving.

In "The Rationality of Caring," Chapter 15, Kari Waerness explains why it is so important to study caregiving; her work adds more fuel to this argument. Waerness studies caring for dependents, a job women typically perform, and concludes that caring work, far from being irrational, contains its own kind of rationality. The rationality of caregiving, however, differs dramatically from scientific rationality. Waerness believes that we must understand the rationality of caring and make qualitative distinctions between caregiving work and other kinds of work conducted in more instrumental settings. Without these distinctions the author insists that we will never be able to create new models of organizing the kind of public systems of care so necessary to modern urban societies and their citizens. In an effort to help create those systems of care, the author thus explores the "rationality of caring" and broadens the definitions that permeate our policy debate. In so doing, she moves from rational calculation and cost benefit analysis to a consideration of human concerns.

The link between "transformative feminism" (Gordon 1991) and caregiving is further strengthened in "Feminism and Caregiving," Suzanne Gordon's final contribution to this volume. In this essay, Gordon responds to a number of feminist critiques of caring theories. Focusing primarily on the work of journalist Susan Faludi, journalist Katha Pollitt, and attorney/author Wendy Kaminer, the essay describes the position of what she calls Lockean feminists. These women often suggest that any discussion of caring and caregiving will entrap women in the prison of Victorian femininity and will discourage men from shouldering their fair share of caregiving responsibilities.

Gordon debunks this notion by analyzing its underpinnings in liberal enlightenment theory. Rather than attacking those who critically analyze the content of caregiving and who try to elaborate a rigorous theory of caring, she believes these feminists simply mimic traditionally male devaluations of caregiving activities. She further insists that men will be unable to appreciate the value and importance of caregiving and share its burdens without such an analysis. It is not a sophisticated analysis of caring practice but the societal devaluation and persistent invisibility of caring practice that is the greatest obstacle to female emancipation and male caregiving, whether in the home or in caregiving professions.

When long-time feminist activist Judith Dushku writes of her socialization in the women's caregiving network in the Church of Jesus Christ of Latter-Day Saints (Chapter 17), she will surely surprise those who believe that religion and its caregiving obligations and networks inevitably oppress women. This revealing personal essay contradicts many comfortable notions about the "nature" of religious commitment.

Dushku, who is an active church member and an active feminist, explains how her education in caregiving within the church has led her to join other women to pose an increasingly powerful challenge to the male hierarchies that govern the Mormon religion. Her essays shows what a complex force caregiving and community can be. In certain cultural contexts, like the one in which she was raised, for certain women, like her sisters in feminism, caregiving can legitimate a belief that women are important, deserve attention, and must be respected. This journey from submission to dissent suggests the political as well as the personal potential embedded in communities of caregiving.

We have included physician Rita Charon's "Let Me Take a Listen to Your Heart" in a section on the politics of caregiving rather than professional caregiving because it explores how power relationships between carer and cared for can shift dramatically. When those who are charged with healing actually attend to the voices and meanings of their patients' experiences, imbalances of power within those relationships are fundamentally changed. If, as feminists once suggested, the personal is political, this very personal essay certainly confirms how a personal transformation in attitude can help to pave the way for more extensive systemic transformations.

More important, Charon's own attempts to find meaning in her patients' experiences through narrative writing is a strategy often employed by those in the caring professions. Patricia Benner, for example, uses this technique to help nurses uncover the value and content of their work. What this attempt to enter more fully into the lives of the cared for indicates is the power of storytelling, of anecdote, of individual particularity, history, and detail. Yet, it is precisely this method of knowing that is put into question by rationalistic, objective data collecting that dismisses individual human experience as "just anecdotal evidence." Charon's insistence on particularity, a commitment exercised within a field that has been increasingly detached from the human and attached to scientific ways of knowing, is thus a profound political challenge in and of itself. Teaching this method to others is an even more potent way of asserting the care perspective as a means of turning sentiment into practice.

References

Gordon, Suzanne. 1991. *Prisoners of Men's Dreams: Striking Out for a New Feminine Future.* New York: Little, Brown.

Chapter 14
Money Managers Are Unraveling the Tapestry of Nursing

Ellen D. Baer and Suzanne Gordon

"If caring were enough, anyone could be a nurse. . . ."

Remember that campaign slogan? It was developed several years ago by the Advertising Council and the National Commission on Nursing Implementation Project (NCNIP) to promote nursing's image. Now it's coming back to haunt nursing.

Today, anyone, it seems, *can* be a nurse. Or, to be more precise, a "care assistant" or "patient care technician" or "multi-skilled caregiver." All across the country, hospitals are trying to contain costs by replacing experienced RNs with unlicensed assistive personnel. Worst of all, this trend is being promoted by nurses who have ties to large management consulting firms. Nursing vice presidents are implementing these changes, and staff nurses are training and supervising their own replacements. And nursing leaders, distracted by promises of an expanded role for advanced practice nurses, aren't raising strong enough objections to this alarming development.

Undoubtedly, nursing is making progress on certain fronts. Seizing the moment, advanced practice nurses are capitalizing on health care reform to solidify their positions in primary care and some tertiary care settings. Nursing educational institutions have expanded their advanced practice programs. Home and community nursing care providers have sought hospital referral connections and membership in vertically integrated network alliances. Nurse researchers have once again reminded the public of the myriad findings that support nurses' competence in these new roles.

An earlier version of this essay appeared as Baer and Gordon, "Money Managers Are Unraveling the Tapestry of Nursing," *American Journal of Nursing* (October 1994): 38–40, copyright © 1994 by the American Journal of Nursing Company. Reprinted by permission of the *American Journal of Nursing*.

Much of this activity is appropriate and wise, but not when it obscures what is happening to bedside nursing and ignores critical questions for nurses and patients alike.

Is nursing prepared to tell the public that continuous bedside nursing care is not so vital after all, after years of asserting precisely the opposite? Do nurses have to trade their preeminent role at the bedside in order to become major players in community or primary care? Can't nurses do all of these things? Isn't there enough money in the health care system — a system that now consumes close to a trillion dollars a year — to pay for the whole array of patient care services nurses are qualified to deliver?

For 100 years, nurses have articulated the importance of expert bedside nursing care for hospitalized patients. Nursing has progressed from functional care to team nursing to primary nursing, continually refining the ideal concept of patient care. Nursing scholars, ethnographers, and even some journalists have studied that care. They have described its complex nature, illuminating not only the technical aspects but the emotional and cognitive content as well. And they have documented its positive impact on patient outcomes.

After World War II, nursing shortages converged with vastly improved medical science and technology. Social science researchers tried to analyze nursing functions to figure out when a registered nurse was necessary at the bedside and when a less-trained person could be used instead. In the 1960s, nursing leaders began to seek entry-into-practice regulations through state legislatures. The legislation never passed (except in North Dakota). All groups were stymied by the difficulty of unbundling nursing practice.

The questions that plagued earlier shortages and debates about entry into practice continue to this day. The problem of explaining the complexity of nursing to politicians, policy makers and the public persists. Why? Because nursing is a profession that provides patients with so many different services, functions, and activities simultaneously.

Nursing is a tapestry woven from countless threads into an intricate whole. At one moment, a nurse may be involved in a sophisticated clinical procedure that demands advanced scientific and technological education and judgment. The next moment, or even concurrently, the nurse may perform what many people would consider a trivial or menial task, such as making a bed, giving a bedbath, handling a bedpan, or feeding a patient.

Nurses' work is also characterized by the kind of interrupted labor feminist historian Laurel Thatcher Ulrich describes in her book *Good Wives* (1991). The nurse will take care of one patient, return to another, or perhaps move onto a third, doing all levels of activity synchronously.

Our society looks at this interrupted labor, and the so-called menial tasks included in it, and finds its diffuseness frustrating rather than fascinating, an invitation to demean and devalue nurses' work rather than to examine its richness and texture. What society fails to understand is that the seemingly menial tasks give nurses the opportunity to explore the mundane details of a patient's daily life, which often make the difference between safety and danger, illness and health, even life and death. The fact that many of these tasks do not demand nurses' total attention allows them to spend time checking monitors and IV lines, assessing skin color and pulses, talking to patients, providing comfort, or teaching self-care activities.

Nurses use these exchanges to develop a subtle baseline sense of the patient that allows them to know intuitively, often at a glance, when an important change has occurred. That is precisely nursing's beauty and uniqueness. Yet it is also what makes nursing so opaque and so vulnerable to market-driven consultants and administrators.

When management consultants hired to save money arrive at hospitals, they see what we call the tapestry of nursing and are distressed by its intricacy. They are unable to grasp that nursing interweaves simple skills with complex judgments, "people sense" with intellectual prowess, fact-finding with patient teaching. Instead of seeing the tapestry as an invaluable whole, these "money managers" try to unravel it thread by thread. "Let's see now," the consultant asks, "what does a nurse do that someone else could do cheaper?"

With saving money their first priority, financial consultants deconstruct the bundle into its parts and delegate the pieces to someone they can hire for less money. Once these fragments have been assigned to less costly workers, administrators feel free to lay off RNs, maintaining only a few as supervisers.

In an attempt to appeal to staff nurses, money managers argue that by liberating nursing from what they call menial tasks they are elevating nursing practice to a higher level. Once removed from many aspects of direct caregiving, the nurse, they say, will "manage" the patient's case. This language reveals how little consultants know about or value the direct patient contact that is the hallmark of bedside nursing and the key to quality care.

It also suggests the gender issues that are embedded in the devaluation of nursing. Much of so-called women's work—mothering and teaching, for example—is characterized by the same kind of interwoven skills and interrupted labor found in nursing care. These qualities invite trivialization in our society. This thinking runs so deep that even many feminists encourage talented women to pursue careers in fields that are considered men's work, reinforcing the idea that women's work is less demanding and less valuable. We now see this pernicious notion applied to nursing, as consultants and managers argue that the farther a nurse is from the bedside, the more valuable she is.

While this bizarre idea may appeal to those who have the least contact with patients, it is clear to bedside nurses and patients that distancing experienced nurses from patients jeopardizes care. Sadly, this is a fact in which money managers, who increasingly control the health care system, have little interest. As recent successful legal actions against HMOs and other investigations into managed care have demonstrated, executives will sacrifice direct patient care to generate greater profits.

This attitude permeates the money managers' approach to home, community, and primary care as well. One HMO executive recently told a class in health care administration that if nurse practitioners save money, his company will use them. But if patients object and prefer physicians, he wouldn't argue with the customer and would jettison nurse practitioners if that were the commercially expedient option.

If nursing leaders and advanced practice nurses look the other way as bedside nursing gets dismantled, what will happen to hospitalized patients who are sicker than ever and need expert nursing care? What will happen to nursing's public image if patients are abandoned in this way? Remember, when nurses are not there to answer call lights or are too overwhelmed to give quality care, nursing will be blamed, not hospital administrators and their management consultants.

If bedside nursing fails to survive, who will support advanced practice nurses when they are under seige in state legislatures, Congress, or the community, as they surely will be in this cost-obsessed environment? And where will tomorrow's advanced practice nurses come from if bedside nursing is allowed to disintegrate?

Nursing's moral claim is that it provides holistic, continuous, expert patient care. This vision is being compromised by attitudes that prevail today. Behaving once again like an oppressed group, nurses blame each other for the kinds of Hobson's choices with which they are faced, instead of blaming the money managers who are decimating health care. Nurse executives condemn staff nurses for demanding and getting salary increases that they say are pricing nursing out of the market. Staff nurses fault nursing directors for allowing hospital management, once again, to save money through cuts in nursing budgets. Home care and advanced practice nurses accuse each other of costing too much.

Everyone seems to ignore the fact that improvements in wages and working conditions came in response to a recent and quickly forgotten nursing shortage. And they seem to forget that the improvements worked: they attracted a new generation of talented young people as well as second career adults into nursing. Now that hospital nursing positions are drying up, we can expect another nursing shortage in a few years. Meanwhile, the patient is getting lost in the shuffle.

Throughout its divided history, nursing has struggled with controversial reporting structures, contested management strategies, conflicting educational systems, strife-ridden attempts to organize practice licensure, dissension in the ranks, and fractious relationships with other professions. While understandably yearning for an expanded role in health care, nurses must not give up the fight to control *all* areas of nursing practice. A division between bedside nursing and advanced practice must not be allowed to become a fault line on which nursing's house could crumble. Nurses must not participate in the unraveling of the tapestry of nursing.

Now is the time for nursing to assert, as a unified profession, with one clear voice, that only qualified nurses can give safe, comprehensive patient care. Now is the time to act. Write to your representatives in Congress and your state legislators. Call your newspapers. Ask your association or union to conduct informational picketing in front of your hospital. Provide public relations seminars that explain the importance of expert nursing care at the bedside. Circulate the American Nurses' Association's brochure, *Everyone Deserves a Nurse.* Educate the public. Make them aware that bedside nursing is in jeopardy—and when nursing is in jeopardy, so is patient care.

The money managers are on the march. The delivery of quality patient care by nurses at the bedside is under siege. And if this siege is successful, nursing as we know it will be destroyed.

Reference

Ulrich, Laurel Thatcher. 1991. *Good Wives: Image and Reality in the Lives of Women in Northern New England, 1650–1750.* New York: Vintage Books, 1991.

Chapter 15
The Rationality of Caring

Kari Waerness

In order to find better models for caregiving work, this article develops an analysis of the concept of caring. The focus is on caring for dependents, and it is argued that this kind of caring, typically a responsibility for women, is based on a specific kind of rationality. The "rationality of caring" is different from scientific rationality, which is aimed at controlling the environment. It also transcends the categories of rationality and instrumentality as opposed to emotions and expressiveness. It is suggested that the search for new models of organizing the public care system must pay attention to the specific qualities inherent in caregiving work.

While rationality has been a central issue in the social sciences since the beginning of those fields, caring is a concept that until recent years has scarcely received any attention in the sociological literature. What it means to care for others and how caregiving services are to be carried out in the welfare states of the western world today is attracting the interest of social scientists—in part because of the challenges emerging from feminism for the search for a women's perspective in social theory, and, in part because of the more recent shift in social policy debate dealing with the public services. In the Scandinavian countries, for example, public opinion shows a declining confidence in professionalism and increased socialization, once considered to be the cornerstones in the development of the welfare state. Instead, a belief in so-called "community care" is spreading rapidly because it is supposed to be cheaper and morally preferable to public caregiving services.

The feminist critique of sociological conceptualizations and theories

An earlier version of this essay appeared as Waerness, "The Rationality of Caring," *Economic and Industrial Democracy, an International Journal,* 5, 2 (1984): 185–210. Reprinted by permission of Sage Publications Ltd.

that do not adequately reflect the position of women in society is highly relevant for understanding this shift or change of direction in social policy thinking. The enthusiasm with which "care by the community" or "informal caring networks" has been discussed in public debate is rarely matched by a clear analysis of either the conditions for or the consequences of methods and measures for its implementation. In fact, the knowledge that can be applied to this new policy option is very limited because there are few systematic theories in sociology on the study of reproduction and the social order. There is no conceptual framework that can be applied in analyzing experiences and activities transcending our traditional sociological dichotomies like public/private, home/work, labor/leisure. This makes it difficult to formulate a theory of caregiving work.

Lacking a ready-made conceptual framework, some empirical facts will be used as a starting point in our discussion to suggest a basis for a more thorough understanding of the factual changes going on in the organization of caregiving work and of the changes in beliefs concerning optimal caregiving.

One fundamental fact, of course, is that the responsibility for caring is still ascribed on the basis of gender—as a part of the formation of "femininity." What this means for women today is that they are faced with the task of caring for the children, the ill, the disabled, and the elderly in the private sphere while at the same time trying to achieve more command over their own lives and a greater measure of economic independence. The new ideology that informal care is better than public care contributes to reinforce these problems (Finch and Groves 1980).

However, the increasing transfer of caring responsibilities from the private sphere has meant that public services have become a very important part of the female labor market. Even if the high-ranking professional and administrative positions in this sector are mostly filled by men, and a great number of the newly created jobs for women are unskilled and low-paid, the importance of public services for the welfare of working women has to be carefully evaluated.

Such an evaluation seems especially important in a situation where we are confronted with the idea that it would be better to replace these services with different kinds of informal caring. The sociological description of the growth of public caregiving services as "an emptying of the functions of the family" or as "deprivatization of social reproduction" is, from a woman's perspective, very inadequate and needs to be reexamined and qualified. In addition to the fact that a great deal of research has documented that most of the caregiving work still is performed on a family or private basis (e.g., Moroney 1976; Waerness 1978; Sundström 1980), informal resources very often have to be mobilized both to make use of existing social services and to substitute for their shortages. Most often women are the ones who have to cope with the deficiencies of the welfare state services. Besides, many of these services have not first and foremost replaced informal caring, but instead gradually changed its content, as an increasing number of professional educators, advisors, and consultants have invaded the private sphere (Stacey 1981, pp. 174–75).

I think the most educated guess social scientists can offer to the question of community care is the following: any idea of a massive replacement of public services by unpaid and informal caring arrangements is unlikely to be realized in the foreseeable future.[1] More probably, in societies like ours, the demand for public care will continue to increase, as a result of changes in the age distribution of the population, changes in family behavior, and women's increasing demand for paid employment. Unless there should be more stigma attached to the use of public services, it also seems reasonable to expect that the number of people who consider public caregiving services to be among the social rights connected with their status as citizens in the welfare state will steadily increase.[2]

As a result of the development of the welfare state, informal care in the private sphere can more adequately be viewed today as a supplement rather than an alternative to public care. Suggested policy alternatives that aim at transferring more caregiving work from the public to the private sphere are based on the assumption that informal structures for providing care already exist and simply need to be activated. This assumption is, however, unrealistic. Social scientists should, therefore, first and foremost, concentrate their research and analysis on the possibilities for a more rational use of currently available resources for public care. By "rational" in this context, I mean, rational in relation to what most of us in our everyday life perceive as the essential values in a "caring relationship."

The recent trend in favor of more community care is at least in part a consequence of many people's experience that the public care system lacks the very qualities necessary to transform "services" into "caring." In view of the challenge posed by those who, for other than economic reasons, question the legitimacy of many welfare state services (e.g., Illich 1976), there is a great need to find better models for organizing caregiving work. To develop such models, it seems necessary to study not only the exploitative nature of women's traditional caregiving work but also the positive qualities inherent in it,[3] as well as why the latter seem to get lost when caregiving is professionalized and socialized. To be able to carry this analysis further, however, more theoretical attention must first be given to the concept of "caring."

Caring: Both Labor and Feelings

Conceptual and theoretical tools from our sociological tradition are inadequate to analyze a phenomenon like caring. Thus it seems reasonable to use a dictionary definition of caring as a starting point. In broad terms, caring is a concept encompassing that range of human experiences that has to do with feeling concern for and taking care of the well-being of others. This definition tells us that caring is both about activities and feelings. "Feeling concern" and "taking charge" have both practical and psychological implications. We often choose the words "care for" to convey a sense of the bonds that tie us to other people in a wide variety of social relationships. We "care for" our friends, our lovers, our children, our parents, our clients, our patients, sometimes our neighbors, and sometimes even people we come into contact with at chance meeting places. Caring is about relations between (at least two) people.[4] One of them (the carer) shows concern, consideration, affection, devotion, toward the other (the cared for). The one needing care is invaluable to the one providing care, and when the former is suffering pain or discomfort, the latter identifies with her or him and attends to alleviating it. Adult, healthy people feel a need to be cared for by others in many different situations. Worn out, dejected, tired, depressed—there are many adjectives to describe states in which what we need or desire is for others "to care for us." In such situations we may feel that we have a *right* to have our need for care met. This means there must be others who feel that it is their duty or desire to honor this right. Persons to whom we are attached through the ties of family, love, or friendship most often are the ones we expect to feel this obligation or desire.

In principle, caring for healthy adults might be based on equal give-and-take relationships between people who have personal ties to each other. This kind of informal care can be based on *norms of balanced reciprocity* in personal relations; that is, help, support, and favors can be exchanged between people in symmetrical relations. When we say that people "care for each other," we have this kind of reciprocity in mind. However, as caring first and foremost tends to be associated with women, *much* of the caring women do for their husbands, older children, and other adult members of the family does not imply this kind of reciprocity and should therefore, in terms of activities, be defined rather as *personal services.* When women provide these services, it can often be experienced as something they are "forced" to do, not as a result of their concern for the well-being of others but as a result of their subordinate position in the family. When providing help and services to persons who cannot perform these activities themselves—young children, the ill, the disabled, the frail elderly—the situation is different. In such relations, the receiver of care is the subordinate in relation to the caregiver. These groups are dependent on some people who feel an obligation or desire to *care for others*.

To provide good care in such relations means that the caregiver at all times performs the activities necessary to satisfy the immediate needs of the cared for. At the same time, most dependents have to meet certain demands and challenges in order to prevent lapses in their development or recovery. Therefore, good caring should be performed in a way that, as far as possible, reinforces the self-sufficiency and independence of the receiver. The dependent is neither to be overprotected nor to be neglected.

Whether we analyze caring as "labor" or as "love," it seems highly important to make theoretical distinctions among (1) caring for dependents, (2) caring for superiors and (3) caring in symmetrical relations. In both emotional and practical terms, it can be assumed that these different categories of caring relations give rise to different problems for women in their struggle for greater independence and autonomy.

These distinctions also make us attentive to problematic situations where women have to choose for whom to care—the weaker or the stronger. Both in women's family roles and in many of the traditional female occupational roles, there is a great risk of confrontations with such dilemmas.[5]

Caring for dependents, those members of society who by normal social standards are unable to take care of themselves, is the field of caring that most clearly is a concern both for social policy and for feminists. In the rest of this paper, I therefore limit most of the discussion to problems connected with caring for dependents, involving people who take on active caring on a consistent and reliable basis. This kind of caring I define as caregiving work, whether it is paid or unpaid, no matter whether it takes place in the public or in the private sphere.

The Scientification of Reproduction: A New Kind of Male Control over Women's Caregiving Work

Traditional arguments for ascribing caring functions to women, in addition to the unquestionable fact that only women give birth to children, is also founded on a perception of women as more intuitive and emotional than men. With the modernization of society, however, this ascribed "natural inclination" was no longer assumed to be sufficient for women to become "good" carers in either the private or the public sphere. In addition, it was thought that they ought to acquire *some* formal knowledge based on science. Scientific work, however, was not for women. Either they were considered to be intellectually incapable of doing re-

search, or scientific work was assumed to be detrimental to their biological function. (It is interesting to note that no one seems to have argued that it is "illogical" that only members of the gender not qualified
for practicing care should be capable of giving expert advice on how
it should be carried out.) We also find stated explicitly, if not so often,
that the defining criterion of scientific knowledge, objectivity, is essentially masculine. George Simmel is one representative for this opinion:

The requirement—of correctness in practical judgement and objectivity in theoretical knowledge—belong as it were in their form and their claims to humanity
in general, but in their actual historical configuration they are masculine
throughout. Supposing that we describe these things, viewed as absolute ideas,
by the single word "objective," we then find that in the history of our race the
equation objective=masculine is a valid one. (quoted in List 1983, p. 6)

The scientification of reproductive work, which in the Scandinavian
countries started in the second part of the nineteenth century, meant
that women became subordinated to a new kind of male authority—the
authority of scientific knowledge. On the one hand, the emergence of
this new kind of authority meant a substitution or a decline of other
kinds of authority—the authority of the husband/father and of the
clerical profession. On the other hand, this scientification also implied
that women lost positions of authority and control. The case of the increasing power of the medical profession, still the most authoritative in
the field of reproduction, is the most important one in this respect. The
traditional lay health care system consists of autonomous healers of both
sexes, and the whole field of pregnancy and childbirth once belonged
to the sphere. The history of midwifery, being somewhat different in
various western countries, still tells us that the increasing influence of
doctors everywhere led to the midwives' losing status and autonomy
(Ehrenreich and English 1973; Oakley 1976). At the same time, the
medical profession's control over health care created new subordinate
roles for women. Both mothers and nurses became medical auxiliaries,
executing what the doctors prescribed (Donzelot 1979, pp. 9–47).

Much research has documented that this increasing scientific control
over reproduction should not be described as an unambiguous development of progress and humanization. In the fields of obstetrics, child
care, health, psychiatry, and care for the mentally retarded we find
everywhere examples of professionals at times confounding traditional
practices that the experts of later times evaluate as better than the new
ones their predecessors prescribed on the basis of "what we know from
science."[6] The same has been true for domestic activities such as keeping
house, cooking, and cleaning. Textbooks on domestic science and infant
care written by male doctors and published in Norway during the last

hundred years clearly give the impression of the belief in the omnipotence of science and the impotence of women, even if the latter belief is not explicitly stated in the books published in more recent decades. An illustrative example of this phenomenon can be found at the time when the first attempt to make housewifery into domestic science was made.

The first two textbooks on housewifery based on scientific knowledge published in Norway, about 1860, were followed by a great public debate among members of the male elite about the quality of women's work in the household. Some years earlier a woman, Hanna Winsnes, had started to write such textbooks, based not on scientific knowledge but on her practical experiences as a housewife in a large bourgeois family household for more than forty years. When her books are compared with "scientific" ones, the modesty of Hanna Winsnes sharply contrasts with the arrogance of the male authors. Only in the textbook intended to be of special help to the poorest housewives does she moralize in an authoritarian manner. On the basis of today's accepted standards for good practices, however, Hanna Winsnes's books are still qualitatively better than those written by male "scientists." Many of her recipes, for instance, even if too bothersome for modern housewives, *could* still be used with relatively good results for a healthy and palatable diet.

The same does not hold for the "scientific" books. Their recipes are mostly too inaccurate to be of much help to the inexperienced cook, and many of their general recommendations are the reverse of what is considered to be correct according to current standards. The male authors use much space to argue, in a very arrogant style, why women's traditional practices (also Hanna Winsnes's) are basically wrong, suggesting that women therefore need some formal knowledge in order to be better housewives. Notwithstanding the praise they received from their contemporary critics, these scientific textbooks were soon forgotten. Hanna Winsnes's books, on the other hand, in spite of much criticism from the male elite, sold thousands of copies over a period of more than fifty years.

The recommendations of experts in the field of children, on subjects ranging from breast- and bottle-feeding, toilet-training, weaning, eating, sleeping, to more general problems of discipline and punishment, have also changed very much with time. To a certain extent it has also been found that what experts considered the only right thing to do at one time they later consider to be totally wrong. Whatever the content of the advice, however, it has often been expressed in such an authoritative manner that a mother who does not manage to follow it may get the impression that this will permanently harm her children.

Evaluating the present state of knowledge on this subject the Newsons admit that there is not a sufficient body of well-substantiated evidence about the facts and consequences of child rearing on which to base sound practical advice to parents. There is no lack of theoretical speculation, but so far very few theories of child rearing have been subjected to the inconvenience of being reconciled with the empirical evidence. Whatever the reason may be for this unfortunate state of affairs, the situation can hardly have arisen simply because the subject has no importance: indeed, it is probably because it has such immense importance that the professional advisers and pseudo-experts have flourished in such profusion. (1976, p. 14)

As some professionals in recent years have become more modest in their roles as advisors, the arguments for the necessity of parents' education have shifted. As science has documented the importance and value of some of the traditional practices that were earlier denounced, "parents' education" is now seen as necessary because of the assumed decline of the extended family and the increasing lack of informal caring networks.[7] In addition to the more modest experts, we still have professionals believing in the omnipotence of science. Rudolf Schaffer seems to be one of them:

There is, in fact, no reason why bringing up the under-fives should not also be guided by firm knowledge scientifically established rather than depend, as happens at present, on fashion, prejudice and what grandmother says. The parent-child relationship need be no more immune from properly conducted objective inquiry than the movements of the planets or the structure of DNA—even if its analysis presents problems of far greater complexity. (Schaffer 1977, p. 11)

We have very little factual information on how mothers react to the experts' different and often contradictory recommendations. However, the number of experts invading the private sphere has steadily increased, and formal training in school and employment teaches women to act according to the dominant kinds of rationality in the public sphere. The question whether this is counter-productive to their developing the skills and attitudes necessary for "rational caregiving" therefore becomes important. Most mothers today probably agree with the scientific experts that "natural inclination" is not sufficient to handle the problems they face in caring for their children. How much help they have from formal knowledge and professional advice, however, is an unanswered question. The studies of Oakley (1974) and Holter et al. (1967) support the assumption that Helena Lopata's conclusions, based on a study of American metropolitan housewives, holds for western women in general[8]:

The social role of mother does not produce many women who express full confidence in their ability to perform it at desired levels. In fact, the more educated the American metropolitan woman, the more conscious she is of the complexity of this role and of the difficulties involved in competent child-rearing. The relational emphasis of this type of mother, combined with a societal focusing of responsibility on her and awareness of the importance of the home for child development, make for worry over actions designed to best meet the goals of the relation. The physical care of the offspring is no longer a major source of concern, as it was for the lower-class antecedents of the modern woman; she quite competently handles preventative and curative situations of child health. It is her desire to provide the offspring with the best available resources for the development of their personality and potentials, coupled with the inadequacy of the sources of knowledge which she can utilize, which creates the greatest degree of concern for the new American woman. (1971, pp. 375–6)

That more theoretical knowledge does not always improve the quality of caregiving work should not lead to the conclusion that less knowledge would be better. Instead, we have to ask *what kind* of knowledge is relevant in order to deal with problems that cannot be mastered by finding the perfect techniques or by acting according to bureaucratic rules, but where the quality of the work still depends on the actor's training and skills.

Wittgenstein, when discussing a somewhat different problem in *Philosophical Investigations*, illuminates what seems to be a crucial problem also when discussing notions of learning and teaching in the context of caregiving:

Is there such a thing as "expert judgment" about the genuineness of expressions of feeling? — Even here, there are those whose judgment is "better" and those whose judgement is "worse."
Correcter prognoses will generally issue from the judgments of those with better knowledge of mankind.
Can one learn this knowledge? Yes: some can. *Not, however, by taking a course in it, but through "experience."* — Can someone else be a man's teacher in this? Certainly. From time to time he gives him the right tip. This is what "learning" and "teaching" are like here. — *What one acquires is not a technique; one learns correct judgments.* There are also rules, but they do not form a system, and *only experienced people can apply them right. Unlike calculating rules.*
What is most difficult here is to put this indefiniteness, correctly and unfalsified, into words. (Quoted in McMillan 1982, pp. 41–42, emphases added)

To the extent that scientific knowledge becomes an absolute gauge of what counts as knowledge, Wittgenstein reminds us that this can be detrimental to practices that earlier belonged to the nonscientific sphere. In the realm of caregiving, where we have a long tradition of male scientific arrogance in evaluating women's practices, this problem today seems to be highly relevant.

The ambivalence with which women writers confront the phenomenon "science" is probably not only a result of the continuing exclusion of women from the business of science. I agree with List (1983) that the roots of this ambivalence go deeper. Science's rationalist culture and the models of behavior it propagates are contradictory, if not hostile, to the feelings women see as their own. A central task of feminist research, in my opinion, then, is to look at the context of caregiving work and evaluate the use of conventional scientific concepts and models, which may well account for the fact that important problems remain over-looked. Furthermore, in this field, female social scientists can use their personal experiences from everyday life to suggest alternative models. These alternatives can contribute then to a change in social theory and research which will better reflect the realities and interests of both women and the weakest members of society. A new image of the social actor and a reconceptualization of "rationality" emerging from women's studies seem to be promising outcomes.

The Sentient Actor and the Rationality of Caring

Both on the basis of my personal experiences from caregiving in the private sphere and from doing empirical research on caregiving work, I find it reasonable to argue the following. There exists something that should be called "the rationality of caring," of fundamental importance for the welfare of the dependents, and at the same time different from and to some degree contradictory to the scientific rationality on which professional authority and control in the field of reproduction is legiti-mated. Titmuss verges on this problem when he writes the following about patients' situation in the modern hospital:

Why is it not understood that courtesy and sociability have a therapeutic value? *Most of us in our home know this instinctively, but somehow or other it gets lost in the hospital.* (Titmuss 1963, p. 126, emphasis added)

Apart from the fact that courtesy and sociability are probably of greater importance in situations where therapy no longer has any effect, one important reason this knowledge is forgotten could be that the value of kindness and politeness cannot be calculated. I further disagree with Titmuss that we know anything about caring *by instinct*. In some way or another it has to be learned. Even if emotions are important for our caring for others in the private sphere, it seems evident that the ability to care in a "proper" way depends on something which can be learned and for which there are rules for proceeding, and that therefore some kind of rationality is involved.

To accept a conceptualization like "the rationality of caring" is to go against the mainstream of western philosophy and sociology, which deals with rationality and emotionality (or instrumentality and expressiveness) as two mutually exclusive qualities of human action—a mainstream that traditionally has defined women as less rational human beings than men. Weber (1966), for instance, even if arguing that emotions are important, still posits a model of social action that defines action based on emotion, like action based on ignorance and tradition, as nonrational.[9] This raises two problems: a confusion between rationality and lack of emotion, and the implication that emotions and feelings are not positively required by the rational action of individuals or by the smooth functioning of institutions (Hochschild, 1975, p. 284).

In the normal discourse of everyday reasoning, however, this dualistic image of rationality and emotionality is not always self-evident. Probably most people experience emotions and feelings as active and legitimate ingredients in behavior that they at the same time define as rational. The *New Webster's World Dictionary* does not support the assumption of the mutual exclusiveness of emotionality and rationality, showing that it has not been totally accepted in our everyday language. One definition of "rational" is the following: "The ability to reason logically as by drawing conclusions from inferences; *often* connotes the absence of emotionalism." To assume that some kind of rationality is operating also in activities and relations where emotions are of crucial importance, therefore, does not seem idiosyncratic according to how rationality can be interpreted in everyday life, even in a rationalized culture like ours.

Arlie Hochschild (1975) argues that we need a new image of the social actor in addition to the images that hitherto have dominated much of the social sciences. The first image is that of *conscious, cognitive actor.* This image portrays people as consciously wanting something (e.g., money and status) and consciously calculating the merit of various means to reach this end. The second image, established by Freud, is that of *unconscious, emotional actor.* Here the actor is guided by unconscious motivations and does and thinks things whose meanings are better understood by the social scientist than by the actor. As Hochschild points out, these two images do not *deny* affective consciousness; images deny nothing.

However, it is a commonplace insight of the sociology of knowledge that we collectively construct social reality, that what we define as real, is real. Because of the authority, prestige, and influence of scientific institutions in modern society, science not only describes but also prescribes social situations and forms of social actions. So, for instance, if we believe in the scientific understanding of head and heart or emotions and rationality as antithetical, we act on the basis of this definition and organize our lives so as to confirm this belief. Our experience then provides further evidence that our definition is correct and the duality goes on and on. It therefore seems important to include in the social sciences an image of a social actor who is *both* conscious and feeling. Hochschild suggests the *sentient actor* as a third image necessary to remind social scientists that human actors must be seen as more than bloodless calculators or blind expressers of uncontrolled emotions. In order to analyze phenomena like caring and caregiving, which seem to fall in a no-man's land when we focus on either the conscious cognitive actor or the unconscious emotional actor, this image of the sentient actor seems adequate.[10] Furthermore, this image gives meaning to a conceptualization like "the rationality of caring."

To get a better understanding of how the rationality of caring differs from scientific rationality, we can analyze how "learning" in the context of motherly care, as an ideal type in the Weberian sense, differs from "learning" in the context of science. In the context of science, one understands from the position of an outsider, and learning means to develop the ability to formulate a body of principles based on what is common to many phenomena and therefore independent of the peculiar and individual. One learns from books and theories, and shows that one knows something by being able to subsume the important points in a neat system of laws. In science, one searches for predictability and control, the dominant criteria according to which scientific success is measured.

In the context of motherly care one has to think and act on the level of the particular and individual. This means one has to understand from the position of an insider, and the kind of generalized scientific knowledge one may have, at best, seems very insufficient in guiding one's practices. Moreover, "as the child grows it requires different things from its mother and this means that she can never perfect her techniques, but must remain flexible and capable of adapting to a changed situation" (Kitzinger 1978, p. 34). Or in the words of McMillan:

> it is vital for mothers to be aware that there are many things in life which can neither be learned from books nor understood from the position of an outsider. It is only because we realize that acting with rigid consistency is not always a sign of reasonable and appropriate behavior that we do not think a mother is stupid when for example, we see her from one day to the next, making delicate adjustments in the care of her infant which other people would not think worthwhile. (McMillan 1982, p. 54)

The point that all those who advocate standardizing and making scientific our methods of childrearing seems to miss is the following: in the context of everyday life, it is foolish to seek "certainty" in one's personal relations. The aim to provide women with scientific certainty that their method of childrearing will be successful is pseudo-science because the relation between individuals is, by definition, something that cannot be subsumed under any kind of statistical generalization. Once that is done, the aspect of individuality vanishes.

It is therefore not surprising that mothers seem to be extremely hesitant about concocting theories about how other people should bring up their children, and that many of them are still skeptical about the advice thrust upon them by "experts."

Expertise in childrearing, according to the rationality of caring, is dependent both on practical experience in caregiving work and on personal knowledge of the individual child in question. When mothers are exchanging advice and support concerning problems of child care, they can therefore at the same time insist that it is easier to bring up the second child than the first, and still say that each child has to be treated quite differently. To search for the kind of precision inherent in scientific rationality therefore seems foolish or wrong in the context of caregiving.

To illustrate the point of how working according to the rules of scientific rationality in some contexts can be counter-productive to what could be defined as rational behavior, the work of a cook can be compared with the work of a chemist:

The use of a chemical balance in the kitchen would not make an inferior cook a better one because in the kitchen the role that the accuracy of measurements plays is not comparable with its importance in a chemistry experiment. For example, while it is obviously important to mix the ingredients in the right proportions if a good cake is to be made, it is possible to juggle with them in order to obtain a certain effect in a way that would be quite unacceptable in an experiment. Moreover, the reasons why someone may be a bad cook, in contradistinction to being a bad chemist, may have nothing to do with inaccurate measurements. In some cases it may actually result from following a recipe rigidly and not knowing how to adapt it to suit one's own particular tastes and circumstances. Such knowledge, however, depends on practice and on the help of those who are experienced cooks. (McMillan 1982, p. 49, emphasis added)

These arguments about concrete activities like cooking may seem trivial or obvious, at least at the level of everyday reasoning.[11] In planning public caregiving services, a similar attitude to the importance of personal knowledge and a lack of rigidity should be considered reasonable or rational. To the extent that such evaluations should be taken into account, it follows that professional and bureaucratic control has to be diminished. That the professionalization and bureaucratization of the public care system still seems to be increasing, tells us that such evaluations may be contradictory to the principles on which the whole ideology of public planning is based, and therefore not so easy to implement.

From various empirical studies of public caregiving services, however, it seems that the image of the sentient actor is a perfectly adequate one for understanding the behavior and attitudes of the caregivers in the lower positions in organizational hierarchies (Abrahamsson and Söder 1977; Liljeström and Özgalda 1980; Ressner 1981; Viklund 1981). The same image emerges from my own study of homehelpers (Waerness 1982, pp. 136–80). The work of these homehelpers was organized in such a way that the individual employee provided flexible and versatile services and help to a few clients over relatively long periods of time. The most satisfying feature of these homehelpers' jobs was said to be their personal attachment to the clients. In fact, this aspect seemed to be the main reason they felt happy about their job and wanted to stick to it. These middle-aged and elderly women argued that their experience as a housewife in their own family for many years was the most important prerequisite for being able to do a good job as a homehelper. Even those who had special formal training for this occupation doubted it had any value, apart from heightening the status of their job.[12] Working on the basis of their competence as housewives, however, often meant they had to break the official job instructions. Often they had to work for more hours than they were paid, and sometimes they even had to do things that were directly forbidden according to the rules. They also expressed very clear opinions about the negative aspects of their job. The isolated working situation, which meant they had no colleagues with whom to share problems and experiences, and the lack of influence compared to the more professionalized working groups in the social services were regarded as very negative features of their work role. They also had a very clear understanding that their conduct as employees in many ways could be evaluated as foolish, according to the general norms for rational behavior on the labor market. Still, they gave priority to doing what seemed right according to the rationality of caring.

Public authorities feel compelled today to change the current organization of the homehelp service, in part, to secure the individual homehelper the same rights as other employees on the labor market, and, in part, because of the diminishing supply of middle-aged housewives who both are willing and feel competent to work under the same conditions as in the past. The authorities admit that it may be difficult to find measures to change the organization without changing the service in such a way that it becomes less personal and comprehensive.

In their study about wards in institutions for the mentally retarded, Abrahamsson and Söder (1977) used flexibility in work as an indicator of "good caring." The work was said to be flexible to the extent that the behavior of the staff varied over time and in relation to the individual needs of the mentally retarded person involved (Söder 1981, p. 48). To be capable of working in this way, I assume, the individual caregiver had to be both conscious and feeling, that is, a *sentient actor*. In investigating the relationships between flexibility in work and different organizational characteristics of the institutions, this study shows that decentralization of power was the factor most strongly correlated with flexibility in work. Wards where the staff had influence over work-related decisions functioned with greater flexibility than wards where decision-making powers were centralized. The way work was coordinated was also found to be of importance. Wards where work was coordinated by formal planning and detailed instructions were often working in a routinized, nonflexible way. More access to experts of any kind, a remedy planning authorities generally believe is for the better, showed no direct correlation with the degree of flexibility in work. Still more important, it could be shown that a more professionally trained staff did not result in more flexibility. On the contrary, formal training seemed to promote a tendency to more routinization, a finding so surprising in relation to accepted truths that it needed further comment:

It must be reasonable to assume that increased knowledge on the part of the staff should lead to more flexibility at the workplace. When we still do not find more flexibility on wards with a high proportion of educated personnel, we have to question the content of the education. Only to insist that education is for the good seems meaningless as long as one does not specify what kind of knowledge the caregivers need. (Abrahamsson and Söder 1977, p. 80)

One explanation for the fact that professional training did not further flexibility could be that this kind of learning socializes individuals to think and act according to the values inherent in scientific rationality and in such a way that the values inherent in the rationality of caring become degraded or suppressed. In other words, the conscious cognitive actor becomes more of an ideal than the sentient actor. Because the head-heart duality is accepted in all sciences, it is probable that any kind of formal education based on scientific knowledge will to some degree promote a more instrumental attitude towards work, at the expense of the expressive.

What studies of medical education say about this problem probably has some relevance for most formal education in the field of caregiving. Merton and Barber (1967) describe the doctor's role as one of "detached concern." They refer to the combination of detachment (an instrumental trait) and concern (an expressive trait) as a perfect example of sociological ambivalence in that it involves an oscillation between conflicting norms:

The therapist role of the physician . . . calls for *both* a degree of affective detachment for the patient *and* a degree of compassionate concern for him. . . . Since these norms cannot be *simultaneously* expressed in behavior, they come to be expressed in an *oscillation* of behaviors: of detachment and compassion, of discipline and permissiveness, of personal and impersonal treatment. (Merton and Barber 1967, p. 96, emphases added)

The degree to which formal education for caregivers in subordinate positions leads to a strengthening of the belief in the duality of rationality and emotion can explain why the educated caregivers become less able or willing to give individualized care than the ones with no formal training at all.[13] Changes in the work roles of the nurses support this view. In trying to achieve professional and academic status, leading nurses everywhere tend to favor the development of formally acquired knowledge. This one-sidedness has led to a devaluation of the informally acquired and intuitive kind of knowledge and skills which are learned through practicing bedside care (Alvsvåg 1981; Martinsen and Waerness, 1979). More "nursing science" is therefore not a solution to the problem of strengthening the values inherent in the rationality of caring, at least as long as this science is based on the generally accepted notions of scientific knowledge and learning.

Schumacher (1978) argues that there are many problems in human life which cannot be solved through scientific reasoning, for which such reasoning in fact leads to answers that appear to be the exact opposite of what is needed. He proposed calling these problems *divergent*, in contrast to *convergent* problems to which the scientific methodology of problem solving is adequate. Most of the examples of divergent problems he mentions belong to the realm of caregiving. What he argues about divergent problems in general therefore seems to have great relevance for the problems emerging from the increasing professionalization of caregiving work.

Divergent problems offend the logical mind which wishes to remove tension by coming down on one side or the other; but they provoke, stimulate and sharpen the higher human faculties without which man is nothing but a clever animal. A refusal to accept the divergency of divergent problems causes these higher faculties to remain dormant and to wither away, and when this happens the "clever animal" is more likely than not to destroy itself.

Man's life can thus be seen and understood as a succession of divergent problems which are inevitably encountered and have to be coped with in some way. They are refractory to mere logic and discursive reason, and constitute, as it were, a strain-and-stretch apparatus to develop the Whole Man, and that means to develop man's supra-logical faculties. All traditional cultures have seen life as a school and have recognized, in one way or another, the essentiality of this teaching force. (Pp. 147–48)

Better Caregiving: A Question of the Possibilities for Delimiting Professional and Bureaucratic Power

Scientific rationality is related to people's fundamental need for autonomy and control, and has constantly celebrated new victories as more and more spheres of life in modern society have become rationalized. At the same time, this rationalization has meant that other fundamental human needs, above all the need for care and closeness, needs we have learned to label "feminine," have become devalued. In order to be "real persons" with self respect and worthy of the esteem of others, modern men have to define themselves as "independent." The fact that "there is an element of dependence in every relationship, even with a dog," as Freud expressed it, and that helplessness and dependency are part of life itself for all of us—in childhood, illness, and old age—may in part be hidden and repressed as long as the caring function is left to an invisible, oppressed women's culture. Women still provide most of the caregiving work as unpaid family work, and the bulk of the helping that in western societies is reported as community care turns out on closer scrutiny to be care by close female relatives, a point which seldom is clearly stated (Abrams 1977).

As women to an increasing degree have become socialized to the dominant values in a rationalized society, their "dual life" in the "welfare-service society" does implies not only a heavy daily workload, but also means that they have to cope with the antithetical expectations of instrumentalism and expressiveness (Glennon 1979, pp. 160–64). This coping is the more difficult as these dual expectations are present in both women's family roles and most of their paid work roles.

It seems reasonable to assume that the scientification of reproduction has had an independent effect on most women's feelings of insecurity and lack of competence in all kinds of caregiving in the private sphere, whether they are well integrated in an informal female network or not. This is a point that many advocates for more community care as a solution to the crisis in the public care system seem to miss. As Stacey and Price (1981, pp. 100–132) have pointed out, the autonomy of women in the domestic sphere has gradually been so reduced that younger women today scarcely have a private domain in which they feel able and competent. Today's emphasis on more community care as a basis for a hierarchical and professionalized public care system, to the extent that it could be realized at all, would therefore most probably have the following consequences. The tendency of professional caregivers working as advisors and consultants would be strengthened and still more of the practical tasks would be left to subordinate and unpaid female members of the family. Furthermore, the presence of nonstigmatizing public services in the welfare state has been shown to be important for dependent people, as it allows them to maintain a kind of balanced reciprocity in their family relations. When dependent people have access to such services, the chances are greater that they can be on good, affectionate terms with their family members. Because they are not totally dependent on family members, they can receive help and support which they value very positively from them (Nordhus 1981).

Research from several countries has documented that a wish to maintain what Rosenmayr and Kockeis (1965) call "intimacy—but at a distance" seems to be the kind of relation a growing number of aged people prefer to have with their children (Shanas 1979). This desire may seem to be a typical attitude among the aged and disabled, not only in family relations but in relation to the public care system as well. The fact that the homehelp system, a caregiving service that moves on the borderline between the domestic and the public sphere and is very little professionalized, has become so popular, may be an indication of this development.

Studies of women's self-organized caregiving work on "the hidden market" also show that caregiving work can be paid. At the same time, much importance can be attached to ensuring that the relation between provider and receiver is to be comprehensive, personal, and characterized by equality (Gullestad in press). For example, clients can prefer to have their daughters or daughters-in-law as homehelpers, paid by the social services. Or non-related homehelpers can be regarded as "daughters" or "friends" (Teeland 1978, pp. 170–171; Schorr 1962, p. 419). Such attitudes toward combining personal attachment and payment in a relation are mainly found among working class women.[14] Middle class women are more likely to regard the paid caregiving relations on the hidden market more in terms of contractual employer-employee relations (Gullestad 1984).[15]

To deplore payment of informal caregiving on the grounds that the introduction of market values damages the quality of care is thus a typical middle class evaluation. In both the private and the public sphere, much of the paid caregiving of working class women, both today and in earlier times, contradicts this evaluation. On the other hand, not all kinds of private and unpaid care are of "good quality." When focusing on the problems of today's public services as being too impersonal, rigid, and insensitive, it is easy to forget the problems of oppression, injustice, violence, abuse, and moralizing that can arise in private and personalized caring relations. When public authorities today appear to accept the idea that the care for those who mainly need human consideration, warmth, and a bit more time[16] is better left to voluntary organizations than to the public care system, they seem to have forgotten the working class historical experiences with voluntary work in the form of charity.

However, the greatest problem within the public care system today is that there is too much detachment, not that there is too much concern. From the little evidence that exists, "more concern," in fact, is not primarily a question of whether caregiving is being paid for or not.

Strengthening the values inherent in the rationality of caring, is, therefore, in today's welfare state, not a question of replacing public *paid* care within informal *unpaid* family care or voluntary work. Rather, it seems to be a question of what possibilities there are to reorganize the public care system in such a way that practical experience in caregiving work and personal knowledge of the individual client can be an independent basis for greater influence, at the expense of professional and bureaucratic control and authority.

As virtually all prophets—or as they now are called, futurologists—seem to agree that the future will see an ever increasing reliance on specialized knowledge and skill and on applying that knowledge to the solution of practical problems by specially trained persons (e.g., Bell 1968), such a change may seem rather utopian. Freidson, as late as in 1973, argued that the tendency of many other occupations to organize around a professionalized service would increase in the future. Post-industrial society, in his opinion, would be the professional society. However, the growing skepticism in recent years toward further professionalization as a means of solving the ills of the capitalistic welfare state may imply that there is a chance this trend could be counteracted.

Since some representatives of the prestigious medical profession now admit that "the time has come for a major conceptual shift in the health care policy debate, from viewing lay people as consumers of health care to seeing them as they really are: its primary providers" (Levin and Idler 1981, p. 1), there may be reason to be optimistic. Furthermore, in the face of the substantial shift in the pattern of disease in the western world over the past forty years from approximately 30 percent of all diseases being chronic to the present 80 percent,[17] a shift to which the medical delivery has been unable to adjust adequately, the need for a change seems urgent.

Greater limitation on or diminution of professional and bureaucratic control in the public services requires a fundamental change in the values and interpretational frameworks of the public administration and the political bodies: an acknowledgment that many of the problems in the public care system today are *divergent* problems which cannot be *solved* with any kind of scientific methodology, but which still must be *coped with* on the basis of human actors' knowledge and skills.

More decision-making power for women, on the basis of their personal experiences from practical caregiving work in the private sphere and from working class jobs in the public caregiving services, seems at least to be a necessary condition for this to be realized.

Using Dawe's metaphor of sociology as a conversation in which the prime imperative is that we ceaselessly listen to and converse with the voices from everyday life . . . including our own (Dawe 1978, p. 414), a feminist sociology could be a tool to visualize how concrete forms in the public care system could further such changes and thereby strengthen the values inherent in the rationality of caring.

From what we already know, the organizational principle on which we should insist, in order to improve the situation both for dependents and caregivers today, could be worded like this: "Small, but not too small, is beautiful." This means that neither the small private and intimate family, nor the highly professionalized and specialized public care system, provide the kind of flexible and comprehensive care which seems optimal in relation to both dependents and caregivers' contradictory needs for both autonomy and closeness.

The need for reconceptualization of the notion of rationality has become a central concern for feminist sociology in Norway in recent years. The works of Marit Hoel, Bjørg Aase Sorensen, Kristin Tornes and Hildur Ve have given me great inspiration in my own work on the rationality of caring. I am also very grateful to Ritva Gough at the Swedish Center for Working Life, Stockholm, for her insight into the problems of caregiving which she has shared with me during our many informal discussions.

Notes

1. On the basis of evidence from social policy research, it seems unlikely that such a change should take place in the Scandinavian countries, at least in the short run.

2. Two surveys based on random samples of older people (70+) in the same Norwegian municipality in 1969 and 1981 show this to be the case for care in old age. In 1969, 16 percent of the aged preferred public to family care, while this proportion had increased to 58 percent in 1981. See Daatland 1983.

3. The most well-known feminist analyses in the first phase of the new women's movement focused mainly on the exploitative nature of women's traditional roles, e.g., de Beauvoir 1953; Friedan 1963; Firestone 1971; Millet 1971; Mitchell 1971. More recently, however, feminist writers working from their experiences in this new movement have struggled to redefine the grounds of feminist theory; this has also led to a refocusing on the positive experiences from traditional caregiving in the private sphere, especially that of motherhood (Friedan 1981; Smith 1979; O'Brien 1981). One reason for the need for these new kinds of analyses could be that analyses like de Beauvoir's and Firestone's create visions

of a future society which most women probably do not want to see realized. For a woman to be liberated, she must not, according to de Beauvoir, give birth. Firestone envisions a society where biological reproduction no longer takes place, but has been substituted by the technological means for a totally mechanistic process of reproduction.

4. In the social policy debate on the need for more "informal care," no clear distinction is made between "self-care" and "caring for others." These two concepts are, however, related to the contradictory values of independence and self-sufficiency on the one hand and responsibility and consideration for the well-being of others on the other. A clear distinction is necessary to make clear that these two sets of values often give rise to quite opposite priorities, both in everyday life and in the distribution of scarce resources for public care.

5. In the guidance literature for both wives and nurses published around the turn of the century, we find explicit advice on how they should behave in such situations. Most often, women are strongly recommended to obey the husband or the doctor.

6. Because we do not know to what extent women's practices have changed according to the changes in the experts' advice, historical studies tell most about changes in ideology. In the field of obstetrics, however, we have hard data on deaths attributed to puerperal fever and on infant mortality rates, which clearly show that the conversion from midwife to doctor at various points in time heightened the risk of death for both mothers and children (see, e.g., Branca 1975, pp. 74–112).

7. Present public discussion about the need for parental education is not as in former times, related to problems of physical care, but rather to problems of bettering the psychosocial conditions for children's development. How to organize such education without professionalizing the socialization process and without disabling the parents in the attempt to support them is admitted to be a problem (see, e.g., *Psychosocial Conditions for Development in Early Childhood* 1979).

8. Holter et al. (1967) found that housewives' expressed need for information was greatest on topics related to children's development. In general, the expressed need for information was highest among the most educated housewives and in the most urbanized districts. Oakley (1974) finds the social context in which the role of the mother is carried out today very dissatisfying, as social isolation and constant responsibility are general problems for modern mothers of all classes in urban communities.

9. Dawe (1978) argues that one important reason why Weber gave analytic primacy to instrumentally rational action was the scientific aspiration he brought to sociology. As such action was crucially concerned with scientifically precise relationships between means and ends, it was the easiest type of action to understand and explicate in the rigorous and exact terms scientific analysis demanded. Thus, even if Weber acknowledged that actual social actions and relationships are manifested in various combinations of elements of all his types of actions and orientations, he did not analyze them for the various ways in which they manifest such combinations. Instead, instrumentally rational action became the yardstick for analysis of actual courses of action, which were viewed in terms of their approximation to or deviation from that norm. Dawe argues that for sociological analysis in general the resort to science leads to a denial of human agency. To respect, grasp, and articulate the essential autonomy, contingency, and creativity of human agency, in Dawe's opinion, sociology must abandon its obsolete and imperious scientific pretension, "which cuts us off from

the world of which we also are members" (Dawe 1976, p. 409). Instead, Dawe suggests another metaphor for sociology than science: the metaphor of conversation.

10. Arlie Hochschild argues that the image of the sentient actor makes us attentive to the fact that the "social" goes deeper than our current images of the social actor have led us to suppose. Roles and relationships are surely not social patterns that apply only to thought and action, leaving feeling as an untouched, timeless, and universal constant. We therefore should integrate the sociology of the head with a sociology of the heart (1975: 299–300).

11. For someone who has not learned to cook, however, this is not obvious, and in general most of us very often forget how much learning is required for what may seem to be the simplest tasks.

12. In Sweden, a special training format for homehelpers has been organized by many municipalities in order to increase the supply of homehelpers. So far, these training programs have not been very successful. A very high proportion of the women who have received this training say that the actual content of the job as homehelper does not correspond very well with the expectations they got in the training, and that therefore they want other types of jobs (*Pensionärunder-sökningens rapporter om social hemhjälp m.m.* 1947–51).

13. Ve (1983) shows how "the hidden curriculum" in the whole educational system furthers instrumentalism at the expense of the expressive. Apart from the first years in school, where there is some room for the giving of care to each other according to his or her personal needs, the school mainly conveys values connected to instrumentalism. Because it is not clear how this value orientation conflicts with the rationality of caring, this creates special problems for girls, especially from the working class.

14. This class difference among women is related to the descriptions of class differences in general. Researchers disagree in their interpretations of the working class lifestyle, but many have pointed out the greater tendency to expressiveness compared with the middle class (e.g., Bernstein 1975; Sennett and Cobb 1972). To bring sociology closer to the realities both of the working class and of women, we should stop treating instrumentality and expressiveness (or rationality and emotionality) as two mutually exclusive qualities of action and instead treat them as separate continua that vary independently and can be applied to a single action.

15. The importance of the caregiving work of nannies and maids for children in the upper classes is nearly invisible in the research literature. Freud, for instance, when discussing the relations between mother, father, and child, did not problematize very much what children's relations to nannies and servants could mean. As most of Freud's patients came from bourgeois or upper class households, we can assume that in early childhood they were mostly taken care of by servants.

16. This statement was made at a seminar for representatives of voluntary organizations and the Ministry of Health and Social Affairs in Norway in 1976. In the published report from this seminar, no one expresses any objection to this view.

17. These figures are given by Levin and Idler (1981, p. 259) without rendering any account of how it is calculated. In documents from WHO not formally published, I found the same figures.

References

Abrahamsson, Bengt and Mårten Söder. 1977. *Makten och verksamheten: Om villkor och verksamhet vid vårdhemsavdelingar.* Uppsala: Acta Universities Upsaliensis.

Abrams, Philip. 1977. "Community Care: Some Research Problems and Priorities." *Policy and Politics* 6, 2.

Alvsvåg, Herdis. 1981. *Har sykepleien en fremtid?* Oslo: Univsersitetsforlaget.

Beauvoir, Simone de. 1953. *The Second Sex.* New York: Bantam Books.

Bell, D. 1968. "The Measurement of Knowledge and Technology." In *Indicators of Social Change: Concepts and Measurements,* ed. Eleanor B. Sheldon and Wilbert E. Moore. New York: Russell Sage Foundation.

Bernstein, Basil B. 1975. *Class, Codes, and Control.* New York: Schocken Books.

Branca, Patricia. 1975. *Silent Sisterhood: Middle Class Women in the Victorian Home.* London: Croom Helm.

Daatland, Sven Olaf. 1983. "Eldreomsorgen I en småby: De offentlige hjelpetjenester og familiens rolle." *Tidsskrift for Samfunnsforskning* 2: 155–73.

Dawe, Alan. 1978. "Theories of Social Action." In *A History of Sociological Analysis,* ed. Tom Bottomore and Robert Nisbet. New York: Basic Books.

Donzelot, Jacques. 1979. *The Policing of Families,* trans. Robert Hurley. London: Hutchinson.

Ehrenreich, Barbara and Deirdre English. 1973. *Witches, Midwives, and Nurses: A History of Women Healers.* Old Westbury, NY: Feminist Press.

Finch, Janet and Dulcie Groves. 1980. "Community Care and the Family: A Case for Equal Opportunities?" *Journal of Social Policy* 9, 4: 487–512.

Firestone, Shulamith. 1971. *The Dialectic of Sex: The Case for Feminist Revolution.* New York: Bantam Books.

Friedan, Betty. 1963. *The Feminine Mystique.* New York: Dell.

———. 1981. *The Second Stage.* New York: Summit Books.

Glennon, Lynda M. 1979. *Women and Dualism: A Sociology of Knowledge Analysis.* New York: Longman.

Gullestad, Marianne. 1984. *Kitchen-Table Society: A Case Study of the Family Life and Friendship of Young Working-Class Mothers in Urban Norway.* Oslo: Universitetsforlaget.

Hochschild, Arlie Russell. 1975. "The Sociology of Feeling and Emotion: Selected Possibilities." In *Another Voice: Feminist Perspectives on Social Life and Social Science,* ed. Marcia Millman and Rosabeth Moss Kanter. New York: Anchor Books.

Holter, Harriet, Willy Martinussen, and Bjørg Gronseth. 1967. *Hjemmet som arbeidsplass: Studier av husmorens arbeidssituasjon, av veiledningsbehov og veiledningstilbud.* Oslo: Univeristetsforlaget.

Illich, Ivan. 1976. *Medical Nemesis: The Expropriation of Health.* New York: Random House.

Kitzinger, Sheila. 1978. *Women as Mothers.* London: Fontana.

Levin, Lowell S. and Ellen L. Idler. 1981. *The Hidden Health Care System: Mediating Structures and Medicine.* Cambridge, MA: Ballinger.

Liljeström, Rita and Elizabeth Özgalda. 1980. *Kommunals kvinnor på livets trappa.* Stockholm: Svenska kommunalarbetareförbundet.

List, Elisabeth. 1983. "The Science of the Fathers and the Science of the Sons: Reflection on a Feminist Criticism of Science." Working paper, Institut für Philosophie, Graz.

Lopata, Helena Znaniecka. 1971. *Occupation: Housewife.* Oxford: Oxford University Press.

Martinsen, Kari and Kari Waerness. 1979. *Pleie uten omsorg?* Oslo: Pax Forlag.

McMillan, Carol. 1982. *Women, Reason, and Nature: Some Philosophical Problems with Feminism.* Oxford: Blackwell.

Merton, Robert King and Elinor Barber. 1967. "Sociological Ambivalence." In *Sociological Theory, Values, and Sociocultural Change,* ed. Edward A. Tiryakian. New York: Harper Torchbooks.

Millett, Kate. 1971. *Sexual Politics.* New York: Avon Books.

Mitchell, Juliet. 1971. *Woman's Estate.* Harmondsworth: Penguin.

Moroney, Robert M. 1976. *The Family and the State: Considerations for Social Policy.* London: Longman.

Newson, John and Elizabeth Newson. 1976. *Patterns of Infant Care in an Urban Community.* Harmondsworth: Pelican.

Nordhus, Inger H. 1981. *Gammel og avhengig?* Bergen: Department of Psychology, University of Bergen.

Oakley, Ann. 1974. *The Sociology of Housework.* New York: Pantheon.

———. 1976. "Wisewoman and Medicine Man: Changes in the Management of Childbirth." In *The Rights and Wrongs of Women,* ed. Juliet Mitchell and Ann Oakley. Harmondsworth: Penguin.

O'Brien, Mary. 1981. *The Politics of Reproduction.* London: Routledge and Kegan Paul.

Psychosocial Conditions for Development in Early Childhood. Fifth International Seminar on Health Education, Schmallenberg, 25–29 June 1973. International Journal of Health Education.

Pensionärundersökningens rapporter om social hemhjälp m.m. 1979. Stockholm: Socialdepartementet Ds S 5.

Ressner, Ulla. 1981. *Vardarbetarkollektivet och facten.* Stockholm: Arbetslivscentrum (Swedish Center for Working Life).

Rosenmayr, Leopold and E. Kockeis. 1965. "Propositions for a Sociology of Aging and the Family." In *Selected Studies in Marriage and the Family,* ed. Robert F. Winch and L. Goodman. New York: Holt, Rinehart, and Winston.

Schaffer, Rudolph. 1977. *Mothering.* London: Fontana, Open Books.

Schorr, Alvin Louis. 1962. "Current Practices of Filial Responsibility." In *Selected Studies in Marriage and the Family,* rev. ed., ed. Robert F. Winch, Robert McGinnis, and Herbert R. Barringer. New York: Holt, Rinehart, and Winston.

Schumacher, E. F. 1978. *A Guide for the Perplexed.* London: Abacus, Sphere Books.

Sennett, Richard and Jonathan Cobb. 1972. *The Hidden Injuries of Class.* New York: Knopf.

Shanas, Ethel. 1979. "Social Myth as Hypothesis: The Case of the Family Relations of Old People." *Gerontologist* 19, 1: 3–9.

Smith, Dorothy I. 1979. "A Sociology for Women." In *The Prism of Sex: Essays in the Sociology of Knowledge,* ed. Julia A. Sherman and Evelyn T. Beck. Madison: University of Wisconsin Press.

Söder, Mårten. 1981. *Vårdintegration, vårdideologi och integrering.* Uppsala: Acta Universitas Upsalicensis. Abstracts of Uppsala Dissertations from the Faculty of Social Sciences 25.

Stacey, Margaret. 1981. "The Division of Labour Revisited or Overcoming the Two Adams." In *Practice and Progress: British Sociology, 1950–1980,* ed. Philip Abrams et al. London: Allen and Unwin.

Stacey, Margaret and Marion Price. 1981. *Women, Power, and Politics.* London and New York: Tavistock.

Sundström, Gerdt. 1980. "The Elderly Women's Work and Social Security Costs." *Acta Sociologica* 25, 1: 21–38.

Teeland, Laurence. 1978. *Keeping in Touch.* Department of Sociology Monograph 16. Gothenburg: University of Gothenburg.

Titmuss, Richard M. 1963. *Essays on the Welfare State.* Boston: Beacon Press.

Ve, Hildur. 1982. "Ideals of Equality in the School System of the Welfare State." Paper presented at the Tenth World Congress of Sociology, Research Group 32, Women in Society, Mexico City, 16–21 August. Bergen: Center of Women's Studies, Institute of Sociology.

Viklund, Rune. 1981. *Att arbeta I omsorg.* Stockholm: Arbetslivscentrum (Swedish Center for Working Life).

Weber, Max. 1966. *The Theory of Social and Economic Organization.* New York: Free Press.

Waerness, Kari. 1978. "The Invisible Welfare State: Women's Work at Home." *Acta Sociologica* Supplement.

———. 1982. *Kvinneperspektiver på sosialpolitikken.* Oslo: Universitetsforlaget.

Chapter 16
Feminism and Caring

Suzanne Gordon

For the past several decades a growing number of scholars, researchers, activists, and practitioners in the caregiving professions, moral philosophy, gerontology, feminism, sociology, history, and religion have developed a body of thinking in the field of caring. They have attacked the myths that have shaped our sexist and classist images of caring, proposed alternative models of both family and professional caregiving, suggested how we might educate men and women so they would be motivated to give care and better able to tolerate receiving it, and proposed public policies and funding strategies that could help mobilize Americans to fight for the programs and policies we so desperately require as we edge toward the twenty-first century.

Although these ideas, insights and proposals could not come at a more opportune moment, many have either been ignored or attacked in the public debate. Although they are particularly relevant to women who are reeling under the crushing burden of having to both work and care in our society, a significant group of feminists view the field of caring with deep suspicion. Indeed, the very attempt to discuss the problems of caregiving in certain feminist circles has produced a backlash that is gaining momentum throughout America today.

Susan Faludi's *Backlash: The Undeclared War Against American Women,* Wendy Kaminer's *A Fearful Freedom: Women's Flight from Equality,* and her attack on the ethic of care in an *Atlantic Monthly* cover story, feminist writer Katha Pollitt's *Nation* cover story entitled "Marooned on Gilligan's Island" and more right wing supporter of women's rights Diane Johnson's novel *Health and Happiness* are excellent examples of this feminist refusal to explore the complexity of the issue of caregiving. In these

An earlier version of this essay appeared as Gordon, "Feminism and Caregiving," *American Prospect* 10 (Summer 1992): 119–27. Reprinted by permission of the author.

works, scholars and activists who talk about an activity they describe as *central* to women's lives and history are accused of arguing that it is an *innate*, or *natural* female quality and that women are *naturally* morally *superior* to men. Descriptions of history are taken as prescriptions for the future. Thinkers and observers who carefully define what they mean by caring and caregiving and examine and analyze the very difficult dilemmas that caregivers face are said to be vague, fuzzy-headed, soft, and hopelessly feminine. Feminists who try to expose and explore the complexities of the work patriarchal culture has rendered invisible are condemned as proponents of the very nineteenth-century definitions and sentimental images of femininity that they themselves try to demystify.

In their arguments these advocates of women's rights echo patriarchal attitudes toward caregiving that disempower caregivers, legitimize traditional masculine views of caring, discourage—albeit inadvertently—men from sharing the duty of care, and help keep caregivers both female and male alike in their subordinate social and economic place. In fact, the authors in question are so vehement in their denunciations of discussions of caregiving that one feels they are simply intent on keeping caregiving work just what it has always been—invisible.

Like many issues in modern feminism, the debate about caring has a long and complicated history. Many contemporary women—feminist and nonfeminist alike—are understandably nervous about discussions of caregiving. Women's work has long been a problem for the women assigned to do it. Whatever burdens caregiving entails were foisted on women's shoulders—no matter how ill suited or unsupported an individual woman was to perform the tasks and duties involved. Patriarchal societies have not truly valued caregiving, but have instead sentimentalized and romanticized what they insist are women's "superior moral virtues," and "natural" inclination to care for the dependent. This imposition of the duty to care on one sex alone and to turn caring for other human beings into an exercise in self-abnegation has been used to enforce women's dependence on men.

As historians Nancy Cott and Ann Douglas have pointed out, the propaganda of the "cult of domesticity" that arose in the late eighteenth and early nineteenth century insisted that women were the natural repositories of virtue. Their job description as gender was to nurture the family and produce moral individuals (read men) to act in the workplace and public realm. Power could only be gained indirectly, in the family through feminine example. Women, of course, were expected to rejoice in this domestic confinement and respect the limits patriarchal society had imposed on their intelligence, talents, and contributions.

Since the inception of the feminist movement, feminists have rebelled against this domestic sequestration. In fighting for liberation, however, they have been divided about how to achieve equality and how that struggle should affect women's traditional caregiving roles. Divisions on this subject, Nancy Cott explained in *The Grounding of Modern Feminism* (1987), have persisted throughout feminism's long and fractious history; and the tensions that she described in the late 1800s are alive today.

By the close of the century the spectrum of ideology in the woman movement had a see-saw quality: at one end, the intention to eliminate sex-specific limitations; at the other, the desire to recognize rather than quash the qualities and habits called female, to protect the interests women had already defined as theirs and give those much greater public scope. A tension stretched between emphasis on the rights that women (like men) deserved and emphasis on the particular duties or services that women (unlike men) could offer society; as also between the claim that women had to act for their own advantage or for the benefit of others. (1987, pp. 19–20)

Although it is difficult, if not treacherous, to try to categorize neatly a movement that is extremely diverse and has resisted ideological and institutional cohesion around any particular issue, the feminist debate about caring centers on the question of how much or little one should emphasize or minimize gender differences. Since caring has been so consistently contaminated by patriarchal attitudes and actions that have oppressed women, the very mention of the word, as we shall see more explicitly when examining the work of Faludi, Kaminer, Pollitt, and Johnson, immediately triggers a debate about difference. Caring's fate within feminism is linked with how that controversial conversation unfolds.

On this subject and many others, the most powerful and popular voice in American feminism today is that of what I call Lockean feminism. Lockean feminists—whether they acknowledge it or not—are part of the long tradition of individualism elaborated by the English political, psychological, and moral theorist John Locke, whose influence on American liberalism has been incalculable. Contemporary articulations of Lockean individualism base individual identity and worth on the possession of individual rights and property; emphasize the pursuit of success and power in the marketplace; promote self-control through psychological, social, and political theories that stress disengagement from others and radical self-reliance and autonomy; and contain only the most limited concepts of moral obligation to those others who might pose pressing claims on the self.

In the Lockean tradition, particularly as it has been expanded upon by contemporary thinkers like John Rawls, fairness and justice play a crucial role. The moral good is transparent: individuals should have the right to pursue their own life plan but should not take more than their share or override the rights of others. And they should act fairly and rationally when in or near positions of power. Abraham Lincoln stated this position succinctly when he said that the purpose of government, like that of an all-powerful traffic cop, is to "lift artificial weights from all shoulders; to clear the paths of laudable pursuits for all; to afford all an unfettered start and a fair chance in the race of life."

For Lockean feminists, this doctrine of rights and fairness—the creation of a level playing field on which to compete—is the essence of feminism. In *Backlash*, Susan Faludi faithfully echoes the Lincolnesque position when, totally ignoring the raucous history of a multifaceted social movement, she blithely asserts that

feminism remains a pretty simple concept. . . . Feminism's agenda is basic: It asks that women not be forced to "choose" between public justice and private happiness. It asks that women be free to define themselves—instead of having their identity defined for them, time and again, by their culture and their men. (1991, p. xxiii)

Freely choosing Lockean feminists struggle primarily for formal equality with men in the world of work, politics, and culture. They tend to fear that discussions of difference—particularly of caring—will derail women's progress in this realm, ushering in a return to the cult of domesticity and women's entrapment in the home and caring professions. They base many of their statements about absence of gender differences on excellent feminist research, like that conducted and collected by Maccoby and Jacklin, Eccles and Jacobs, and Lykes and Stewart among others. This kind of research, Rachel T. Hare-Mustin and Jeanne Marecek explain in a very illuminating paper entitled "Gender and the Meaning of Difference," reveal that male-female differences are not as "universal, dramatic, or enduring" as has often been asserted (1992, p. 23).

Feminists who minimize differences are very wary of the subject of morality, not only because they worry that the duty to care has been traditionally imposed on women alone, but because, like most modern self-interest maximizers, they find any notion of self-sacrifice abhorrent. Many Lockean feminists, on the other hand, are profoundly committed to the principles of universal benevolence and justice. This commitment is expressed in the language of economic justice—an essential abstraction, which, however, may be inadequate (though certainly not useless) in helping us contemplate crucial personal and social decisions.

The commitment to equality, Lockean feminists adamantly insist, means that women should be liberated to pursue whatever personal or professional choice they desire. Presumably this freedom to choose extends to the choice of staying at home to raise children or a career in the so-called helping professions. Not so. It soon becomes evident that there is a definite hierarchy of choices, and that the favored new ones involve elite, high-paying jobs in traditional masculine fields and activities. Liberation quickly becomes measured in terms of how far women have traveled away from work in the home and caregiving professions. Indeed, Lockean feminists seem to associate teaching, nursing, and social work so much with femininity that they no longer even acknowledge that those professions were in fact feminist achievements.

Almost all Lockean feminists would, nonetheless, argue that women's liberation depends on some resolution of the problem of caregiving. They propose workplace and public policies that allow women and men unpaid or paid time off to take care of newborns or adopted children, family leave to take care of sick or dying relatives or spouses, and more flexible work arrangements like job sharing, part time jobs, and flextime work schedules. Because the problem of eldercare does not yet seem to have posed a serious obstacle to many of the most vocal Lockean feminists, and certainly has not dramatically inhibited the ambitions of those baby-boomers who have followed them, most have concentrated on the dilemmas of childcare. But when eldercare is mentioned they support similar policies for the care of the elderly.

Institutional solutions to caregiving that provide working mothers and daughters with surrogate caregivers are highly favored. In the service of this goal, Lockean feminists at least pay service to the fact that professional providers—nurses, teachers, and family day- and eldercare providers—should receive better pay and improved working conditions. And they insist, of course, that part of the real solution to caregiving lies in getting men to share in the duty to care.

Because Lockean feminists, however, seem to associate caregiving so much with female exploitation, it is difficult to imagine how they could bring themselves to join caregivers in their struggles for equality, encourage the study of caregiving work to discover its positive qualities and lessons, or investigate the moral practices that motivate human beings to engage in caregiving work. As we shall see, some of their comments on caregiving are so derogatory that it is hard to understand why anyone reading or hearing them would consider a career in traditional women's work a legitimate choice; why citizens should sacrifice a night out or weekend away to better fund caregiving work or provide social support for family and community caregivers; and why men would want to devote themselves to activities that many women now seem to deem valueless.

A second group of feminists, what Faludi and many others have called "relational" feminists and Rachel Hare-Mustin and Jeanne Marecek call "Alpha bias" feminists, tend to overemphasize gender differences. Jean

Baker Miller and her colleagues at Wellesley College's Stone Center, Nancy Chodorow, Mary Field Belenky, and Mary Daly fall into this camp, as does Carol Gilligan, although to a sometimes greater and sometimes lesser degree. Hare-Mustin and Marecek express it best when they write that "Alpha bias is the exaggeration of differences" (1992, p. 30). Although feminist psychodynamic theorists disagree about the origins of gender differences, they view them as universal (at least within contemporary western culture), highly dichotomized, and enduring.

These "relational" feminists have made invaluable contributions to our understanding of female and male socialization and have encouraged female self-confidence and solidarity. And their work has added immeasurably to exposing the limitations of those radical individualistic theories of moral and psychological development that have inhibited the human possibilities of both women and men. "Relational" feminism, however, frequently verges on a subtle form of biological essentialism and may encourage the creation of a women-only culture that can hamper women as they try to reconcile equality and difference, as well as the care and justice perspectives.

"Relational" feminists are sometimes subtly or overtly resistant—more in practice than in theory—to broadening discussions about how men can integrate into their work and personal lives the qualities and practices these feminists describe and analyze. And some appear to favor waging psychological rather than confrontational political struggles. Moreover, some seem reluctant to explore what happens to gender differences and caregiving when women are resocialized in highly competitive, individualistic institutions (like most of the major ones in our society). Such investigations, obviously, underscore how quickly gender differences can be neutralized depending on social context.

In their essay on equality and difference, Hare-Mustin and Marecek discuss another school of feminism they call constructivism, which offers, they say, "a way to reconceptualize ideas and data about gender. The constructivist view is that the 'real nature' of male and female cannot be determined, thus attention should be focused on representations of gender instead of gender itself." Whether the last group of feminists I will consider—what I call transformational feminists—would all define themselves as constructivists is unclear. Nonetheless, they reject a rigid choice between equality and difference.

Because they are feminists, these thinkers and activists focus on women's experiences. They believe, however, that the capacity to care is not determined by gender but rather resides in all human beings. Social arrangements and relationships shape and govern caring behavior and the conditions under which caregiving is performed both inside and outside the home. Those who work in the caring professions might add that a study of women's behavior in nursing, teaching, or social work can reveal not only how caring some women are, but how uncaring women can be: how easily they, too, can exhibit competitive, controlling behaviors and even discriminate against "male usurpers" trying to advance in a woman's world. The examples of those courageous, empathic men who have chosen to be nurses, kindergarten teachers, or eldercare providers also challenge sex role stereotypes as explicitly and effectively as those of females who have become lawyers, bankers, or physicians.

Central to the theories of these transformational feminists is the idea that caring, as Nel Noddings has argued, is not something that one person does to another. Caring exists in relationships and flourishes or sours depending on the social context. Nor are the empathetic activities so critical to caring relationships instinctual processes, requiring only fusion with the one cared for. Caring is an emotional and cognitive process that requires education, knowledge, reflection, and the ability to detach from—as well as connect with—another. The knowledge and education the expert caregiver needs may be gained in the workplace, the home, or the community, as well as in an academic institution, but it is a prerequisite of what Patricia Benner has called the *skill* of involvement and is mobilized by caregivers with different levels of commitment and expertise.

Most important, scholars and activists in the burgeoning field of caregiving clearly distinguish the content of the critical human activity from the patriarchal and individualistic myths that have so distorted its image. The core activities of caring, they argue, should not be confused with the prejudices and institutional arrangements that patriarchal, individualist cultures have imposed on it and that often lead to caregivers' apparent self-immolation and self-abnegation. The fact that caregiving was one of the areas in which women's subjection to men was affirmed, and that caring work has been traditionally devalued and underfunded, should not be used as evidence to prove that it is inherently inferior and fundamentally more exploitative than much of the work men have performed in the marketplace.

If women address the complex problem of caregiving in our society, transformational feminists believe they will not inevitably travel down a slippery slope at whose bottom lies a complete reversal of all advances toward female emancipation and equality. Flight is not a solution to women's caregiving problems. The solutions are moral, pedagogical, and political and involve engagement and dialogue. That is why the liberation of women from patriarchal attitudes, an end to sexism, and the achievement of true equality depends not only on the progress of those feminists who work to secure women greater access to traditional male jobs, privileges, and rights but also on the progress of feminists who have tried to analyze and research the insights, skills, and practices women have developed because of their *socialization* and their work in the home and caring professions. By making this invisible work visible to a wide public, these feminists hope to help expand women's professional horizons while simultaneously seeking greater respect and financial rewards for women's traditional activities in the home and helping professions.

Faludi, Kaminer, and Johnson seem oblivious to any distinctions between feminists who are concerned with caregiving and who have analyzed the limitations of the Lockean individualism.

In *Backlash* Faludi argues that "the last decade has seen a powerful counter-assault on women's rights, a backlash, an attempt to retract the handful of small and hard-won victories that the feminist movement did manage to win for women." This ubiquitous and ever present backlash, the *Wall Street Journal* reporter contends, is

sophisticated and banal, deceptively "progressive" and proudly backward. It deploys both the "new" findings of "scientific research" and the dime-store moralism of yesteryear; it turns into media sound bites both the glib pronouncements of pop-psych trend watchers and the frenzied rhetoric of New Right preachers. The backlash has succeeded in framing virtually the whole issue of women's rights in its own language. Just as Reaganism shifted political discourse far to the right and demonized liberalism, so the backlash convinced the public that women's liberation was the true contemporary American scourge. (1991, p. xvii)

Faludi briefly traces the history of backlashes that have followed flowerings of feminist activity in the past and explains that anti-feminist arguments in the late nineteenth century repeated themes that are recycled in the contemporary version. In the 1980s and '90s these arguments have been broadcast by journalists and others who inundate the public with largely unsubstantiated and poorly researched reports that paint feminism as a sinister force responsible for a plethora of female and social ills—from rising divorce rates and male unemployment to female depression and the break up of the family. She believes that American men are susceptible to backlash arguments because, in a classless society, masculinity becomes a substitute for class identification.

Her voluminous compendium of the war on what she depicts as a very shaky female citadel includes some excellent reporting on right wing antifeminist activists, grumpy Hollywood producers and directors, Madison Avenue and television network airheads, plastic surgeons and cosmetic companies, and pop psychologists, as well as the difficult struggles of women in the workplace. She laments the fact that women have been too quick to abandon their principles and movement and makes a heartfelt plea for a greater appreciation of feminism's importance. But apart from this she offers little analysis and few strategies that could help women fight off the backlash.

Faludi's thesis—that a major backlash against feminism has presented a serious obstacle to women's struggle for equal rights—is indisputable. The author has rightly been applauded for her verve and righteous indignation (in our society, there can never be too much of that), and for collecting the fragments of evidence and presenting a coherent case to the public. Many sympathetic reviewers have, however, regretted the fact that Faludi indicts not only the enemies of equal rights but advocates like Carol Gilligan—to name the most notable example. Most reviewers seem to consider this to be a regrettable accident or oversight.

Faludi's attack on Gilligan and what she calls "relational" feminists, is not accidental but stems from her ideological stance. Throughout the book, for example, her reporting on the kind of journalistic superficiality and overkill so endemic to contemporary media culture is marred by her own tendency to exaggeration (one sadly, but not surprisingly, promoted by many in publishing today). She consistently presents feminism as a frail and rather uncomplicated flower. Its past and present victories are not simply hard-won but "small" or "tiny," while the backlash is nameless and faceless, omnipresent, and overpowering.

Seemingly incapable of making "qualitative distinctions," Faludi's backlash includes not only direct attacks by males provoked by the advances of the women's movement but many instances of institutional sexism as usual. Her judgments can be indiscriminate. When feminist activists choose to expand on the feminist agenda to attract new recruits and allies by referring to "family issues" rather than "women's rights," she regards this as a retreat not an advance. Even a movie like *The Accused*, which finally brought the issue of gang rape to the attention of a mass public, is metamorphosized into a feminist failure. She contends that the film "should be mourned" as a depressing artifact of the times—because it tells us only how much ground women have already lost. By the end of the '80s, a film that simply opposed the mauling of a young woman could be passed off as a feminist statement. (1991, p. 139). "(Reading this, I found myself—to my horror—echoing Camille Paglia: "What does this woman want?")

Because her imagination is conspiratorial rather than historical, Faludi does not seem to view the current assault on women's progress as part of a larger conservative attack on all progressive forces but portrays it as unique to women. Her analysis, and the impatience in which it is rooted, may be a function of youth—or of membership in a profession allergic to most attempts to appreciate the historical difficulties inherent in the kinds of massive, social changes that women have, in fact, wrought. Whatever the cause, it does not allow her to understand either the magnitude of feminist success (even the advent and victories of Lockean feminism are social developments of major importance) or the problems that any social revolution as powerful as ours inevitably creates.

Wedded to a conspiracy theory of history, Faludi furthermore seems desperate to find as many conspirators as she can possibly unearth. Since the logic of conspiracies requires not only willing recruits but fifth columnists as well, enter Gilligan and the "relationalists." To a Lockean feminist hostile to family and caring concerns, they are the perfect enemies within. In a chapter entitled "The Backlash Braintrust: From Neocons to Neofems," Faludi thus issues her importunate caveat: that an influential group of researchers, and popular writers have "helped spread anti-feminist sentiments across the political spectrum." These backlash braintrusters include women identified with "liberal and leftist causes" who have also "crowded onto the backlash dais" (p. 202). She intones that ominously.

In fact, some of the backlash experts were even women who claimed to be feminists. Some classified themselves as second generation "neo-feminists," speaking up for "mothers' rights." Others brandished membership cards from the early days of the women's movement; they were feminist writers of the seventies now issuing revisionist texts. And then there were the unwitting and unwilling messengers—feminist scholars, who watched in dismay as their studies of gender differences were distorted by the backlash's burgeoning staff of zealous interpreters." (p. 202)

Her main targets in this chapter are Sylvia Ann Hewlett, Betty Friedan, and Carol Gilligan but Germaine Greer and Susan Brownmiller also receive a good lashing, and there is brief reference to my own book, *Prisoners of Men's Dreams*. All are equated with the most indefatigable opponents of female emancipation—George Gilder, Allan Bloom, Robert Bly, Michael and Margarita Levin, and Warren Farrell. Friedan, for example, is not only accused of being an unpleasant egomaniac, but assailed for the profamily positions she espoused in *The Second Stage*. This section is larded with the kind of language that serves no analytical purpose but only helps reinforce the notion that feminists really are antifamily. Friedan, Faludi says, "stomps" on feminism, calls for a "murkily defined new order that is heavy on old Victorian rhetorical flourishes" and generally "retreats into a domestic haze" (pp. 322, 325). I am no fan of Betty Friedan and have been very critical of her work, but this is irresponsible and damaging to feminism itself.

After dispensing with Friedan, Faludi goes on to thrust and parry at her main enemy, "relational feminists." She believes a consideration of "women's special needs" or qualities will boomerang.

"Special" may sound like superior, but it is also a euphemism for handicapped. . . . Most relational scholars no doubt believed they could bring back the cult of domesticity on their own terms. These academics hoped to push for women's "special rights" without jeopardizing fundamental civil rights and opportunities. All the same, in their tributes to the "domestic arts," their sometimes self-righteous homages to female moral superiority, and their denigration of "simple-minded equality," they risked clothing old Victorian conceits in modern academic dress. (p. 327)

The "relational" scholar she pursues most relentlessly is Carol Gilligan. Ironically, she spares Jean Baker Miller and her Stone Center colleagues from the sting of her rhetorical whip. Perhaps she is only familiar with Miller's early and only book, *Toward a New Psychology of Women*, rather than her later papers and Stone Center Colloquoia and offshoots. These feminists are far more preoccupied with difference, specialness, and sometimes even superiority than Gilligan.

Faludi repeats some criticisms of Gilligan's early work, *In a Different Voice*. Gilligan's critics have questioned the size of her sample and her lack of social and class analysis. More important to Faludi is the fact that Gilligan's work has been used by antifeminists "to bolster their arguments that independence was an unnatural and unhealthy state for women" (p. 330). Such antifeminists include the authors of *Smart Women/Foolish Choices*, *Being a Woman*, and *The Failure of Feminism*.

In a particularly mean-spirited passage, Faludi denies Gilligan her own equal right to respond to such conservative abuses. She cites a strongly worded contribution to the feminist journal *Signs* in which Carol Gilligan deplored the misuses of her work (Gilligan 1986). But Faludi does not forgive Gilligan for elaborating an ethic of care and responsibility. "Her regrets," she writes of Gilligan, "don't really matter. The general public does not subscribe to *Signs*. And the damage has already been done" (p. 332).

Faludi's critique of Carol Gilligan's work could have been interesting, and some of the problems she raises are legitimate. They have, in fact, been partially addressed in Gilligan's later book—the co-edited collection, *Mapping the Moral Domain* (1988). Unfortunately, Faludi seems unfamiliar with that text. Her own secondary sources seem to include only critics of Gilligan and none of the research and scholarship her work has inspired—a body of thinking that qualifies, corrects, and expands on many of her insights.

Rather than doing her homework, Faludi is content to put words into the mouths of the relational feminists she seems to abhor. These feminists Faludi reports "offered dewy-eyed visions of female domestic confinement." They "romanticize" and "celebrate" rather than "explore" women's traditional socialization, and urge on us a "cult of domesticity" in their tributes to the "domestic arts." Yet none of the feminists who are the most active and respected in this field use the terms she mobilizes, like soldiers on a search and destroy mission, to portray their own far more complex and sophisticated arguments.

Like many other journalistic critics of caring, Faludi does not seem to have any historical grasp of the meaning and function of the nineteenth-century cult of domesticity. In contrast to the real advocates of the cult of domesticity, neither "relational" nor transformational feminists ask women only to play roles in the family and caregiving professions, but to play many roles in many professional settings. They do not ask women to produce moral individuals but themselves to reflect and act on their definitions of the good. Their focus is on understanding motivation and professional and personal practices so that men—not only women—can be educated to learn "the skill of involvement."

Transformational feminists—who have been active in the fight for improved human services, education, child- and eldercare, and health care—most emphatically do not counsel women to be dependent and participate indirectly in society. Quite the contrary, they ask women to take direct action themselves, personally, politically, and professionally to promote *both* social justice and caring. To them caring is often considered to be a subversive, not adaptive, activity that will challenge, not provide a haven from, the tyranny of the marketplace and the negative consequences of radical individualism. This is a far cry from the nineteenth-century vision of feminine purity, dependence, and sheltered living.

Perhaps Faludi is unable accurately to assess what her caring sisters do believe because she seems to find little of value in the work women have done in the home and caring professions. This may explain why a book that examines the impact of backlash on women's emancipation in very diverse workplaces contains no investigation of how it has shaped women's struggles in the caregiving professions. There are many feminists among the nurses, teachers, and childcare workers who make up the ranks of her so-called relational feminism. Their lives, work, and ambitions have also been adversely impacted by the conservative policies of the 1980s and '90s. But we learn nothing about their struggles. In fact, Faludi's attack on relational feminism demonstrates how very complicated feminism really is and always has been and how easily feminists themselves can replicate the "masculine" values their culture and their men try to impose on women's choices and lived experiences.

The disdain some feminists display toward the full range of women's choices also infuses attorney Wendy Kaminer's *A Fearful Freedom: Women's Flight from Equality* (1990). Kaminer takes issue with feminists who are concerned with family, community, relationship, and caring. "The private concerns of women—children and family—and the costs of careerism are defeating the drive and desire of many to participate equally in public life" (p. 7). Even the most minimal examination of women's different historical and contemporary experiences, she contends, will inevitably impede their march toward equality.

Criticizing Carol Gilligan and what she calls "protectionist feminists," Kaminer dismisses the attempt to "cultivate a 'morality of responsibility' instead of a 'morality of rights,'" and denounces all their talk of cooperation and collectivity. "Feminists who put their faith in sisterhood, have difficulty reconciling their demand for jobs and economic equality with the fact that jobs are awarded competitively" (p. 7) she comments, summarily rejecting the ideal of sisterhood that once fueled the feminist movement.

Speaking in the tones of the battlefield general rather than the political organizer, Kaminer argues that women, out of "practical necessity," must talk about cooperation and maintain "some sense of solidarity," or "none or few of the spoils traditionally monopolized by men would be available to any women at all" (p. 7). But her individualistic Lockean framework, as we see when we examine women's behavior in our ruthlessly competitive marketplace, simply provides no structures of collective accountability and moral motivation.

Adopting the pragmatism, and cynicism that passes for wisdom in this conservative era Kaminer observes:

In an ideal world, competition would, no doubt, give way to cooperation. People would simply agree on the allocation of resources, caring as much about their neighbors as about themselves. In the meantime, women who want power will have to join the fray and fight for it. (p. 7)

Because she seems to reject even the ideal of a more cooperative commonwealth as well as collective action to achieve it, liberation becomes a scramble to the top that inevitably pits women not only against men but against each other.

Throughout *A Fearful Freedom,* Kaminer constantly devalues women's experience and history in the domestic sphere. "Like immigrants who want to preserve their culture and be Americans too, women are caught," between "feminine values" and a "masculine world." (p. 10). True enough. But according to her, this "woman's culture" is utterly trivial—"the private world of children and shopping and female friendships" (p. 10). Being better at "washing dishes and socks." (This tactic is becoming more and more popular among some advocates of women's rights. In an essay entitled "Against Caring" Hilde Nelson warns nurses away from a caring ethic (1992). She contends that feminist educator Nel Noddings's analysis of a feminine ethic articulates "rather nicely the traditional woman's work of mothering, tending the family, gardening, and cooking. It spoke to the 'lived experience' of countless suburban housewives" (p. 8).

Given this image of the indolent, 1950s suburban housewife lunching at Lord and Taylor with her comrades in consumption, it is no wonder that Kaminer presents the male workplace as the Mecca to which female pilgrims should journey. Discrimination "maintains a dual labor market" that "denies them (women) 'masculine' jobs." In her conception of the marketplace, "masculine jobs" are, however, not simply better paid and more respected, they are also the ones "requiring stamina and strength, and the capacity to command." (p. xv). Instead of explaining that women's work demands the same, she implies that it prepares us to be weak, subordinate, and obedient.

Entirely hostile to caring commitments, Kaminer opposes rather than tries to reconcile caring with the struggle for rights and social justice. "Rights," she bluntly asserts—as if these rights had an existence independent of those who administer or implement them—"are more trustworthy than judges or social workers, and the displacement of rights by a commitment to 'caring' is a prescription for discretionary injustice" (p. 16). She does not seem to understand that those critics of the limitations of the rights and justice perspective do not "deny the crucial importance of justice and rights in affirming the wisdom and value of the voice of care" philosopher Alisa L. Carse writes in this volume (p. 85). Rather, like Carse, they may choose to "defend the need to retain a sturdy rights conception within ethics, but affirm at the same time the need for an ethic more demanding than the ethic of justice—one which gives an essential place to 'care' through norms of character and citizenship (for all people), traditionally thought more appropriate for women than for men" (this volume, p. 85).

Kaminer, like Faludi, is legitimately concerned that women not idealize caring or suggest that women are "naturally endowed" to care and thus morally superior to men. But caring is again misconstrued in this text as well as in her article in the *Atlantic Monthly*. "In a modern day version of Victorian True Womanhood," Kaminer writes in that magazine, "feminists and some anti-feminists pay tribute to women's superior nurturing and relational skills." Incredibly, she argues, "Believers in gender difference tend not to focus on changing the cultural environment to free men and women from stereotypes, as equal rights feminists did twenty years ago, instead they celebrate the feminine virtues" (1993, p. 59).

Making invidious distinctions between "equal-rights feminists and "caring feminists" (distinctions that often disappear when one examines the record of "caring feminists" who have long championed and fought for equal rights), Kaminer accuses "caring feminists" of arguing that differences between men and women are "natural," of promoting visions of "women caring, sharing, and nurturing their families as naturally as they breast-feed." (1990, p. 213) Lumped together with a mysterious and often anonymous group of "protectionist feminists," caring feminists are accused of fighting for special maternity benefits, maternity leave, and "mommy-track jobs," when most advocate universal programs like parental leave and universal health care and education, and have vocally rejected the so-called mommy-track. Most important, Kaminer believes that voluntarism should govern our obligations to others. Because she believes that all men freely choose their jobs and careers as well as to care or not, women should do the same. Thus she formulates the happy fiction that all sacrifices can be freely chosen and that women should use freedom of choice as their guiding moral principle as they reflect on their approach to their personal relationships and care-related dilemmas.

This claim that there are two kinds of feminists—those concerned with the tough problems of discrimination and equal rights and those concerned only with the softer side of life—caring—is at the heart of Katha Pollitt's (1992) attack on Nancy Chodorow, Sara Ruddick, Carol Gilligan and myself. Pollitt insists that writers and activists who explore culturally constructed female differences are in fact pandering to men, that "men like them because, while they urge understanding and respect for 'female' values and behaviors, they also let men off the hook" (Pollitt 1992, p. 802).

Similarly, Pollitt feels that analysis of caring work is a kind of clever gimmick used to reassure women that patriarchal oppression is a figment of their imagination and that social transformation is unnecessary:

By arguing that the traditional qualities, tasks, and ways of life of women are as important, valuable, and serious as those of men (if not more so), Gilligan and others let women feel that nothing needs to change except the social valuation accorded to what they are already doing. It's a rationale for the status quo, which is why men like it, and a burst of grateful applause, which is why women like it. Men keep the power, but because power is bad, so much the worse for them. (p. 804)

Indeed, those who study an ethic of care, and by extension the work of caregiving are seen the ultimate betrayers of the feminist cause,

Once again, women are defined by their family roles. Child-raising is seen as women's glory and joy and opportunity for self-transcendence, while Dad naps on the couch. Women who do not fit the stereotype are castigated as unfeminist—nurses nurture, doctors do not—and domestic labor is romanticized and sold to women as a badge of moral worth.

Novelist and essayist Diane Johnson's comments on and descriptions of caregiving contain similar devaluations of caring. In her article "Iron John and His Friends" (1992), Johnson seems to doubt that it is possible to value caregiving and those who do it. In a brief section on my book, *Prisoners of Men's Dreams*, she fears that an analysis of the nonexploitative aspects of caregiving "merely rephrases the same age-old definition of womanliness that has always been used to devalue them (i.e., women)" (p. 16).

Citing Thorstein Veblen, she proposes that caregiving tasks "arise from the condition of servant and concern themselves with servile attendance on the persons of other people" (p. 16). Women, she insists must stop "staking out these mostly thankless jobs as if they were desirable and to be done only by females." Men, she contends with the utmost certainty, will do caregiving work when it is better paid.

In her 1990 novel *Health and Happiness*, Johnson vividly dramatizes this sexist definition of caregiving in her description of life in a "top-flight" San Francisco teaching hospital called Alta Buena. The novel's most important characters are physicians—most of them male—who perform medical heroics and occasionally make mistaken or unethical decisions.

All the physicians in the book have names, but many of the nurses do indeed remain anonymous servants. None of her major characters is a nurse. What is worse, nurses never play a major role in patient care. When one of Johnson's main characters—a young woman suffering from a blood clot—is hospitalized by an impersonal and uncommunicative physician, Johnson assigns the hospital's coordinator of volunteer services to perform the duties nurses perform. While the nurses ignore the patient's agony and anxiety, she is the only one to talk to the bewildered young woman and minister to her needs. Even the nurses on the Intensive Care Unit (ICU)—who would be some of the most technically proficient in the hospital—seem to be little more than inert pieces of medical equipment. ICU nurses are in reality among the most involved in helping patients and their families make decisions about terminating heroic medical treatment. Yet when the mother of one of Johnson's fictive patients is asked to permit physicians to write a Do Not Resuscitate (DNR) order for her terminally ill son, nurses stand idly by emptying bedpans and distributing medication.

To add insult to injury, Johnson's only vaguely developed nursing figure is described in the most stereotypical manner. In a real hospital, "head" nurse Carmel Hodgkiss would be in charge of coordinating complex patient care. Her assignment at Alta Buena? To coordinate the gossip about physicians' love lives. She was the one, Johnson writes, "who best kept track of love and sex at Alta Buena" (p. 7).

After reading this book, one would never know that nurses are highly trained professionals; that caring involves emotional, cognitive, and technical skills; and that hospitals are, in fact, nursing institutions to which patients are admitted because they need skilled nursing care following medical interventions. (Of course, with the kind of nursing care her nurses provide, Alta Buena's mortality rate would have soared off the charts.) The real health care universe is collaboration between care and cure, but Johnson does not grasp this important fact. So when the book's female protagonist decides to leave her job cooking in a local Yuppie restaurant for a really important career, predictably she decides to go to medical school and become a physician.

Those who are concerned with caregiving are understandably frustrated at the disregard so many of their so-called sisters display toward activities and occupations that are fundamental to their personal, professional, and political projects—indeed central to the lives of all human beings. It would seem that many women—feminist and nonfeminist alike—have developed a phobia toward the very idea of caregiving. At the mere mention of the word, the red flag goes up, a distorting scrim of fear and prejudice obscures the vision, and the imagination atrophies. In her work, on the cult of domesticity, Nancy Cott (1987) has spoken of the dangers of reading twentieth-century values and preoccupations into the nineteenth century. One might want to extend this warning to feminist theorists and observers who seem intent on reading the values of nineteenth-century celebrations of feminine superiority and purity into many of the late twentieth-century analyses of caregiving.

This misreading seems almost inevitable because so few critics of care seem aware of the rich scholarship produced by those in the field. Since some critics are so wedded to the idea that caregiving involves little more than a pat on the head, the emptying of the societal bedpan, or the ceaseless oozing of empathy, they might even be surprised to learn that such scholarship exists. (When I mentioned nursing research to one typically Lockean feminist, her incredulous reply was, "Nursing what?")

The implications of this feminist caring problem are significant and must be addressed in the larger public and feminist debates. Politically correct feminism now allows discussion of women's need for better childcare and eldercare services, more part-time and flextime work, and more male participation in caregiving. But Kaminer, Faludi, Pollitt,

Johnson, and many others do not seem to comprehend that caregiving is a human necessity throughout the lifespan. They simply fail to grasp the magnitude of the caregiving problems our urban industrial societies have inadvertently created.

Institutional solutions to these problems are, of course, essential. But the important effort to provide societal support for caregiving—as Charles Taylor, Patricia Benner, and Nel Noddings, among many others, insist—must be supplemented by the education necessary to produce caregivers who will be motivated and skilled enough to really care for others. Curious, intelligent, competent men and women will never be willing to dedicate the years necessary to learn the necessary skills, knowledge, and wisdom if we continue to confuse service to others with "servile attendance" on their personal needs. Corporate leaders and politicians will never give men and women time off work to care for others if they think that caring is simpleminded head patting and good listening. If this traditional masculine disrespect and disdain for such activities continues unabated—even among women—we will never convince politicians and taxpayers to allocate funds for institutional services and desperately needed support for community and family based caregiving.

Even a positive resolution of the abortion debate is dependent on an appreciation of the complexity of caregiving. Because most right-to-lifers share the traditional patriarchal conception of caring, they can cavalierly decree that any woman can adjust to the demands of childrearing and caring. To them, it is that magical stream of estrogen—not social support and the willingness and desire to learn how to care and be responsible for another human being—that ensures a lifetime supply of love, nurturing, patience, and parental wisdom and understanding.

Today many feminists encourage and applaud men who share caregiving in the home and helping professions, but some simultaneously look down on women who may freely choose to work in the home as mothers or who become nurses, teachers, childcare providers, or social workers. But if all feminists do not genuinely honor the full range of the choices women make, how can they ask men to change? If work in the family wraps one in a "haze of domesticity," in a "cult of domesticity" that muddles our minds and blunts our talents, why would any man who could avoid it volunteer for this kind of social lobotomy?

Most critics of care propose a simple solution that they insist will resolve this conundrum. Elevate the salaries of caregivers, they say, and more men will enter the helping professions. Like Diane Johnson, they do not seem to understand that negative images of caring—not just pay and benefits—influence career choices. Nurses at the kind of major, urban medical center she describes would earn as much as $50,000 to

$60,000 a year (more than twice as much as the average American male earns). Yet only 3 percent of America's 2.1 million nurses are men—a huge gender gap that is the rule even in the most prestigious hospitals and medical centers. Most public school kindergarten teachers, with the same amount of education and experience, earn as much as high school teachers. Yet men make up over 30 percent of the nation's high school teachers, and 16 and 2 percent respectively of elementary and kindergarten and pre-K teachers.

Prejudice—not simply low salaries—has kept men out of the caring professions. "When a man says he wants to be an elementary school or kindergarten teacher, people think he's asking for a demotion," my daughter's elementary school principal—who taught third grade for years and was the only male in his school—recently told me. Prejudice also inhibits male caretaking in the home. Men in countries like Sweden rarely make use of generous parental leaves to take time off work for childrearing. Few men have full-time responsibility for their elderly parents (and most elderly parents refuse to accept hands-on caregiving from their sons).

This situation is the legacy of prejudice, not just low pay and poor working conditions. It does not suggest that recruiting men to either caregiving in the home or helping professions involves a Victorian romanticization of caregiving. But it certainly involves a realistic appraisal of the importance, difficulty, and complexity of this work.

The feminist project of making women's traditional invisible work visible has never constituted an attack on independence or equality. Feminists concerned with caring focus on women not because they believe caring is an innate female quality but because, as feminists, they view the world through the lens of female experience. Moreover, any discussion of caregiving must recognize the fact that women have done, and still do, most of the caregiving in our society.

In order to achieve equality and alter this unequal distribution of labor, it is necessary to follow a number of different paths. By making the invisible visible, feminists are trying to demonstrate that women's historical and contemporary work inside and outside the home is as demanding and important as any that men have done, and that it also furnishes lessons, attitudes, and skills that are as critical as those learned in the male marketplace. This revelation, such feminists hope, will encourage men to share caring and society to value it.

By inadvertently or intentionally keeping caring work invisible, advocates of women's rights undermine women's prospects for equality as well as the professional and personal aspirations of some of the very women they insist they are trying to protect. It is, of course, predominantly women—millions on millions of them—who out of choice, not simply coercion, continue to care for others in hospitals and nursing homes, childcare centers, community clinics, schools, rehab and mental health facilities, and homes and communities all over this country.

The feminist assault on care—perhaps unwittingly, but nonetheless assuredly—reinforces the class system that relegates these women to the bottom of the career ladder and allows at least some of their sisters to get near the top. Men, we know all too well, have always depended on the unpaid or ill paid labor of women to support their professional lives. But today an elite group of professional women now also depend on the caregiving services of a large group of working class, working poor, and minority women who are assigned to do the work they will not deign or don't have time to touch.

As I was writing this essay, a good friend of mine who has, like me, "brandished her membership card" since the inception of the feminist movement called me to talk about her elderly father's recent admission to a nursing home. Both her parents are in their eighties, and her father has Alzheimer's disease. During the Christmas vacation, she returned to her family's home to be with her mother and visit her father. She spoke with despair of watching his decline, and with enormous respect and admiration for the care her mother and others diligently administer to this increasingly difficult patient, twenty-four hours a day, day in and day out. She worried about the fact that much of his care was provided by ill-paid Caribbean women whose attentiveness often reflected the lack of regard in which the society holds them and their work.

And, finally, she talked poignantly about helping her mother—a woman she has always found distant and angry—sort through the accumulated debris of a sixty-year marriage. There was nothing romantic about her account of the care she was finally providing a woman who had cared for her for almost two decades. No glowing embers of spiritual light emerged from the innumerable bags of garbage she dragged to the Salvation Army twice a day; she experienced no dramatic epiphanies as she watched her father waking up from sleep, disoriented and fighting wildly as his attendants tried to calm him down.

But, as she ended our long phone conversation, she concluded that she found some surprising satisfaction in the work she had done with her mother over those long and emotionally draining days. This was the first time, she said, she had ever experienced true affection and connection with her mother. "There are rewards in this after all," she said as she soberly contemplated the experience.

I cannot help thinking of my friend's story, my own as a mother and daughter, and those I have listened to and observed in my work with caregivers. The attitudes conveyed in the work of anticaring advocates of women's rights like Kaminer, Faludi, Johnson, and others are disturbing not only because of the intellectual distortions and almost willful misinterpretations they contain, but because they leave us with no way to account for, analyze, and, yes, promote one of the major activities that sustains human existence and society.

There may very well be no nine-second sound byte with which to explain what constitutes caring in each and every instance. But without it, as everyone of us knows and most feminists used to acknowledge, we cannot make it through life. It may not count for much in the "free" marketplace, but it is not just another trivial pursuit. Most important, if men and women struggle to assume its burdens, obligations, and joys more equitably, and try to create a society that provides genuine social support and rewards for caregiving, considerations of the subject are not fated to hamper the progress of women toward equality.

References

Carse, Alisa L. 1991. "The 'Voice of Care': Implications for Bioethical Education." *Journal of Medicine and Philosophy* 15 (1991): 5–28.
———. 1996. "Facing Up to Moral Perils: The Virtues of Care in Bioethics." This volume, pp. 83–109.
Cott, Nancy F. 1987. *The Gounding of Modern Feminism.* New Haven, CT: Yale University Press.
Davidson, Nicholas. 1991. *The Failure of Feminism.* Buffalo, NY: Prometheus Books.
Douglas, Ann. 1977. *The Feminization of American Culture.* New York: Knopf.
Faludi, Susan. 1991. *Backlash: The Undeclared War Against American Women.* New York: Crown.
Field Belenky, Mary et al. 1986. *Women's Ways of Knowing: The Development of Self, Voice, and Mind.* New York: Basic Books.
Friedan, Betty. 1981. *The Second Stage.* New York: Summit Books.
Gilligan, Carol. 1982. *In a Different Voice: Psychological Theory and Women's Development.* Cambridge, MA: Harvard University Press.
———. 1986. "Reply" (In a Different Voice: An Interdisciplinary Forum). *Signs* 11, 21 (winter).
Gilligan, Carol, J. Ward, and J. Taylor, eds. 1988. *Mapping the Moral Domain: A Contribution of Women's Thinking to Psychology and Education.* Cambridge, MA: Harvard University Press.
Gordon, Suzanne. 1991. *Prisoners of Men's Dreams: Striking Out for a New Feminine Future.* Boston: Little, Brown.
Hare-Mustin, Rachel T. and Jeanne Marecek. 1992. "Gender and the Meaning of Difference: Postmodernism and Psychology." In Hare-Mustin and Maracek, eds., *Making a Difference: Psychology and the Construction of Gender.* New Haven, CT: Yale University Press.
Johnson, Diane. 1992. "Iron John and His Friends." *New York Review of Books,* January 16, pp. 13–17.
———. 1990. *Health and Happiness.* New York: Knopf.
Kaminer, Wendy. 1990. *A Fearful Freedom: Women's Flight from Equality.* Reading, MA: Addison-Wesley.

————. 1993. "Feminism's Identity Crisis." *Atlantic Monthly* 272, 4 (October): 51–68.

Miller, Jean Baker. 1976. *Toward a New Psychology of Women.* Boston: Beacon Press.

Nelson, Hilde. 1992. "Against Caring." *Journal of Clinical Ethics* 3, 1: 8–14.

Pollitt, Katha. 1992 "Marooned on Gilligan's Island." *Nation* 225, 22 (December 28): 799–807.

Rawls, John. 1971. *A Theory of Justice.* Cambridge, MA: Belknap Press of Harvard University Press.

Chapter 17
The Mormon Caregiving Network

Judith Dushku

Several months ago, a phone call interrupted the everyday chaos of my domestic life. It was a woman from my church. Her voice conveyed suffering and the fact that she needed my ear. My dog and four teenage children were clamoring for my attention, but I pulled up a stool for what I knew would be a long talk. I care deeply for this friend. Much later, I was headed for the car to go to work when I remembered I had promised to loan my van to a church sister who needed to transport a group to visit the hospital. So off I headed—blocks out of my way—so we could trade keys and she could pick up her charges. Finally I went to work.

That same afternoon, during my second week of teaching summer school and two weeks before my kids finished their school semester, the phone rang yet again. A woman with a Texas accent introduced herself. "Hello, Professor Dushku, I am working on an asylum case for a wonderful Ghanaian woman and I need your help. Will you please assist me with this case?" she hastily announced.

I knew why she had called. I teach African politics. Ten years ago I had written a document for a lawyer friend about political circumstances in Ghana. The lawyer used this to prove that his client deserved asylum in the United States. He won the case and my name had ended up in the footnotes. Since then I have had several requests to assist immigration lawyers with clients from Africa. I write about groups that have experienced discrimination, suggesting which groups are likely to suffer persecution. I accepted the early cases, but lately I have declined others because the research is too time consuming.

I explained all this to the Texas lawyer, but she pressed on: "This is such an interesting case, because it not only involves traditional tribal

An original essay.

ties and affiliations with political factions in Ghana, which you wrote about before, but it also is about religious persecution. My client believes she can prove that she has a 'well-founded fear of persecution' on the basis of her recent baptism into the Mormon Church, which was followed by documentable discrimination at the hands of local police."

Damn it, I thought, feeling the same pull that compelled me to lend my ear to my troubled friend and my car to another church woman. It's quite simple: I am bound by a sense of responsibility for anyone in need within the Mormon community in which I was raised. It is as natural to me as the obligation to feed my kids. At fifty-one I am sometimes still surprised at how quickly I shoulder this obligation whenever I feel I am being "called to serve." "Now you have me hooked!" I explained to the lawyer from Texas. "I cannot refuse to help this sister, since I am a Mormon woman. I want to help in any way I can."

The Texas lawyer had no idea that I was a Mormon or that Mormons felt this obligation to "share one another's burdens," but she happily told me the details of the Ghanaian woman's claims, and I began to plan my research on Ghana and reorient my writing schedule.

I did the work and ten days later I sent off the document, with a familiar sense of satisfaction and goodwill mixed with a sense of frustration. How, I often wonder, can I allow these callings to totally overwhelm my life and compel me to such exertions of energy and time? I have lived my life with these contradictory feelings when I am alerted to the needs of a "sister," which is what we call one another in our church.

While I nearly always heed the "call," and am nearly always glad that I did, thinking about it has often led me to question the whole process of caregiving in the church. Am I being manipulated in some way? Are the results of my actions ones I would have chosen? Do I give my life over to others to manage, and leave the important choices about what I do with my time to others? Do I, and other Mormon women, define our worth in our religious community by the quantity and quality of service and caregiving that we render? When we suffer from flagging self-esteem, do we sometimes redouble our efforts to serve because it guarantees us a secure place in the community of the Latter-Day Saints? Do we all "lose ourselves by being defined by others' needs," out of a need to feel accepted? And does this ultimately undermine our sense of value independent of such service?

These are not the only questions I have asked myself as an active and devoted member of the Mormon church and community. I am a feminist, and, perhaps most fundamentally, I constantly question my allegiance and commitment to a church that is in many ways indifferent to women and even hostile to their interests. As one who has long been involved in progressive politics, I am consistently challenged by my church leaders' positions on race, gender, and politics. Only recently, for example, the church excommunicated a number of feminists who are old and dear friends. As I write, I do not know whether or when my turn will come. Reflecting on this absurd reality, I wonder at how I and so many good Mormon women continue to reliably give so much of ourselves to this institution.

Yet I am simultaneously drawn to this very church by the strong caregiving and women's support and feminist community it has nourished. For most of its short existence, the Mormon church has earned a reputation for intransigent misogyny. It has, however, also encouraged and sustained a woman's organization that has taught women to value one another and to value caregiving practices as well. Through the women's Relief Society and the institution of what is called "visiting teaching," women are taught to care for one another and to take caregiving seriously. Unlike the situation in other religions where women are taught to care almost exclusively for men and children, in the Church of Jesus Christ of the Latter-Day Saints women are taught to care for each other. Throughout their lives, women are assigned a rotating series of "visiting teachers" who help them on a monthly or, if necessary, weekly or daily basis. The teacher is also taught—she receives care and attention from a rotating series of women who are in turn assigned to help her.

Women and men are all, moreover, taught that caregiving is not just sentiment but practice, not just a natural, intuitive process, but a set of skills that must be taught and learned. The institution of visiting teaching and the Mormon attitude toward caregiving embeds women in an ongoing structure of obligation and caregiving relationships that legitimate the idea that it is a social good not only to give help but to ask for and accept it.

One could easily argue that this structure of caregiving is only a gimmick to attract and entrap people in an authoritarian institution, that it is a mechanism of social control used to keep women in line and give them a false sense of importance in a church whose hierarchy systematically deprives them of a leadership role.

Much of this is true. But to focus only on the misuses of caregiving is to take far too narrow a view—one that conforms to stereotypical views of both women and caregiving which contend that the commitment to care is a conservative social force. The Mormon women's caregiving network demonstrates that caregiving can lead to what Suzanne Gordon has called a politics of transformation, not merely one of adaptation. With or without intending it, the women's structure in the church has created a system that celebrates women and enthusiastically affirms their worth. The church has placed an emphasis on the importance of attending to the needs and aspirations of women by charging so many of us with the important work of reaching out to our sisters. This has imbued at least some of us with values that have—in this era of female emancipation— led us from a politics of charity to a politics of dissent. It is the caregiving system that has so long nourished women that has, in fact, helped us to mount a significant feminist challenge to precisely those positions and values that have led so many non-Mormon women to criticize the Mormon church.

Those outside may be surprised to learn about a thriving Mormon feminism. The first question many women ask when they hear us mention Mormon feminism is "Mormon what? Isn't that an oxymoron?" And, indeed, some of us laughingly call ourselves "oxymormons." But I know hundreds of Mormon women who consider themselves feminists. In Salt Lake City an unofficial Mormon feminist group—the Mormon Women's Forum—was organized in 1988. For the past twenty years, I have belonged to a Mormon feminist group—Exponent II—that is based in Boston, Massachusetts. Many of us take feminism, even radical versions of it, very seriously and see it as the shaping ideology of our lives. At the same time we continue as believing Mormons within the mainstream of the church, serving one another and trying to protect ourselves and each other from its damaging antifeminist attitudes. While other aspects of Mormonism may tie different ones of us to the organization, many women say that it is largely this vast women's service system—reflecting as it does their definition of Christianity—that binds them to the church. They say they identify so strongly with women and the issues of women's lives because they have been nourished by a theology that promotes the idea that serving women is very important business that deserves our highest level of creative commitment as Christians. And in a complementary dynamic the supportive environment provides a place where women grow strong.

Thus, in addition to the official church system for serving women, some female members have built women's groups within the Mormon community but outside the official organization. There is no way to know how numerous these groups are, and it would be a mistake to assume that they are all feminist in their orientation. Some may have developed out of book groups or parenting support groups. Many members of these independent groups consider themselves part of a powerful feminist tradition that existed within the church in the nineteenth century and that has sustained and promoted feminist goals since that time. Although such groups have been officially denigrated by Mormon leaders, most women in them have chosen to keep their ties to the church and to continue to serve in its official women's organizations. They have, however, felt a need to maintain their safe discussion groups away from the watchful eyes of the central leadership.

Exponent II, the group of New England-based Mormon feminists I have already mentioned, has for twenty years produced a feminist newspaper with the same name, named after a nineteenth-century feminist newspaper called *The Woman's Exponent*, officially published by the Mormon church in Utah in the 1880s until 1910. While consciousness-raising groups formed in the secular world have come and gone (and women from Exponent II have been involved in some), the group has continued to meet for twenty years with most of the original members, and the paper still comes out regularly. My active participation in both this group and the official women's network makes it possible for me to maintain an enduring commitment to change the aspects of the church that are so troubling to me.

The hundreds of Mormon women I regard as like-minded feel like loving allies in a shared desire to remain in the church, support its natural feminist programs, and at the same time transform the church's women-demeaning practices and attitudes. The fact that we have given care to and genuinely care for one another as women in the church makes our determination to change things urgent and compelling. Indeed, I believe that the feminist and caregiving communities that exist within the church—often intertwining, sometimes separating—create a powerful bond of affection and a mutual obligation which is the foundation for some of the most profound of political challenges.

Let me describe how the church's community of caregiving operates and how it has strengthened me and other women I know over the years. Then I will describe how it has helped connect women who have gone on to sustain a strong vision of a feminist support network within Mormonism.

My story about the Ghanaian woman is not unusual in my religious culture and typifies the ways I and any Mormon woman in this community of caregiving react under similar circumstances. This Mormon sister whom I felt called to care for so was not "one of my own people." She was of a different nationality, culture, age, and place. I knew so little about her that to people outside of my faith my rush to her aid might appear a strange response. But, in the context of the Mormonism that I know and in which I grew up and have been immersed since my birth in 1942, it makes perfect sense.

While I was born in a predominantly Mormon town in Idaho, I grew up in non-Mormon communities far away from Utah and Idaho. My parents sacrificed to make sure that I participated in every program the Mormon church sponsored and recommended for young people. This was central to my identity as an unusual kind of Christian when I was growing up in Kansas, California, and Michigan. I was generally proud of the network of kindness and service that outsiders noticed with respect. Sometimes I resented my parents' willingness to inconvenience our family for the sake of others with so little warning. Other times I complained when these compassionate acts of caring were greeted with little gratitude. But part of the message I was taught at church and at home was that the gratitude was unnecessary—that caring for others well and with love was a reward unto itself. I believed it.

When I left Michigan in 1960 for college at Brigham Young University in Utah (the official Mormon college), I expected to continue in this pattern of caretaking of "my sisters." In my dorm I was surrounded by young women with the same expectations. We held meetings and worked out a system of caretaking in the dorm through which each student had someone to look after and was assured, in turn, that someone in the dorm would look after her needs. Through periods of intense homesickness and some other disappointments in the culture of BYU, I do remember my dormmates acting as ready caretakers over the next few years.

BYU was oppressively conformist in other ways, and I was very unhappy with the rigid restrictions and the attitude of negative judgment toward young women that pervaded the atmosphere of the university. I had never heard of feminism and had no conscious sense of BYU as a place that discriminated against women as a group. Nonetheless, I suffered because no professor or administrator ever encouraged me to do anything that felt like growth and positive "taking charge of my life." Instead, they encouraged me to be passive and to marry. These pressures to do things I felt were not in my best interest led me into a secret rebellion, which I considered necessary for my psychological survival. At the same time I felt guilty for failing to marry. I thus experienced a great sense of liberation when I was accepted for graduate study in Boston in 1964.

I did some serious rebelling from some of Mormonism's other rules and obligations over the next decade, as I moved from graduate school into the work force and became a professor of political science and an activist in leftist politics. But my readiness to show up to care for any "sister" I was told was in need remained a constant throughout this period of an otherwise creatively turbulent life.

I tried to expand the circle from time to time and assigned myself to non-Mormon people. I mobilized caretaking skills that I had internalized to work in the "Great Society" programs during the Johnson years in Boston's "inner city." Describing myself as a troubled believer in Mormon theology, I went through brief crises in faith when I was tempted to leave Mormonism behind. Nonetheless, the assignment and opportunity to care for other people and feel part of a strong and reliable network that promised the same care to me kept me tied to this complex institution. Since I was single, lived away from the midwest and west where I had family and friends, and moved with burdensome frequency from one Cambridge student apartment to another, this network of caring and caretaking was a tremendous comfort.

I remember trying to communicate to my kind and humane revolutionary friends—so energetic in their commitment to establishing better institutions in our society—that there were components of my religious community which worked wonderfully in accomplishing some of the very goals they pursued. These good revolutionaries and communalists had great ideas but none of the skills for genuine cooperative living and group caregiving that I felt I had learned in my life. I acknowledged the racism that clung to Mormonism and was humiliated at being associated with it. I acknowledged its authoritarianism and was embarrassed by my willingness to tolerate it in order to reap other benefits from the network. But I still believed that if I could erase the warts from Mormonism's culture of caring I could offer it as a practical model for building institutions like those envisioned by my friends. I spent hours yearning for a way to tell the story of the Mormon caring system I found so moving. I tried to introduce methods and skills that I had learned growing up into our discussions for building communes that worked. People responded positively, but the job of initiating a whole system of caring and caregiving into a community of people who were new to these skills was overwhelming. Our ideas rarely materialized into successful and enduring experiments.

Not only did I engage in a political rebellion against the church, I also rebelled against one of Mormonism's strictest rules, that prohibiting marriage outside the faith. I married a non-Mormon with whom I shared a commitment to the antiwar movement and a passion to racially integrate society and make public schools work in Boston. I struggled over theological issues in the Mormon Church. Yet, again, I can never remember refusing to accept an assignment to reach out to someone who was ill or depressed or in need of an apartment for a night. No matter how busy I was with work, then babies, and then a very troubled marriage, I continued to respond nearly automatically to any Mormon's call to serve until I was in my thirties.

At that point the women's movement inspired me to examine my life and reassess the commitments that bound me to a path of weekly, sometimes daily service to my brothers and sisters in the church. Even as I began to examine its costs for me and other women, I wanted to keep caregiving in my life. I wanted to understand why so many Mormon women—who were also reexamining their relationship to the church—felt the same way.

The feminist group called Exponent II helped me to do this. In the early 1970s, I joined a radical feminist consciousness raising group in

Cambridge and at the same time I helped start what became the Exponent group of Mormon women, also in Cambridge. Both groups shaped my early years in the movement. The radical-secular-feminist group was made up of brilliant women who were writers and academics and activists. Over the next five years I always looked forward to our meetings. But the group never provided a supportive place in which members could really try out new ideas and strategies. It contained too many factions and cliques. The group seemed unable to sustain all of its members emotionally.

I have since known other women who remind me of those close feminist associates. They continue to offer me great ideas and tell me about fascinating new books and articles about feminism, socialism, psychology, and culture. I appreciate them and still love their company and the chance to interact with and learn from them. But I don't think of them as the people I could call on when I am grief stricken or depressed, or when I have issues with my teenager's drug use or my parents' changing lives.

For that kind of support I looked to the other group that I joined in the 1970s—the Exponent group of Mormon feminists. That group talked, read, shared ideas from the literature of the time, argued and challenged one another, and planned for a better society. What was different was its members' commitment literally to carry life's little burdens for one another. It seemed easy for us to combine the emotional and intellectual notions of support. This is perhaps what makes us different from other women in secular American society. The commitment to serve is central to the way Mormon women identify themselves.

The closest examples I have observed of this outside Mormonism have been in Africa and Nicaragua. In both places women's groups discuss women's issues and often write and publish literature on these subjects. But they do not separate the personal issues from their political feminist ideology. To think and talk together about ideas means that you also work together to help each other get life's practical work done well. They hold each other's babies while manuscripts are being xeroxed. They pick up a woman friend's groceries for her while they are shopping for their own, knowing that this will save that woman a trip. While trying to arrive at a cogent political analysis and strategies for political change, they accept each other's life sustaining work as their own.

Women in many Third World countries commonly respond to one another this way. And so do women in this Mormon network. Caregiving is a powerfully implanted value which continues to compel each new convert or carefully socialized new generation of Mormons even in congregations in huge urban settings far from Mormonism's origins in the West. Indeed, for those of us who live far from the seat of Mormonism, the obligation to care for a sister in need seems even stronger. It is part of our expression of our belief and affiliation with Mormonism wherever we live.

If one examines the Mormon church and the culture of Mormonism that surrounds it, the reasons for this are obvious. In the Church of Jesus Christ of Latter-Day Saints, women are told from their youth that their greatest calling is "motherhood," but that close on its heels is the calling to "serve one another." I believe most observers of Mormons and most Mormons themselves would agree that the expectation to respond to a call to serve rests most heavily on women. It is part of a doctrine that promotes the idea that women are "by nature," more willing to sacrifice themselves for others and have certain virtues or qualities that make service come more "naturally" to them. Mormon women thus internalize values that encourage them to think of themselves as specially chosen to enjoy the blessings of service. Women are taught this formally and informally in the Mormon church and throughout the culture of Mormonism in numerous ways. Hymns, talks, poetry, and all kinds of activities reinforce these values. While many LDS people do not believe this, it is clear that service callings go more frequently and casually to women.

The centerpiece of weekly meetings in the century-old Relief Society is a well-developed curriculum that includes four areas for development considered essential for all balanced women. One of the four areas is called "compassionate service," a term used since the end of the nineteenth century to include all volunteer service within the church. The four subject areas are discussed on a rotating basis at Relief Society meetings, held every Sunday in every Mormon meeting house in the world. Lesson books are written in Salt Lake City and distributed gratis throughout the worldwide church to ensure that every congregation keeps roughly to the same schedule.

Normally lessons on "compassionate service" are taught every fourth Sunday of every month of every year. Some lessons talk about the scriptural and theological justifications that give compassionate service such a high priority in our lives. Others are very practical and stress specific ways to serve and show caring and love. Embedded in these well-written lessons is the notion that caregiving is a skill that anyone can learn, and that it is done best by those who are instructed in the procedures as well as inspired and consistently encouraged to practice it.

These lessons include discussions about food preparation for bedridden people, for example, I remember one that explained why a variety of colors in food is emotionally stimulating and pleasant for housebound and bedridden people, and that presented ideas about food decoration and presentation. Having never studied nursing or dietetics, this was revealing and useful to me. And, of course, there was a time when I used this advice.

I have had lessons on supporting families with handicapped children, caring for mentally ill adults, effective volunteer work in group homes, supporting adolescents trying to lose weight and stay healthy, standing by women who have been abused and are going through periods of anger and distress, knowing when to refer depressed sisters to more professional help, hospice-type care for the terminally ill, and help with moving through the grieving process.

In addition to monthly lessons on the subject, local conferences allow us to share experiences about our compassionate service and encourage one another in this calling. The church publishes booklets and talks with suggestions for effective caregiving. These often relate women's positive experiences with such service. I have been struck by the amount of research and thought that has gone into the variety of lessons on effective caregiving. Similarly impressive are the number of ways women reexamine the question of why we help others and to what end.

A very specific program that involves all female members of the Church also promotes caretaking. This "visiting teaching" program has its roots in the pioneer days, first in Illinois, then in early Utah. There women were designated to visit, teach, and assist assigned sisters in their congregations (called "wards") and to "bear their burdens." In the middle of the nineteenth century this program was sometimes quite informal and at other times more formalized. But as the church moved into the twentieth century the program was more and more routinized.

While men are chosen as home teachers and asked to serve families, each ward bishop calls a woman to be the Relief Society president and organize the day-to-day service to women. In each ward, the president of the Relief Society calls women to accept a stewardship for other women and to agree to visit and support these designated women for a year or more. The program is impressive in scope. Several million women all over the world go out, usually in pairs, to visit several million others— usually visiting them at least once a month, but more if there is illness or other pressing need. All visits are reported to a supervisory woman and, if a visiting teacher is unable to make her visit, someone else is asked to fill in. From time to time there have been debates over whether phone calls could replace face-to-face visits. Currently the personal visit is favored, but with less rigidity than five years ago.

An elaborate bureaucracy is set up to accomplish this work of assignment and oversight. Women hold meetings and spend valuable time discussing which women would be best to offer another comfort and a sense of unity. We discuss ways to follow up on reported difficulties discovered in particular homes. In a typical ward where many women do not work during the day, the Relief Society leaders spend hours each week coordinating care and making sure that all female members get a quality visit. This endorses the ideology that women's domestic lives are very important.

This program also provides critical support to deeply troubled women. I have a good friend who is a survivor of early childhood sexual abuse and has had years of difficulty coping with life. She found a therapy group and a therapist that offered her help. With the financial aid of the church, she signed up for group therapy. However, after she started the group, it moved to a town twenty-five miles away which was inaccessible by public transportation. This hit her hard and she became more depressed. Her visiting teacher, who met with her regularly, asked the bishop to "call" a second visiting teacher to assist in getting her to her group therapy sessions. For a year the two women picked up my friend and transported her twice a week to and from her group. It was a critical piece of help and caregiving.

The visiting teacher program cuts across class, economic, ethnic, and age group lines. Assignments are made with the unity and integration of the ward as part of the goal. Barriers to this exist, however, because the wards are limited to geographically defined neighborhoods that often do not have a highly diverse mix of people available.

In gatherings of Mormon women the visiting teaching program is often a topic of discussion. What is the impact on women who spend a lifetime serving other women and their families? What is the impact of having other women serve us over a lifetime? Most see many positive effects. Each visiting teacher feels she is valuable. She feels her presence makes a critical difference in another person's life. She feels trusted to solve problems and be creatively helpful, often in times of real crisis. She gets feedback on her successes which affirms her powerful role in improving someone else's life. The process is mutually affirming and empowers the server and the served.

Women also note a sense of spiritual affirmation that comes from participation in this program. Each Mormon has a story of some act of kindness or service to recount. In the retelling, it is assumed that the visiting teacher could only have acted so sensitively and so punctually and with such clarity of purpose because God inspired her to do so. This belief that women serve well because they are good people, involved in a good program, and personally led by God is a heady feeling that works well to continue to elicit lifelong loyalty to and participation in the program.

As a mother who has always worked full-time, I have had mostly positive experiences from this program. When my sister was dying, I was an emotional wreck and my children were in shock. My sister had left the church years before her final illness, but had still welcomed visiting teachers into her home. When she was dying, both her visiting teachers and mine brought food when appropriate, housed out-of-town family and guests, picked visitors up at airports, sat by my sister's bed when hospice nurses were unavailable and the family was in transition, and arranged for a funeral dinner. I will never forget the kindness of visiting teachers during that desperate period.

Nor will I forget my visiting teacher's response when I chose to divorce my husband twelve years ago. That was not a popular or acceptable thing to do in Mormon circles. (Divorces are officially allowed, but normally women are encouraged to accommodate to a bad marriage until there is no recourse and probably until her husband leaves her.) My visiting teacher felt uncomfortable with my decision and told me so. Nonetheless, when the time came and I officially announced that I was filing for divorce, she told me she prayed to know what I needed. She was inspired, she said, to know that I needed to be congratulated and celebrated. So she did her best to do just that. No sighs, no pitying looks, no intimations of negative judgments, only smiles and cheering all around, followed by offers of practical help with kids when my husband was moving his stuff out of the house. Considering her values, her response moved me deeply.

Since all of us who have spent any time in the church have been visiting teachers, we all have experience with both visiting others and caring for them and with being visited by other women. We all have stories to tell. Some of them, of course, are negative, but my assessment is that most are positive. One woman I know had recently moved to Boston to be with her husband who had a year's appointment at Harvard. She had taken a sabbatical from her long-time teaching job in Utah. Her children were grown. When she arrived in Boston she had offered herself to the visiting teacher program as an extra person with time on her hands. Although she had skills and opportunities to do other things, for the whole year she chose to fill her days with visiting teaching assignments. She is a feminist and a long-time supporter of our Mormon women's newspaper. She told me her choice to be a full-time visiting teacher resulted partly from her faith and partly from her feminism (if the two can be divided). She wanted to support Mormon women in any way she could. It was, she concluded, an inspired choice, and she was glad there was a system in place for her to join when she arrived in Boston. Her enthusiastic willingness is typical of the kinds of motives that make the program work.

Sometimes the obligation to serve becomes too much of a burden. For women with serious time constraints, or for women who simply choose to do something other than service, the pressure to serve cheerfully and compassionately at all times becomes an impossible weight. In our Exponent II discussion group we have grappled with the question of how this pressure affects women's feelings of worth. We have often discussed the ambivalence Mormon women feel when they attempt to dedicate their lives to a career, thus abandoning a life where they are perpetually available to give care. We debate the gender bias inherent in this situation.

Mormon men are expected to serve their brothers and sisters in the community as well. Many do extraordinary things and spend long hours responding to their callings. But because women are officially discouraged from seeking employment outside the home, and are therefore assumed to be on call all day, they are more likely to be asked first. Moreover, men are allowed to place limits on their availability because of their full-time work. No one ever questions men who put family-supporting, "breadwinning" work above service, even if their work clearly fulfills personal or economic rather than family needs or ambitions.

This gender bias also gives men the privilege of taking over from women, and even excluding women from, their caregiving assignments when their visiting teacher has uncovered tricky ethical or legal issues in a particular family. At that point women with long-established relationships may be shoved aside because men are deemed to have superior knowledge and wisdom that takes priority. Women also complain that male leaders sometimes criticize their service-related decisions. This raises serious gender issues.

Mormon feminists like myself and those I work with have not papered over these serious problems. Indeed, our challenge is simultaneously to eliminate gender bias and the kinds of coercive pressures and negative judgments leveled against those women who choose different paths, without diluting the Mormon program of caretaking. So many of us have known the benefits of belonging to the church and of being in this community that we want to preserve its positive aspects. We similarly want to preserve our shared theology and culture. Mormon women tend to be very close. We feel that we have learned how to be intimate because of the visiting teaching program. While we know that intimacy-building skills exist in many places and cultures, most of us feel that these skills are abundant in our culture and we credit Mormon upbringing with teaching them to us.

In our Exponent group these issues are constantly debated. Indeed, it is in part our analysis of the gender biases in our caregiving programs that has led us to question broader church attitudes toward women. From the gendered definitions of caregiving, we have moved on to challenge other ways the church limits women's lives. While we continue to support the idea of women caring for one another and participate in the visiting teaching program, we have asked women to expand their sense of available life choices. We urge women to make it clear to children of both sexes that service is an option and that women should not be the one to shoulder most of the caregiving obligations. We believe our ability to pose this challenge has been fueled by our traditions of mutually supporting one another in making each other's lives work better.

Our goal is to keep this dissident network alive, to encourage more of authority and to make caregiving more the work of men as well. While offering our energies to sustain the caregiving community that does so much to support us and make our lives richer, we continue to make gains. We thus support every collective strategy that can lead to the organization of independent groups of Mormons who share views on a more liberated church culture and church organization. Hopefully these groups will serve as buffers that protect Mormon activists who might otherwise be isolated and vulnerable to pressures and prejudices from within the main body of church membership. To these groups, we clearly express our positive feelings about the general supportive and communalist kind of Christianity that Mormonism offers to its members.

Indeed, I believe non-Mormon academics and researchers could fruitfully examine the culture of Mormonism, particularly assessing its impact on women. I suspect most would find that the women's caregiving system within the church is one of its principal successes. It exemplifies the practical and actual institutionalization of ideas of Christian feminism. In a world in which thoughts about the construction of such a feminism are mostly theoretical and seldom realized, objective analyses of the role of a theology of mutual responsibility and a "law of stewardship" would be most helpful to faithful insiders who admit to having made the kind of compromises we have made. The more critically I have analyzed caregiving within the church, the more confident I am that Mormon feminism and the Mormon women's caregiving network provides an exemplary and surprising model.

Chapter 18
Let Me Take a Listen to Your Heart

Rita Charon

There are some things that I learned through this experience about what's important to me as a patient and what the medical staff can do to help or to make things worse. There's a line that divides people who have passed over into the condition I'm in. There's no way I can convey to you the feeling of the death sentence and how it changes your life. In situations where odds are really very poor, how important it is for doctors and medical staff to foster a patient's feeling of control and of hope. Empathize. Put yourself in the shoes of your patient as much as possible. Get as close to your patient as you can.

—Jonathan J. King

Who can teach health professionals about compassionate care better than sick persons themselves? Dr. Jonathan J. King, a professor of computer science at Stanford University, died of a rare form of liver cancer in 1991. He died in his forties, his sons six and twelve years old, his work only begun. Throughout his illness and his courageous attempts to get better, he gazed at us health professionals, piercing the mystery of our work, recognizing our suffering as we care for sick and dying patients. This man, in the center of his own anguish, thought of us. Not bounded by his suffering, he reached over the line that separates the sick from the well to teach us what he had learned. We celebrate his memory, and we mourn him.

Dr. King realized, in his generosity and compassion, that we who care for sick and dying patients suffer ourselves. If all of us who surround sickness can recognize and accept our own burden of pain, we are better able to tolerate and ease the suffering of patients and their families. An example from child psychology helps to understand our position. When infants are young, they take part in parallel play. Two infants will

An earlier version of this essay was presented as the First Annual Jonathan J. King Lecture, Stanford University Medical Center, November 1991, and appeared in *The Pharos of Alpha Omega Alpha*. Reprinted by permission.

play happily side by side, but one infant's play has nothing to do with the other infant's play. Their play does not connect them. Only as they mature can they participate in true mutual play, in which their activity together achieves meaning. Similarly, health professionals and patients often engage in parallel suffering, in which the suffering of the patient and the suffering of the caregiver are not related. Only as the health professionals mature can they grow beyond their own pain to join patients in their suffering, achieving meaning through true intersubjectivity.

How, though, can caregivers achieve this ability to recognize, understand, share, and therefore lessen the suffering of patients? How can they acknowledge and then set aside their own considerable suffering in order to join the patient in care? They first must respect the powers of sickness and dying. The dying person stands irrevocably apart from the healthy. In the seventeenth century, John Donne wrote, *Devotions Upon Emergent Occasions*, "As Sicknesse is the greatest misery, so the greatest misery of sickness is *solitude*" (1975, p. 24). Sick and dying people must endure isolation—as a matter of custom, as a means of sparing the well, and, finally, as an estrangement from their healthy selves.

Illness is secret, hidden, and frightening. Good taste, it sometimes appears, dictates that the sick person be discreet, covering the sights and smells of illness from the healthy lest they be offended. The sick person is made to feel responsible for keeping the tragic news to him- or herself. Why has it taken so long for people with disabilities to get access to public spaces if not for the queasiness that the healthy can feel at the sight of the ill?

This cultural need to hide sickness is not as powerful as the inner feeling of sick people that they inhabit a different world from that of the healthy. "Illness is the night side of life, a more onerous citizenship," explains Susan Sontag in *Illness as Metaphor* (1979, p. 3). Nothing strips illusion away from life as powerfully as illness: the sick person cannot bask in intimations of immortality. Alone in their knowledge of mortality, sick people struggle to be in the world with the well, who are deceived about the most fundamental feature of life: that it ends and does not often end easily. Since the well do not know this, the sick must endure a burden, for the sake of the well, of either frank self-deception or the keeping up of a false front. Those of us who accompany sick and dying people can offer a critical element of care by doing without the false front, for our courage to face the worst can contribute to the patient's fearlessness, honesty, freedom, and, oddly, hope. For hope comes home to the sick person who no longer must say "I'm not feeling myself," who can reconcile the healthy with the present self, and who can heal the divide that sickness brings.

Many health professionals work in hospitals, where sick and frightened people come for cure, for care, and for comfort, and where many persons die. Oftentimes, patients come to our hospitals at the end of a long search, referred from a community far away, in search of the specialist or the advanced capability not available elsewhere. We can be, that is, our patients' final hope. In order to grapple with the kinds of suffering we witness in hospitals, we need to consider the nature of these extraordinary places.

Our hospitals are powerful strange islands of pain and magic. Children believe that their grandparents disappear into them, lost beyond being found. Smart, capable grown-ups regress when they have to go to hospital. To outsiders, hospitals are dream sequences where alien languages and customs are used, where rules that apply everywhere else are suspended, where human interchange is replaced by a peculiar set of commands: take off your clothes, hold your breath, don't move. The boundaries that customarily exist between public and private or between acceptable and taboo break down. Behaviors that would be basis for legal action in the outside world, that would be called sexual abuse or assault and battery, are permitted. As surgeon and writer Richard Selzer says, "I feel that one must not gaze into the body, that it is an evil deed for which punishment awaits" (1976, p. 24). How often do we close a door lest someone see what we are doing—undressing a wound, dissecting a cadaver, administering pain?

Visitors to our island see frantic yet highly organized activity on the scale of a space station or a medium-sized town. Workers in protective clothing—face masks, puffy paper shoes, whole body pajama suits, goggles—walk as if they always wear these costumes. Alarming signs abound on walls: "People with pacemakers or metal replacement joints do not proceed." "Absolutely no dead animals are to be stored in this freezer." Visitors are thrown by the awful smells, the sights of wounded people, the sounds that should be private. Strangers in their pajamas lie on stretchers in elevators. People with body parts marked with red crayon wait silently in a room labeled Radiation Treatment. Disease is the signifier on this island; no healthy visitor can feel at ease.

Anyone can tell the insiders from the outsiders. You don't need to see the hospital ID badge or white coat or blue smock. Insiders move in and out of messy situations with ease. They look without flinching at people with great scars or disfigurement. They calmly give directions to the emergency room to people wheezing, bleeding, or seizing. They may unexpectedly break into a run, guided by the overhead pager reciting the location of a cardiac arrest. When a beeper beeps, all their hands go to their waists.

We who work in hospitals are considered different by others. We can't talk about our work to those who do not work with us. People will call us and ask us what to do in the case of illness, as if mere physical contact with such places confers expertise or authority. Hospital workers become the referral system for those outside it, for if the hospital worker doesn't know the answer to a question, he or she—whether a worker in the mail room or maintenance or the chemistry lab or the emergency room—will have access to those who do. Medical students often go through a crisis during the summer after their first year of school when they go home for vacation and get phone calls from Aunt Katherine who just found out she has breast cancer and should she have an operation or the chemotherapy? Or from a high school friend who calls to ask about the early signs of AIDS. They solemnly realize that their lives are transformed. They were not prepared in medical school for the secrets they will be told, the intimacies they will reach with friends, relatives, and strangers, and the help that these people will expect from them. Experienced hospital workers know that because we work in hospitals people tell us things they otherwise wouldn't tell us. They tell us because they know we will help them. And we listen.

We listen. When a doctor examines a patient, he or she may say, bent over the bared chest with stethoscope in hand, "Let me take a listen to your heart." The heart has much to tell the listener. Permission to listen to it must be requested, for the secrets of the heart belong to the patient. We say, "take a listen," reminding ourselves that in listening there is an expropriation. When we listen—either to the murmur of the heart that signifies serious disease or to the story of an illness that a patient entrusts to us—we are obtaining something of great meaning, something toward which we have a responsibility. It may be a responsibility to replace a mitral valve, or it may be a responsibility to be moved by the story we hear.

What is it that we hear? We hear about suffering. We hear about lives that are transformed by disease that came for no reason, to people who have done nothing deserving punishment. The disease causes great physical and emotional pain, ends working lives, puts family life in turmoil, and may lead to financial ruin. We hear from patients and their families the sense of unfairness, anger at the capriciousness of a universe that would make one ill at the start of one's child's life, that can invade a life forcing aside all other concerns: work, commitments, and love. Slowly, slowly a sick person faces the disease—first denying it, then giving it a name, then realizing that it will end his life.

If we are to respond in caring ways to the suffering of others, we have to understand it and let that suffering come close. Dorothy Soelle (1975) and Warren Reich (1989) have described suffering as evolving through three phases: mute, expressive, and transforming. The first phase after a sudden loss is mute suffering. Initially not able to put the suffering into words, the patient will try to minimize the problem, will feel ashamed of it, and will wonder if it was deserved. During this mute time, the sufferer feels assaulted by the pain or loss and frantically seeks a way to continue to be himself or herself despite the ravages of suffering. The suffering takes over the person's self, leaving no room for autonomous action.

A patient of mine, Mr. Castellucci, always comes early for his appointments. He worries about his sugar, his insulin, and his cholesterol. He feels guilty that he does not watch his diet carefully and eats out a lot since his divorce. His daughter is sick again, in and out of the hospital for her lupus. He watches her kids, gives her money when he can, and spends some weekends at her apartment.

He used to work in a textile plant loading and unloading trucks, a physically demanding job. He lost his job during the summer, and at age 52 he cannot find a new job. He goes to the union office every two days with nothing to show for it. His unemployment and health insurance will run out. Already marginal and held together by his work and his little circle of buddies at the bar and the diner, being unemployed threatens everything that defines him.

He called me last week, tentatively, apologizing for taking up my time, to report that he had had a seizure. Alarmed, I arranged for immediate admission and an emergency head CT scan. The CT showed a tumor. He accepted this news stoically, saying he hoped it would get better and that he would do everything the neurologist said to do, not realizing what this will mean—the biopsies, the probable diagnosis of cancer, the operations, the radiation, the hopelessness.

Mr. Castellucci is built like a lineman, neck like the trunk of a tree, hands like shovels. I sense that he is close to his limit for tragedy. Much has happened to him—his wife has left him, his daughter is sick, he has lost his job, and now he is threatened with a tumor. Although Mr. Castellucci continues to appear stoic and composed, I can imagine that his fear is out of bounds. I want to hold this big tough man. I want to console him. I want to let him cry about the unfairness. "No wonder," I say to him, "no wonder you feel so bad."

As we undertake the diagnosis and therapy for his tumor, he will move into the next phase of suffering, the expressive phase, that phase which allows for the possibility of change. At some point, the person who suffers regains a voice and can tell of the inner pain, the anger, the blame, and the sense of having been betrayed. This telling requires a listener. Once the suffering achieves the status of language, it can—with the help of the listener—be examined, put into order, and understood. Only when the suffering is expressed can it be claimed and, once claimed, its meaning can be sought.

In the Bible, Job laments:

And now the life in me trickles away,
   days of grief have gripped me.
At night-time, sickness saps my bones,
   I am gnawed by wounds that never sleep . . .
My skin has turned black on me,
   my bones are burned with fever.
My harp is tuned to funeral wails,
   my flute to the voice of mourners. (Job 30:16–17, 30–31, Jerusalem Bible)

A young woman, a designer, came to see me for the first time with a complaint of an earache. She had been to several doctors and ear specialists, and had taken antibiotics, decongestants, and x-rays. The pain had gotten worse. It had spread all over her neck and face. She rubbed the right side of her face as she spoke, agitated and tearful.

I went through my routine, asking about past hospitalizations, medications, and allergies. I asked, as all doctors do, about the health of her family members. She chose to start with her father, telling me that he had been operated on for cancer of the lung two years ago and that this year he had developed cancer of the jaw, requiring another operation. She was an only child, her mother was unable to face her father's illness, so my patient was the one who was seeing her father through this serious time. As she described her father's illness to me, she rubbed the right side of her face to show me where his cancer was. "You know," I said, "that's the same gesture you used in describing your own pain." She stopped. She placed her hand in her lap. Her agitated motions for the first time ceased. "I didn't know that," she said. "I didn't know that it was related to my father."

I examined her and did some blood tests, but she needed no treatment. She continued in her own psychotherapy, now aware that her physical suffering was repeating the illness of her father.

Now, she told me that. I had to listen attentively and let everything she told me register. In her gesture and in her narrative of suffering, that is, in her expressiveness, she gave me what I needed to help her. She no longer has the earache, although she still suffers with her father in his disease.

In the next phase of suffering, that of transformation, the person achieves a new identity by discovering the meaning of suffering. In *Man's Search for Meaning*, Victor Frankl says that "Suffering ceases to be suffering in some way at the moment it finds a meaning" (1971, p. 179). Carlos is a young patient of mine with meningomyelocele, or spina bifida. He has been paralyzed from the waist down since birth. Until recently, he lived with his mother and siblings where he was treated, in his words, "like a potted plant." He has told me of the great suffering he endured as a child in a home where his parents fought, often physically, in his presence, and he, disabled, was unable to come to the defense of the one being hurt. He attended public schools in the days before mainstreaming, where he and other children with physical or cognitive disabilities were assigned indiscriminately to so-called special classes in which little teaching or learning went on. He recalls how his artistic talent and his gift for creating worlds of fantasy released him from the boredom of these classes.

Despite the indifference of the school system and the patronization of his family, Carlos grew to know himself and his strengths. Around his thirtieth birthday, he moved out of his mother's house into his own apartment in a city building designed for the disabled. He and I waged a long, successful battle to get him fitted with long-leg braces that allowed him for the first time in his life to get out of his wheelchair and to experience the world, as he said, "with height." An accomplished artist and magazine illustrator who is no stranger to the erotic and the intimate, Carlos has found supportive friends, lovers, and fellow activists for disability rights. Transformed by his suffering, Carlos has found both his freedom and the meaning of his losses by looking his suffering full in the face, by not flinching from the pain of his predicament, and by identifying with the self who could accept and then transcend the pain dealt him.

Sick persons, then, can suffer mutely, can express the suffering's toll, or can be transformed through the agency of suffering. However, what happens to us health professionals as we see patients who suffer? "I am a prisoner of perception, a compulsory witness," says the protagonist of Saul Bellow's *Herzog* (1964, p. 72). The most powerful response to suffering is compassion, that ability to experience with someone else what he or she is suffering and to accompany another on a journey of suffering. The compassionate witness will be able to recognize the pain in another and thereby to act on behalf of the one suffering. However, suffering does not automatically call forth compassion. Rather, the witness must work very hard to achieve that state. Why is compassion sometimes absent in the face of suffering? What can we do to bring it about? An unsentimental examination of patient care reveals that there are structural, social, emotional, and existential barriers to genuine compassion in health care workers. Rather than leave health professionals feeling guilty that they are not always in states of compassion toward their patients, let us examine some of the barriers to that care.

The structure of hospitals and health care often thwarts our best intentions. The nurse who is assigned ten patients instead of the customary six has to ignore call bells, let patients wait for bedpans, pain pills, and meals. This nurse will get the antibiotics hung, will respond to crises like chest pain or high fevers, and will give medically essential treatments. Will she answer questions of a frightened spouse? Will she notice a patient's tears? Will she stand vigil, even for a moment, with a grieving family at the bedside of a terminally ill patient?

Haven't we all sat behind a desk at the nurses' station when a family member approaches tentatively, asks softly, "Where can I get a blanket for my father, my father is cold?" In the middle of writing a note or paging an intern, we wave the son or daughter away vaguely, toward someone else who might have the time to escort the person to the linen closet. We suspect that there might not be an extra blanket there at all. Clerks at the front desk of the emergency room have to face patients and their families who rage, "We've been here for four hours, my grandmother can't breathe, do you want to wait until she dies?" What is the clerk to do? He or she knows that the sickest patients get taken inside first, that the nurses and doctors make those judgments, and that the staff and the patients have to accept their decisions. What does it do to the clerk to have to say over and over, "There are sicker people in front of you, we'll see you as soon as we can."

Saying no to the blanket-seeker or to the patient waiting in the emergency room erodes something within us. Every time we have to deny people simple human services, every time we have to walk by a room with a distraught person inside calling out, "Nurse, nurse, someone help me," a part of our gentleness and kindness dies off. We steel ourselves against hurtful things about which we can do nothing. Our naive willingness to help and our innate human sympathy are replaced with executive necessity. One does what has to be done, be it to stick a needle in an antecubital fossa, to debride a burn, or to tell someone that their tumor has spread. We develop a complex set of boundaries between ourselves and hurting patients, allowing for the distance required for us to act.

Social factors as well as these structural ones interfere with our ability to act compassionately. Not all patients bear their suffering nobly, and none is noble always. No more saintly than healthy people, patients can be cranky, manipulative, demanding, and cowardly. Throughout illness, patients rail against their sickness, use their sickness as excuses, and exhaust the patience and generosity of their caregivers. Some illnesses are caused by things the patients do—drink alcohol, smoke cigarettes, or use drugs or guns. I once heard an intern refer to a city hospital in New York as the "hospital for self-inflicted diseases." Some illnesses are exacerbated because patients do not follow medical advice. So-called noncompliant patients confound the people who would care for them, making the care appear to be a charade.

Three weeks ago I walked toward a nurses' station in Presbyterian Hospital, past the visitors' lounge. Standing in this public space with television blaring a game show were three people: a black woman appearing to be in her mid-fifties, a third-year woman medical student, and an intern in his second month of doctorhood. I knew the medical student as a woman who had had some difficulty in her first two years of school and who had seriously considered quitting medicine. The intern I knew to be a young man with high ideals and uncommon generosity who had worked during medical school in a shelter for homeless persons. Both the medical student and the intern were white. I passed this lounge as the older woman cried out loudly, clutched her head, then sobbed uncontrollably. The intern stood ineffectually beside her rhythmically patting her shoulder, the medical student stood a few paces behind them watching with a look of alarm on her face. Any of us would have recognized the scene with biological accuracy. The intern had just told the black woman that her loved one had died. The intern, within a few minutes, was at the nurses' station asking for a blank death certificate. The woman was by herself in the lounge, the medical student anxiously orbiting the intern.

Now. Why was this done so horribly? There is often no private room, first of all, where such conversations can take place. Is there a consultation room, a praying room, a patient's family room on each floor of a hospital? Must one look for an empty clean utility room at such occasions, or ask the nurses on break to vacate the coffee room? What do we learn about our work from the fact that there is no room for grieving, for comforting, for the privacy of sudden loss?

In addition to these structural features, there were emotional and existential reasons that the scene in the lounge was so awful. The intern, two months into his professional life, no doubt felt that he had had a hand in this death. No matter if the patient died on the stretcher on the way from Admitting. Any doctor will doggedly believe that he or she is responsible for bad outcomes. As doctors age, they develop a sense of fate that somewhat absolves them from the extraordinary depth of guilt and remorse that the young ones feel. Interns go about their work convinced that they have caused death, pain, suffering. The tragedy is that this intern, like most, will not recognize the palpable hurt he caused the woman in the lounge but will anguish over his order to have run the D5-normal-saline at 125 cc an hour instead of at 80. The mistakes, that is, are hunted up in the technical realm and not in the realm of meaning.

This intern will know that there was something awful about the scene in the visitors' lounge, but he will not have the guidance to learn how he could have done it better. The medical student, powerless in the circumstances, will be that much more convinced that medicine is a brutal enterprise and will be that much less able to see its capacity for comfort. Meanwhile, the black woman in the lounge has just lost her husband or her lover or her child. For the rest of her life, she will date events as having happened before or after this moment. No doubt, the intern had his next admission down in the emergency room to work up. No doubt, the student had blood to hang or labs to check. But despite these competing claims for time, they could have found the woman a chair, offered her some privacy, and asked her, "Is there anyone you'd like me to call for you?" or "Shall I sit with you for a while?" We their teachers let them down. We teachers need to find ways to bring the intern and the student back into the visitors' lounge, into genuine human contact with the suffering woman.

Those of us who care for sick patients know about the things that separate us from them. I help to run support groups for interns at my hospital, letting interns talk among themselves about the things that make their work difficult. I am sure that nurses, therapists, social workers, and other health professionals would talk about similar things. My interns talk about the stress of being with sick and dying patients. They talk about feeling powerless to truly make things better. Up for thirty-six hours at a stretch, they are too tired to even feel satisfaction when they do accomplish something for their patients. Instead, their patients' inevitable declines feel like judgments on themselves. If only they were smarter or stronger or faster or more capable, they would be able to fix things, to cure disease, to give people back their health.

Along with the sadness and sense of powerlessness is a sense of rage. It is not rational, and it often is not conscious. The intern can feel very angry at the sickness, angry at the risk to his or her own safety, and angry at the endlessness of the tasks at hand. When a patient spikes a fever in the middle of the night, an intern can feel that it was done in spite. What intern has not said, "I'll be home by seven tonight, promise, I'll be home for dinner." Seven comes and there is another fever to work up or that blood gas was worse than the last one or a nurse calls to say, "Valeri says he's got chest pain." The intern disappoints those waiting for him at home, mad at the fever, mad at Valeri, mad at the $pCO2$ for being 55.

Our own lives can create a barrier to compassionate care in the form of transference, that is, the ways in which we project our personal relationships onto patients. A patient may make me unduly sad, not because he has end-stage congestive heart failure but because he reminds me of my father. My own autobiography is called into play, and my own feelings of sadness and loss complicate my ability to care for this gentleman. If I fail to recognize my projection, I will not be able to offer him effective care.

Many of us have had illness in our own families. Many of us are health care professionals because of illness in our families, in attempts to master the complicated sense of helplessness or at least to do better than was done to us. We know the phone call in the middle of the night from the intern or the nursing supervisor. We have traveled those journeys in the dark to the intensive care unit because things suddenly looked bad. Even though we know the great fearfulness that accompanies these journeys, the end of a personal road, the loss and the regrets, we keep these to ourselves. In our understandable need to protect our own feelings and in order to be able to do our work, we must make distinctions between the pain of others and our own pain. But however professional we become, it won't stop—the aching in the back of the throat, the knowledge that what we are all given is to feel pain and make do. We can only look, see it, and mourn our collective fate. Even though our personal experiences with sickness and loss may bring us closer to those who suffer, they also sometimes force us away, lead us astray, or prevent us from recognizing the claims of others.

How, then, to do better? Once we have examined the factors that make patient care difficult, can we find ways to increase our compassion? Compassion, like suffering, has been described in three phases—mute compassion, expressive compassion, and transforming compassion.

The first phase occurs in the space prior to language. Silent witness is offered to a suffering person, the witness unable to put into words his or her response. We all remember patients from the start of our careers—patients whose suffering we witnessed silently. The first patient I interviewed as a second year student was an elderly diabetic man who had had his right leg amputated years before and was now hospitalized for amputation of his left leg. I remember being shocked by the brutality of it: "Is that all we can do for him, to cut off his legs?" I asked myself. I remember leaving his room in tears, not having done my medical student interview. There was nothing I could say in the face of his loss, but my tears were for myself and not for him. My response to his suffering, however powerful, did nothing for him. In other circumstances, silence can be the most powerful response of compassion in the face of unspeakable suffering.

Compassion beyond silence can be more affirming than mute compassion. Expressive compassion allows the response of the witness to achieve language, and that language is useful to the patient. The listener who is tuned to the patient, as Job's flute is tuned to the voice of the mourners, is able to give voice to the patient's feelings and to move the patient from a mute suffering to a voiced one. That is, if the listener is attentive enough to put words to the patient's feelings, that verbalization may radically help the patient. This phase of compassion requires an active listening, an attention to that which is said and that which is withheld. Such a listener develops a habit, similar to the careful reader of fiction or poetry, of asking, "Why is she telling me this now?" "What is being left unsaid?" Henry James (1981) describes the reader in terms that equally apply to the compassionate listener: "To lend himself, to project himself and steep himself, to feel and feel till he understands, and to understand so well that he can say" (p. 136).

Expressive compassion brings the listener into the signifying world of the teller, allowing the teller's images and metaphors to achieve meaning and giving space for the story to emerge, however chaotically or hesitantly. The responsibility of this listener is to believe that the story has meaning and to hear it out to the end, in whatever language is available to the teller. Here is the point: the listener blessed with expressive compassion helps the teller to find words for the tale. In so doing, the listener learns what must be known in order to help. The active listening is prelude to action. Once the story is heard in all its complexity, despite the pain it may cause the listener, the one who listens can then act—can do what must be done medically, socially, and emotionally to lessen the suffering or even to end it.

These skills do not come automatically to health care workers. We have to teach ourselves and our students how to bear the suffering of patients, to suspend our own needs or beliefs, and to make room within ourselves for the experiences of our patients. We have to develop our capacities for both hearing and articulating the stories of suffering we witness. I invited Carlos to visit with a group of my second year medical students who are learning how to interview patients. He told them of his illness, his pain and losses, and his recent gains in freedom. He described his feelings when he moved out of his mother's house into his own apartment. He told them about the sources of joy and accomplishment in his life of work and love. While telling his story to my students, he said things that I had never heard, proving that the listeners enable the narrative to be told. Now telling his story does not alter his paralysis and does not give him back that which life has denied him. It does, however, reduce the chaos of the events to tell of them. As a bonus, Carlos's telling provided my students with a lesson that is unavailable but from patients themselves. He deepened their ability to be of help to others.

After my students met Carlos, I asked them to write an account of what he had said from his narrative stance. They agreed that they would describe the day he moved into his own apartment. One student wrote: "My own keys. No one but myself has these keys. Listen to their jingling: God, my hands are so shaky, I can't even fit the key through the keyhole! Okay, calm yourself down, Carlos. Alright, here we go. . . . Look at this apartment! My own. My very own. . . . I am no longer a mindless fixture that others used to take for granted." This student-writer imagined herself into the body of the patient, sitting in his wheelchair at the door of his new home, his hands shaking. Carlos then read all the students' papers, as the students and I had agreed he should. He helped us to understand which students had heard him accurately. Such exercises can strengthen students' expressive compassion, their capacity to recognize and tell, with accuracy, the predicament of their patient. At the beginning of a long and dangerous road toward meeting their patients in compassion, these students must learn from their patients, ultimately their master teachers.

Transformative compassion has the capacity to alter the listener fundamentally. As we accompany patients in their illnesses, we undergo radical transformation ourselves. What ultimately happens to those of us who work within this strange world? Do we change because of our closeness to sickness and death? Yes, we change in fundamental and hidden ways. We learn that people die and that we will die. We learn that death is not easy. We have to learn to hurt people, even though it is for their own good. We develop ways to avoid some of the pain: we take a detour to avoid walking by the ICU waiting room, because there are always strangers crying in the phone booths. It is too painful to be too close to such sadness every day, so we learn to get off the elevator one flight down and walk up a distant stairway.

As we sit in our little examining rooms with patients, or as we lean over a bedside rubbing a back, giving chest PT, or taking a cardiogram, we confront the irreducible burden of living. We look full in the face at the inconsolable sadness, the rage, the betrayal of sickness, of mortality, of loss. Although of course we care for patients who get better, who have reversible diseases, and who leave the hospital better than when they came in, the weight of our work resides in those who do not. Here, in confrontation with serious illness, we have the opportunity to cross over that line that separates the sick from the well, to diminish the isolation that is the feared result of illness, and to accept without flinching the community of the sick. In giving this gift to our patients, we get a much greater gift in return: to become the person who hears, who understands, and who gives in true compassion. We achieve new identities, as persons who can give freely.

Here is what all this means. This is what Jonathan King told us. It means that we who fully witness the suffering of our patients are closer to their pain but also closer to their comfort. Once we allow ourselves to listen with compassion and to let the full implications of their suffering register on us, we are in a position to change the state of affairs. We who witness can give control and hope through our compassion. It will not always lead to cure, and it will not always lead to a change in the medical treatment, but it can lead to a radical change for the patient. It can confer recognition and communion, ending the isolation and strangerliness of sickness.

Let us take a listen to our hearts. Let us acknowledge all that makes compassion so very difficult—the personal memories, the feeling of powerlessness, and the feelings of rage and of defeat. Let us name the fears that prevent us from joining our patients in their pain: the fear of loss, the fear of death, and the fear of making mistakes. We, too, need to be heard as we tell of our pain, as we let ourselves come close to the suffering of others. Our colleagues can listen to us—our fellow workers who themselves are on the same journey. Can we let one another help us? Can we let these feelings come up in the light of day? And then, with our colleagues' help, let us move away from the parallel suffering that isolates us from those for whom we care and find the courage to move toward genuine recognition of the patient's experience of suffering.

There is a great satisfaction waiting for us all. Once we have found that peacefulness, that state of acceptance beyond the fear and beyond the need to protect, then we can help. Imagine, now, sitting in your little room with a patient, a patient in pain and confusion who mourns for his healthy self. You have the power to reach him, to make that massive movement out of yourself into his experience. Do you know what that will do for him? It will let him get his bearings. It will let him tell his story to the end. Your words, your understanding will act as a comfort and a charge—a current of power. Your compassion can free your patient to understand the incomprehensible, to make sense of the tragic, to speak the unspeakable. You, together with your patient, will finally grasp the meaning of what takes place in our lives. Moved by suffering, you will ease that suffering. You will have become an instrument of healing.

References

Bellow, Saul. 1976. *Herzog.* New York: Viking Press.
Donne, John. 1975. "Meditation 5." In *Devotions upon Emergent Occasions,* ed. Anthony Raspa. London: McGill-Quenn's University Press.
Frankl, Viktor. 1971. *Man's Search for Meaning: An Introduction to Logotherapy.* New York: Simon and Schuster.
James, Henry. 1981. "Criticism." In *Selected Literary Criticism,* ed. Morris Shapira. Cambridge University Press.
Reich, Warren T. 1989. "Speaking of Suffering: A Moral Account of Compassion." *Soundings* 72: 83–108.
Selzer, Richard. 1976. *Mortal Lessons: Notes on the Art of Surgery.* New York: Simon and Schuster.
Soelle, Dorothee. 1975. *Suffering,* trans Everett R. Kalin. Philadelphia: Fortress Press.
Sontag, Susan. 1979. *Illness as Metaphor.* New York: Vintage Books.

compassion so very difficult—the personal memories, the feeling of powerlessness, and the feelings of rage and of defeat. Let us name the fears that prevent us from joining our patients in their pain: the fear of loss, the fear of death, and the fear of making mistakes. We, too, need to be heard as we tell of our pain, as we let ourselves come close to the suffering of others. Our colleagues can listen to us—our fellow workers who themselves are on the same journey. Can we let one another help us? Can we let these feelings come up in the light of day? And then, with our colleagues' help, let us move away from the parallel suffering that isolates us from those for whom we care and find the courage to move toward genuine recognition of the patient's experience of suffering.

There is a great satisfaction waiting for us all. Once we have found that peacefulness, that state of acceptance beyond the fear and beyond the need to protect, then we can help. Imagine, now, sitting in your little room with a patient, a patient in pain and confusion who mourns for his healthy self. You have the power to reach him, to make that massive movement out of yourself into his experience. Do you know what that will do for him? It will let him get his bearings. It will let him tell his story to the end. Your words, your understanding will act as a comfort and a charge—a current of power. Your compassion can free your patient to understand the incomprehensible, to make sense of the tragic, to speak the unspeakable. You, together with your patient, will finally grasp the meaning of what takes place in our lives. Moved by suffering, you will ease that suffering. You will have become an instrument of healing.

References

Bellow, Saul. 1976. *Herzog.* New York: Viking Press.

Donne, John. 1975. "Meditation 5." In *Devotions upon Emergent Occasions,* ed. Anthony Raspa. London: McGill-Quenn's University Press.

Frankl, Viktor. 1971. *Man's Search for Meaning: An Introduction to Logotherapy.* New York: Simon and Schuster.

James, Henry. 1981. "Criticism." In *Selected Literary Criticism,* ed. Morris Shapira. Cambridge University Press.

Reich, Warren T. 1989. "Speaking of Suffering: A Moral Account of Compassion." *Soundings* 72: 83–108.

Selzer, Richard. 1976. *Mortal Lessons: Notes on the Art of Surgery.* New York: Simon and Schuster.

Soelle, Dorothee. 1975. *Suffering,* trans Everett R. Kalin. Philadelphia: Fortress Press.

Sontag, Susan. 1979. *Illness as Metaphor.* New York: Vintage Books.

Contributors

ELLEN D. BAER, RN, PhD, FAAN, is a nurse historian. She is professor emeritus at the University of Pennsylvania School of Nursing and visiting professor of nursing at New York University, where she is director of the doctoral program.

PATRICIA BENNER, RN, PhD, FAAN is a professor of nursing in the Department of Physiological Nursing at the University of California, San Francisco. She is the author of *From Novice to Expert: Excellence and Power in Clinical Nursing Practice*, which has been translated into eight languages. She authored, with Judith Wrubel, *The Primacy of Caring: Stress and Coping in Health and Illness*. She is editor of *Interpretive Phenomenology: Caring, Ethics and Embodiment in Health and Illness*.

ALISA A. CARSE, PhD is Assistant Professor of Philosophy at Georgetown University.

JEANNIE CHAISSON, RN, MS is a medical clinical nurse specialist on a general medical floor at Boston's Beth Israel Hospital.

RITA CHARON, MD is a general internist. She is associate professor of clinical medicine at the College of Physicians and Surgeons at Columbia University. She is also studying for a doctorate in English from Columbia University.

CATHERINE A. CHESLA, RN, DNSc is assistant professor in the Department of Family Health Care Nursing at the University of California San Francisco. She teaches family theory and family intervention to graduate family nurse practitioners. She is currently conducting research on families coping with diabetes. Along with Patricia Benner and Christine A. Tanner, she is author of the recently published *Expertise in Nursing Practice*.

ALICE ELLIOTT DARK is a novelist and short story writer. She is the author of *Naked to the Waist*, a collection of short stories. She was the recipient of a National Endowment for the Arts Fellowship in Literature. Her stories have been published in the *New Yorker* and *DoubleTake*. She also teaches fiction writing.

JUDITH DUSHKU is Professor of Political Science at Suffolk University in Boston, Massachusetts. She is one of the founders and editors of the Mormon feminist newspaper *Exponent II.*

DEBORAH GORDON, PHD is research consultant in medical anthropology at the Center for the Study of the Prevention of Cancer in Florence, Italy, and International Affiliate with the Center for the Study of Medicine and Culture, Harvard Medical School. Her recent ethnographic research in Tuscany, Italy has focused around cancer and the local culture of cancer prevention, death and dying, home care and bioethics.

SUZANNE GORDON is an award-winning journalist who has been writing about women's issues, caregiving, nursing, and health care for over 25 years. She is a frequent contributor to the *Boston Globe* and the *Los Angeles Times* Op-Ed Page. She has written for the *New York Times*, the *Washington Post*, the *Philadelphia Inquirer*, the *Atlantic Monthly*, *The Nation*, *Harpers*, and many other national newspapers and magazines. Ms. Gordon is the author of six books, including *Prisoners of Men's Dreams* and the forthcoming *Life Support: Three Nurses on the Frontlines.*

JAMES G. HENDERSON, PHD is a professor of education at Kent State University.

VICTORIA WYNN LEONARD, RN, MS, PHD, FNP is a family nurse practitioner. She currently works in a well baby clinic for low income mothers and their children. Her dissertation, from which this chapter was excerpted, examined the transition to parenthood of first time mothers with career commitments.

RICHARD MACINTYRE, RN, MS, PHD is an assistant professor of nursing at the Samuel Merritt College in Oakland, California. He is a specialist in HIV and AIDS nursing.

NEL NODDINGS, PHD, is Lee Jacks Professor of Child Education at Stanford University. Her latest books are *Philosophy of Education* (1995), and *Educating for Intelligent Belief or Unbelief* (1993).

CHRISTINE A. TANNER, RN, PHD, FAAN, is professor of nursing, community health care systems at the School of Nursing, Oregon Health Sciences University, in Portland, Oregon. She has conducted research on clinical judgment in nursing for over two decades. She is the editor of the *Journal of Nursing Education.* Along with Patricia Benner and Catherine A. Chesla she is author of the recently published *Expertise in Nursing Practice.*

BARBARA TARLOW, RN, PHD is a former nurse. She is an adjunct professor of sociology at the University of Massachusetts Boston Harbor Campus.

COLM TÓIBÍN is a well-known Irish novelist. He is the author of *The*

Heather Blazing, from which this selection comes, *The South,* and *Sign of the Cross.*

KARI WAERNESS, PHD is a professor in the Department of Sociology at Bergen University in Norway.

Index

Abrahamsson, Bengt, 244, 245
African politics, 278–79, 285
AIDS, 141–52
Aristotle, 92, 96
Artistic problem solving, 194, 200
Attention, 92
Autonomy, 168, 169

Baier, Annette, 93, 95, 96, 100
Barber, Elinor, 245
Beauchamp, Tom, 88, 103
Being there, 61–63; contrasted with doing, 42–43 ·
Benhabib, Seyla, 86
Benner, Patricia, 51, 98, 101, 102, 104, 150, 180, 204, 205, 206, 262
Bioethics, 85, 89, 96–99, 102–5; care in, 97–98; and trust, 99–100
Blum, Lawrence, 87, 90, 97
Borgmann, Albert, 51–52, 126, 138
Bourdieu, Pierre, 204, 206
Brigham Young University, 283
Bronfenbrenner, Urie, 23, 24
Buber, Martin, 25, 26, 28, 34, 35, 164

Caregiving, 42, 141–52, 173–88, 223, 231–55, 267; by intimates, 143–44; defined, xiii; Mormon, 278–91; paid, 248; rational, 238; way of life, 3
Caring, 40, 143, 150, 201, 217, 262; associated concepts, 57; defined, xiii, 30, 234–35; empirical study of, 56–82; and feminism, 256–77; and knowing, 50; and mothering, 126; and talking, 63–65; and time, 58–61; and trust, 99; as doing, 73–76; as feeling, 70–72; as rational choice, 50; in nursing, 141–52; in teaching, 168–

71; medical, 41, 292–305; practice of, 41–55, 278–305; rationality of, 231–55; role of cared-for in 30, 31, 34, 47
Carper, B., 205
Carse, Alisa, 269
Child-rearing, 127–28, 238, 242
Chinn, Peggy, 205
Clinical judgment, 203–19
Comer, James, 168
Community care, 231–33
Compassion (barriers to), 298–305
Compassionate service, 286–87
Compassionate stranger, 173–88
Competence, 24; in caring, 47, 51, 162, 284, 286–89
Confirmation, 28, 164, 190–91
Constructivism, 189, 191–93, 198, 261
Continuity, 165, 170
Corcoran, S., 203
Cott, Nancy, 137, 257, 258, 272
Creative writing, 199

Dark, Alice Elliott, 45
D'Avenant, William, xiv
Dawe, Alan, 250
Dewey, John, 25
Dialogue, 163, 190–91
Diers and Fagin, xiv–xv
Dinkmeyer and McKay, 135–37
Donne, John, 293
Douglas, Ann, 257
Dreyfus, Hubert, 47, 49, 204, 205, 206
Dying, 5–20, 173–88, 292–305

Effectance motivation, 24, 31
Ehrenreich, Barbara, 236
Empathy, 91

English, Deirdre, 236
Engrossment, xiii, 35, 38
Ethic of care, 52–53, 84, 95–99, 139, 241–42, 268
Ethical self, 35–38, 164
Etzioni, Amitai, 155, 166
Exponent II, 282, 284, 290

Faludi, Susan, 256, 259, 263–67
Feminist sociology, 250
Feminist theory, 240, 250, 256–77; constructivist, 261; Lockean, 258–77; and Mormonism, 279–91; relational, 260–61; transformational, 261, 267
Finch and Groves, vii
Frankl, Victor, 297
Freire, Paulo, 163
Friedan, Betty, 265
Friedman, Marilyn, 85, 86

Gadow, Sally, 211, 217
Gender, 102–3
Gilligan, Carol, 83, 84, 86, 88, 95, 104, 264, 266, 268
Gloaming, 5–20, 43, 47
Good and goods, 131, 151, 171
Goodlad, John, 168
Gordon, Suzanne, viii, 173–88, 223, 226–30, 256–77, 280
Gouldner, Alvin, 78–79, 81

Hare-Mustin, Rachel, 261
Heidegger, Martin, 46, 47, 126, 205
Held, Virginia, 86, 103
Herzog (Saul Bellow), 298
Hierarchies, 166–67
Hill, Thomas, 86, 87
Hochschild, Arlie, 241
Holmes Group, 165
Holt, John, 32
Hospitals, 293–305
Hume, David, 96

Idler, Ellen, 249
Impartiality, 85–88, 96
Inclusion, 25, 28
Individual, formation of, 48
Individualism, 47, 48, 94
Informed consent, 98
Institute for Education in Transformation, 170
Intuition, 203

James, Henry, 302–3
Job, 296–97
Johnson, Diane, 271–73
Justice, 84, 94

Kaminer, Wendy, 256, 268–70
King, Jonathan, 293
Knowing, 50–51; the cared for, 240–46; the patient, 203–25
Knowledge, 142–43, 239; masculine objective, 236
Kohlberg, Lawrence, 83, 86
Kramer, Maeona, 205

Larrabee, Mary Jeanne, vii
Levin, Lowell S., 249
Little, Margaret, 90
Locke, John, 258; Lockean feminists, 258–77
Longino, Charles, viii
Lopata, Helena, 238

MacIntyre, Alasdair, 44, 125, 218
MacKinnon, Donald, 34
MacPherson, C. B., x
Management (in health care), 226–30
Marecek, Jeanne, 261
Mauss, Marcel, 81
May, C., 215
McMillan, Carol, 242, 243
Mentoring, 201
Merton, Robert, 245
Miller, Alice, 161
Miller, Jean Baker, 266
Modeling care, 163
Moral education, 163–65
Moral intellectualism, 91–93
Mormons, 278–91
Mothering, 124–40, 242
Motivational displacement, 33, 38; as acting in best interest, 68–70
Multicultural awareness, 151
Murdoch, Iris, 86, 90, 92

Narratives, 101–2, 104, 225, 297, 303
Negotiating (and caring), 58–82
Newson, John and Elizabeth, 238
Noddings, Nel, 76, 160, 162, 166, 189, 262, 273
Nursing, 98–99, 102–4, 141–52, 155, 157–59, 173–88, 203–25, 226–30, 271–72
Nussbaum, Martha, 48, 87, 90, 91

Oakley, Ann, 236

Particularity, 87
Pellegrino, Edmund, 95, 98, 99, 100
Pohlman, Edward, 29
Polanyi, Michael, 204
Pollitt, Katha, 256, 270–71
Practice, 44, 47, 125–26, 164, 168, 194
Price, Marion, 247
Principles (moral), 88–91, 96
Professions, 155, 160–72, 181, 267; professional knowledge, 245

Rationality of caring, 231–55
Rawls, John, 53, 86, 258
Receptivity, 22; and sensitivity, 65–68, 100
Reciprocity, 31–35, 57, 76–80, 234
Reich, Warren, 295
Relatedness, 22, 93–95, 139, 143, 170, 233
Responsiveness and responsibility, 34, 38, 46, 100, 268, 279, 295
Reverby, Susan, 155
Rogers, Carl, 28
Ruddick, Sara, 86, 95, 104

Sandel, Michael, 53
Scandinavian care practices, 231–55
Schaffer, Rudolf, 238
Schon, Donald, 204, 213
Schumacher, E. F., 246
Sears, Robert, 29
Selzer, Richard, 294
Sentient actor, 242
Sharpe, Virginia, 98, 99
Sherman, Nancy, 90, 91, 93
Sherwin, Susan, 102, 103
Shils, Edward, 47
Shulman, Lee, 166
Simmel, George, 236
Sizer, Theodore, 78
Skelly, Florence, 138
Smith, Adam, xv

Söder, Märten, 244, 245
Soelle, Dorothy, 295
Stacey, Margaret, 233, 247
Suffering, 292–305
Swanson, K. M., 217
Swidler, Ann, 139
Sympathetic attunement, 91, 92, 96
Systematic Training for Effective Parenting, 135

Tanner, Christine, 203, 204, 206
Taylor, Charles, 44, 45, 46, 48, 50, 52, 53, 137, 273
Teaching, 28, 31, 155, 160–72, 189–202, 301; visiting, 280, 287–89
Technology, 51–53, 178
Thompson, E. P., viii
Time (and caring), 58–61, 79
Titmuss, Richard, 240
Tronto, Joan, 49
Trust, 45, 60, 99–100, 165, 195

Ulrich, Laurel Thatcher, 227
Unequal meetings, 28, 31, 93, 94

Virtue, 101
Vulnerability, 135, 215

Waerness, Kari, 244
Walker, Margaret, 100, 101
Warren, Virginia, 102, 104
Wealth of Nations, xv
Weil, Simone, 161, 162, 170
Welfare state, 231–33
Whitbeck, Carolyn, 44, 137
White, Robert, 24
Winnicott, Donald, 131
Wittgenstein, Ludwig, 239
Woman's Exponent, 282
Wrubel, Judith, 50, 51, 52, 150, 204
Wuthnow, Robert, 81

Zilboorg, Gregory, 29